Mary Beth Williams
John F. Sommer Jr.
Editors

Simple and Complex Post-Traumatic Stress Disorder
Strategies for Comprehensive Treatment in Clinical Practice

Pre-publication
REVIEWS,
COMMENTARIES,
EVALUATIONS . . .

"As the field of trauma practice matures, we are only beginning to appreciate how intricate and multifaceted the realm of trauma and its impact actually is. *Simple and Complex Post-Traumatic Stress Disorder: Strategies for Comprehensive Treatment in Clinical Practice* does a remarkable job of covering much of this extensive territory. It is a valuable resource to which both newcomers and experts in the field of trauma practice will return again and again. From core topics such as diagnosis and standard forms of treatment to areas that have until now been relatively neglected, such as trauma-oriented family therapy, trauma intervention in the schools, trauma among law enforcement officials, and trauma and the media, this impressive book compiles many of the diverse manifestations of trauma, its impact, and its resolution in a single source."

Steven N. Gold, PhD
Professor, Center for Psychological
Studies; Director,
Trauma Resolution
and Integration Program,
Nova Southeastern University

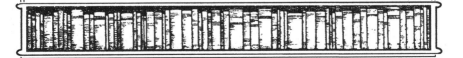

"**W**illiams and Sommer have produced a timely book that expands the boundaries of our knowledge about simple and complex forms of PTSD. Treatment approaches are presented for PTSD and specific trauma populations such as police hostage situations, law enforcement officers in the line of duty, school children, college students affected by trauma, and families suffering traumatic injuries. An important new contribution focuses on the role and responsibilities of media in covering trauma-related events, war, disasters, and intrusions into the lives of victims. This book and its expert contributors break new ground and offer lots of practical advice to scholars and clinicians alike."

John P. Wilson, PhD
Professor of Psychology,
Cleveland State University;
Past President, International Society
for Traumatic Stress Studies;
Co-editor, *Treating Psychological
Trauma & PTSD*

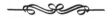

"**A** welcome addition to the literature on treating survivors of traumatic events, this book possesses all the ingredients necessary for even the experienced clinician to master the management of patients with PTSD.

The editors, outstanding leaders in the field, have assembled an excellent group of contributors who cover the range of available treatments for traumatized individuals. This broad range of coverage guarantees the reader a solid foundation in PTSD and establishes an elevated threshold for the no-tion of clinical competence for the field. Topics range from diagnostic and assessment practices written by experts in that arena, to the treatment of adults and children who have been exposed to traumatic events in a wide range of settings and circumstances. Complementing this broad array of topics are chapters defining clinical competence and explicating ethical issues and dilemmas confronting those who treat trauma survivors.

This book also casts a unique focus on traumatic events and the media. This topic is growing in importance as media provides enhanced, immediate, and detailed coverage of the many traumatic experiences that occur worldwide. The impact on the journalists, photographers, and consumers of the media is chronicled in the book, permitting additional attention to this topic from a clinical, research, and editorial perspective. How do we as a society manage these events? What do we expect from the journalists? How do we equip them to manage what they cover? These are pivotal questions raised by the contributors of the respective chapters.

This is an important addition to the libraries of those who wish to become involved in the assessment and treatment of PTSD. While much is known about the treatment of PTSD, much more work remains to be done. This book effectively synopsizes our knowledge of assessment and treatment models and methods."

Terence M. Keane, PhD
Chief, Psychology Service,
VA Boston Healthcare System;
Professor and Vice Chair
of Research in Psychiatry,
Boston University School of Medicine

Simple and Complex Post-Traumatic Stress Disorder

Strategies for Comprehensive Treatment in Clinical Practice

Simple and Complex Post-Traumatic Stress Disorder
Strategies for Comprehensive Treatment in Clinical Practice

Mary Beth Williams
John F. Sommer Jr.
Editors

HMTP

The Haworth Maltreatment and Trauma Press®
An Imprint of The Haworth Press, Inc.
New York • London • Oxford

Published by

The Haworth Maltreatment and Trauma Press®, an imprint of The Haworth Press, Inc., 10 Alice Street, Binghamton, NY 13904-1580.

PUBLISHER'S NOTE
Identities and circumstances of individuals discussed in this book have been changed to protect confidentiality.

Portions of *Life After Trauma: A Workbook for Healing* by D. Rosenbloom and M. B. Williams. Copyright © 1999. Reprinted by permission of Guilford Press.

Cover design by Marylouise E. Doyle.

Library of Congress Cataloging-in-Publication Data

Simple and complex post-traumatic stress disorder : strategies for comprehensive treatment in clinical practice / Mary Beth Williams, John F. Sommer, editors.
    p. cm.
  Includes bibliographical references and index.
  ISBN 0-7890-0297-3 (alk. paper)—ISBN 0-7890-0298-1 (alk. paper)
  1. Post-traumatic stress disorder—Treatment. I. Williams, Mary Beth. II. Sommer, John F.

RC552.P67 S454 2002
616.85'21—dc21

2001039561

To Fred Gosney,
who is making my road in life take on new meaning;

to Bishop Alexander Vallette,
who has shown me that it is never too late to start again;

and to Kaili Nagima Elizabeth
and Naiomi Zhannah Ruth Williams,
my new daughters from Kazakhstan
who are bringing such joy to our lives.

I would also like to acknowledge the help of Fae Deaton,
who volunteered to index the book,
for her friendship and good counsel through the years.

—Mary Beth Williams

To Dean K. Phillips,
a friend and an activist;

to Bill Johnson,
a friend and an advocate;

and to Gordon Sebrell,
a cousin, a friend, and an inspiration;

all Vietnam veterans whose lives ended far too early.

—John F. Sommer Jr.

CONTENTS

About the Editors   xiv

Contributors   xv

Preface: Trauma in the New Millennium   xix

Purpose of the Book   xx
Chapter Organization   xxi

SECTION I: INTRODUCTION

Chapter 1. A Short History of PTSD from the Military Perspective   3

Charles M. Flora

Chapter 2. Assessment and Diagnosis of PTSD in Adults: A Comprehensive Psychological Approach   9

William F. Flack Jr.
Brett T. Litz
Frank W. Weathers
Sherry A. Beaudreau

Introduction   9
Diagnosis versus Assessment   10
Taking a Psychosocial History   11
Methods of Assessment   13
Using Assessment Results in Making Clinical
    Recommendations   17
Summary   19

Chapter 3. Approaches to the Treatment of PTSD   23

Bessel A. van der Kolk
Onno van der Hart
Jennifer Burbridge

Introduction   23
The Symptomatology of PTSD   26
Principles of Treatment   33

Group Psychotherapy   39
Concluding Remarks   40

Chapter 4. Psychopharmacological Treatment in PTSD   **47**
    Ronald Albucher
    Michelle Van Etten-Lee
    Israel Liberzon

Introduction   47
Antidepressants   50
Buspirone   59
Lithium   59
Anticonvulsants   60
Benzodiazepines   61
Neuroleptics or Antipsychotic Agents ("Major
  Tranquilizers")   62
Adrenergic Agents   63
Opiate Antagonists   64
Conclusion   64

SECTION II: TREATMENT OF PTSD IN GENERAL

Chapter 5. Cognitive-Behavioral Treatment of PTSD   **75**
    Lori A. Zoellner
    Edna B. Foa
    Lee A. Fitzgibbons

The Efficacy of Psychosocial Treatments   76
Theoretical Considerations in Cognitive-Behavioral Therapy   80
Treatment Overview   80
Case Illustration   85
Summary   92
Appendix: Common Reactions to Assault Handout   93

**Chapter 6. Short-Term Treatment of Simple and Complex
PTSD**   **99**
    Louis Tinnin
    Lyndra Bills
    Linda Gantt

Introduction   99
The History of Video-Assisted Trauma Therapy   99

Principles of Time-Limited Trauma Therapy 103
Applications of Video-Assisted Trauma Therapy 106
Description of Treatment Procedures 109
Conclusion 117

**Chapter 7. Life After Trauma: Finding Hope
by Challenging Your Beliefs and Meeting Your Needs 119**

*Dena Rosenbloom
Mary Beth Williams*

Introduction 119
Impacts of Trauma 120
The Meanings of Traumatic Events and Coping 122
Working Through Traumatic Events 125
Testing Beliefs 126
Discerning the Meaning of Trust 128
Getting Control 129
Believing in Yourself and Others 130
Feeling Close to Yourself; Getting Close to Others 131
Conclusion 133

SECTION III: GROUP TREATMENTS

**Chapter 8. The Development of a Group Treatment
Model for Post-Traumatic Stress Disorder 137**

*Gordon Turnbull
Tosin Clairmonte
Stuart Johnson
Colina Hanbury-Aggs
Bo Mills
Walter Busuttil
Adrian West*

Introduction 137
Post-Traumatic Stress Disorder 138
Etiological Theories 139
The PTSD Group Treatment Programme 143
The Development of the Tradition of Group Approaches 144
Assessment 145
Efficiency 146

Biopsychosocial Strategy   147
Technique   149
Discussion   158
Group Program for Complex PTSD   159
Conclusion   159

**Chapter 9. Developing and Maintaining
a Psychoeducational Group for Persons
Diagnosed As DID/MPD/DDNOS**   **165**

> *Mary Beth Williams*
> *Sandra Gindlesperger Nuss*

Introduction   165
History of the Group   167
Composition and Structure of the Group   168
Group Process   170
Basic Principles in Conducting a Psychoeducational
    Support Group   171
Benefits of Support Group Participation for Members   174
Values of the Leaders   177
Areas of Concern and Ethical Issues in the Group   177
Countertransference and Vicarious Traumatization   180
A Retrospective Look at the Group: What Did It
    Accomplish?   181
Conclusions   182
Appendix: Group Handouts   184

SECTION IV: CHILDREN, STUDENTS, AND FAMILIES

**Chapter 10. Treatment Strategies for Traumatized
Children**   **215**

> *Mary W. Lindahl*

Brief Overview of the Literature   215
Evaluation and Treatment Plan   216
Educating the Child and Family About Trauma   217
The Role of Parents   218
Telling the Story   219
Addressing the Symptoms   221

Does Trauma Have Meaning?   223
Issues of Development   226
Follow-Up and Healing   228
Conclusions   230

**Chapter 11. Provision of Trauma Services to School
Populations and Faculty   241**

J. Horenstein

Introduction   241
Primary Prevention   243
Secondary Prevention   248
Intervention Strategies: A Case Illustration   253
Tertiary Prevention   254
Final Thoughts   256

Chapter 12. Traumatic Stress in Family Systems   261

Chrys J. Harris

Introduction   261
Assessing Family System Trauma   265
Treating Family System Trauma   268
Preventing Family System Trauma   271
Conclusions   273

Chapter 13. Dealing with Trauma in the Classroom   277

Mitzi Mabe

Surveying the Social Landscape   278
The Way of Listening   280
Student-Defined Education: Embracing Mature Realities   281
Giving Audience to Pain: The Civil Balm of the Classroom   282
The Read Out: Addressing Community in the Academy   283
Ultimate Disengagement, Suicidal Ideation, and the Health
    of Grief   287
How to Develop a Class in Writing That Acknowledges
    the Impact of Trauma   289
The Read Out As a Strategy to Correct Abusive
    Relationships   291

Recognizing and Dismantling Obstacles: Supporting
  Teachers' Work   292
Conclusion   293

SECTION V: SPECIAL POPULATIONS

Chapter 14. Police Hostage Situations   **299**
          Lasse Nurmi

The Role of the Police Psychologist in Hostage
  Negotiations   299
Case Setting   300
The Situation   301
Purposes of Negotiation   301
Phases of the Negotiation Process   302
What Makes a Good Hostage Negotiator?   306
Lessons Learned   306
Conclusions   308

Chapter 15. Law Enforcement and Trauma   **311**
          James M. Horn

Introduction   311
The Nature of Trauma   312
The Oklahoma City Model   316
Help to Law Enforcement Through EAPs   320
Conclusion   321

Chapter 16. Trauma Services to War Veterans   **325**
          Charles M. Flora

Treating the War Veteran   325
Community Outreach   326
Psychotherapy for War Trauma   330
Summary and Conclusions   345

SECTION VI: MEDIA ISSUES

Chapter 17. A Primer on Interviewing Victims   **351**
          Frank Ochberg

Introduction   351
A Guide to Interviewing   353

Stages of Response   357
The Humanitarian Role of the Reporter   359
Secondary Traumatic Stress Disorder   360
Conclusions   360

**Chapter 18. Relating to Journalists As Trauma
Clinicians and Researchers**   **361**

Richard Hébert

Why Cooperate?   361
Recognizing Newsworthiness   363
Next Step: The News Release   365
How to Handle the Interview   367
Conclusions   369

Chapter 19. Working with Survivors and the News Media   **371**

*Janice Maxson
Roger Simpson*

Introduction   371
Reporters and Advocates As Partners   372
Network Response Before a Crisis   373
After the Event   374
The Role of Intermediary   377
Coverage in the First Few Weeks   379
Long-Term Concerns   381
Conclusion   383

SECTION VII: CONCLUSION

Chapter 20. Some Final Thoughts on Competence   **387**

*Mary Beth Williams
John F. Sommer*

Index   **399**

ABOUT THE EDITORS

Mary Beth Williams, PhD, LCSW, CTS, is in private practice in Warrenton, Virginia, where she specializes in the treatment of simple and complex PTSD, as well as DID. She has been a school social worker in Falls Church, Virginia, and Frankfurt, Germany. She is a member of the Rapidan Rappahanock Crisis Intervention Stress Management team. Dr. Williams has written extensively in the field of trauma. Her books include *The PTSD Workbook* and *Life After Trauma: A Workbook for Healing.* She is a former President of the Association of Traumatic Stress specialists and a former board member of ISTSS. She trains internationally for various organizations in Kazakhstan, Finland, Australia, Germany, and Slovenia.

John F. Sommer Jr., BS, a Vietnam veteran, is Executive Director of the Washington, DC, office of The American Legion and Chair of the Department of Veterans Affairs Advisory Committee on the Readjustment of Veterans. He has co-authored articles and facilitated research projects dealing with Agent Orange effects on Vietnam veterans. He has also been involved in ongoing POW/MIA investigations, has testified before congressional committees, and has made numerous trips to Vietnam and other areas in Southeast Asia. He is a charter member of the International Society for Traumatic Stress Studies (ISTSS) and is Co-chair of the society's Ethics Task Force/Committee. He has presented nationally on a variety of trauma-related topics.

CONTRIBUTORS

Ronald Albucher, MD, Veterans Administration Medical Center and Department of Psychiatry, University of Michigan, Ann Arbor, Michigan.

Sherry A. Beaudreau, BA, Department of Psychology, Washington University, St. Louis, Missouri.

Lyndra Bills, MD, Medical Director, The Sanctuary, Quakertown, Pennsylvania.

Jennifer Burbridge, MA, Washington University, St. Louis, Missouri.

Walter Busuttil, MB ChB, M Phil, MRCGP, MRCPsych, Consultant Psychiatrist and Clinical Director, Traumatic Stress Unit, Ticehurst House Hospital, East Sussex, England.

Tosin Clairmonte, MB ChB, M Inst GA, Group Analyst and Psychotherapist, Traumatic Stress Unit, Ticehurst House Hospital, East Sussex, England.

Lee A. Fitzgibbons, PhD, Center for the Treatment and Study of Anxiety, Medical College of Pennsylvania, Hahnemann University, Philadelphia, Pennsylvania.

William F. Flack Jr., PhD, Assistant Professor, Department of Psychology, Bucknell University, Lewisburg, Pennsylvania.

Charles M. Flora, Vietnam veteran, Washington, DC.

Edna B. Foa, PhD, Center for the Treatment and Study of Anxiety, Medical College of Pennsylvania, Hahnemann University, Philadelphia, Pennsylvania.

Linda Gantt, PhD, ATR-BC, Trauma Recovery Institute, Morgantown, West Virginia.

Colina Hanbury-Aggs, BSc, MB BS, Dip M T, Primary Debriefer, Traumatic Stress Unit, Ticehurst House Hospital, East Sussex, England.

Chrys J. Harris, PhD, Family and Therapy Trauma Center, Greenville, South Carolina.

Richard Hébert, Health Sciences Writer, Former Communications Director, Center for the Advancement of Health, Washington, DC.

J. Horenstein, MD, CSM M Gen, Paris, France.

James M. Horn, MFS, BCETS, Director, Forensic Behavioral Science Consulting and Training, Stillwater, Oklahoma.

Stuart Johnson, Dip Couns, Adv Cert Psych, Primary Debriefer, Traumatic Stress Unit, Ticehurst House Hospital, East Sussex, England.

Israel Liberzon, PhD, Veterans Administration Medical Center and Department of Psychiatry, University of Michigan, Ann Arbor, Michigan.

Mary W. Lindahl, PhD, Licensed Clinical Psychologist, Associate Professor of Psychology in the School of Education and Human Services at Marymount University, Arlington, Virginia, where she is the Coordinator of the Forensic Psychology Master's Program. She also has a private practice in Alexandria, Virginia.

Brett T. Litz, PhD, Behavioral Science Division, National Center for PTSD, Boston Department of Veterans Affairs Medical Center, and Department of Psychiatry, Boston University School of Medicine, Boston, Massachusetts.

Mitzi Mabe, MA, University of Maryland, Baltimore, Maryland.

Janice Maxson, doctoral student, University of Washington, Seattle, Washington.

Bo Mills, MB BS, DTC (London), Specialist in Psychosexual Medicine and Traumatic Stress, Traumatic Stress Unit, Ticehurst House Hospital, East Sussex, England.

Lasse Nurmi, MA, PhD candidate, Police College of Finland, Espoo, Finland.

Sandra Gindlesperger Nuss, BSW, Counselor, The Aurora House, Falls Church, Virginia.

Frank Ochberg, MD, Director, The Dart Foundation, Okemos, Michigan.

Dena Rosenbloom, PhD, private practice, Middletown, Connecticut.

Roger Simpson, PhD, Associate Professor, School of Communications, and Coordinator, Journalism and Trauma Program, University of Washington, Seattle, Washington.

Louis Tinnin, MD, Trauma Recovery Institute, Morgantown, West Virginia.

Gordon Turnbull, BSc, MB ChB, FRCP, FRCPsych, FRGS, FRSA, Consultant Psychiatrist and Clinical Director, Traumatic Stress Unit, Ticehurst House Hospital, East Sussex, England.

Onno van der Hart, PhD, Mental Health Center, Buiten Amstel, Amsterdam, the Netherlands.

Bessel A. van der Kolk, MD, Trauma Clinic, Brookline, Massachusetts.

Michelle Van Etten-Lee, PhD, Veterans Administration Medical Center and Department of Psychiatry, University of Michigan, Ann Arbor, Michigan.

Frank W. Weathers, PhD, Department of Psychology, Auburn University, Auburn, Alabama.

Adrian West, BA (Hons), Dip Clin Psych, Clinical Psychologist, Ashworth Hospital, Liverpool, and National Crime Faculty, Police Staff College, Bramshill.

Lori A. Zoellner, PhD, Center for the Treatment and Study of Anxiety, Medical College of Pennsylvania, Hahnemann University, Philadelphia, Pennsylvania.

Preface

Trauma in the New Millennium

What is a trauma? Is it the loss of a job for a person who is only months away from retirement? Is it witnessing the murder of a relative? Is it enduring years of physical, sexual, and/or emotional abuse? Is it waiting anxiously for the turn of the clock on the year 2000 to see if the Y2K bug really would lead to devastation and destruction? How many thousands of persons bought generators, canned goods, and other products in preparation for the chaos that they had been told would undoubtedly come? How many thousands of persons on January 1, 2000, sheepishly looked at their stores of goods and wondered "why"? Trauma is in the eye of the beholder in many instances. One person may walk away from a traumatic event virtually unscathed physically to retreat into a world of avoidance and fear. Another person, enduring a similar, if not the same, event, may take up the cause and work to change a circumstance, situation, or even "the world." To be sure, some events are so horrific that they impact, in some way, all who are privy to them. But, if only 10 percent of those exposed to trauma develop some form of post-traumatic stress syndrome, the numbers who have entered into the category of having a need for clinical intervention can be staggering.

It is humbling to sit in a small cafe at 2 a.m. in northern Finland and talk with the lead guitarist of Duo Mennan about what he is learning is occurring in Kosovo at that very minute. The mobile phone rings and it is his father, running for his life. It is humbling to share in the personal pain of a young boy who "took the pain" for the others who are part of him as he (and the other alters) were forced to perform sexual acts for attendees at "parties." It is humbling to watch as resilience grows from the ashes of pain and torture, terror and abuse.

PTSD is now a much more familiar term than it was in 1994 when the *Handbook of Post-Traumatic Therapy* was published. Since that time, countless debates over the efficacy of treatment methods and/or critical incident stress debriefing have taken place. Practice guidelines have been authored by International Society for Traumatic Stress Studies (ISTSS) committees, and new "power therapies" have been created. New organizations and trauma centers have been created to offer services to refugee and nonrefugee populations. The literature of trauma has grown immensely and training programs for trauma therapists are now in existence in the United States and Finland.

PURPOSE OF THE BOOK

This book looks at what constitutes competent practice in the trauma field at this moment in time. It does not focus on distinct differences between treatment of type I (one time) traumatic events and type II (chronic, ongoing) events, as recognized by L. C. Terr (1994). However, it does look at what constitutes competent diagnosis, competent generic practice, competent work with the media, competent hostage negotiation, competent self-help, and other strategies.

The book also offers information to those in the field who want to know "just a little more" about how to offer services to a variety of populations and groups who have been traumatized. As a practitioner, I cringe at the pervasiveness of turf issues and threatened territoriality that engulfs many disasters and incidents. What is important is healing, not whether a referral was written on blue paper or yellow paper! Perhaps, through the chapters in this book, readers will become more familiar with the ways to diagnose and treat those individuals who are most impacted by traumatic events without turning those traumatized persons into perpetual victims.

This book is about healing and the ways to promote healing through the use of individual treatment, crisis intervention, group treatment, and self-help. It is about the resilience of the human soul to go on, even after the most horrific of events. It is an acknowledgment of the strength of many trauma survivors as they "slog through" lakes of tar that seem to stretch endlessly in front of them. When something does "go right for a change," it is a way to help them accept their own abilities and strengths that helped them survive the horrific events of their lives.

In 1994, the editors' first book, *Handbook of Post-Traumatic Therapy,* brought together experts from most regions of the United States in its chapters. This book expands the readership and contributors to a more global level. Contributors come from the United States, as well as other countries (e.g., France, Finland). The language of trauma is truly global in impact and scope; the context of healing also must be similarly global.

CHAPTER ORGANIZATION

According to the *Practice Guidelines* for the treatment of post-traumatic stress disorder of the International Society for Traumatic Stress Studies (2001), the prevailing notion is that treatment of PTSD has a much better prognosis if there is early implementation of clinical intervention, even though few studies support this view. Many individuals who are traumatized suffer from PTSD for extended periods of time and could be classified as suffering from chronic PTSD or a disorder of extreme stress. The treatment modalities offered in this book take into account both groups of individuals, although more attention is given to the more chronically traumatized than to individuals experiencing a one-time disaster or disastrous event. These individuals, again according to general belief and as reported by the guidelines, are more difficult to treat. Because many persons diagnosed with PTSD also have other comorbid disorders, including depression, anxiety, panic, bipolar disorder, and substance abuse, it is the hope of the editors and chapter authors that the treatment methods presented here will also help in the treatment of those disorders as well.

The book is divided into seven sections. Section I provides more of an overview of issues surrounding the history, diagnosis, and general treatment of PTSD in chapters by Flora, Flack and colleagues, and van der Kolk, van der Hart, and Burbridge, respectively. Also in that section is the chapter by Albucher, Van Etten-Lee, and Liberzon describing psychopharmacological treatment.

Section II looks at more specific treatment approaches for all trauma survivors. Zoellner, Foa, and Fitzgibbons describe cognitive behavioral treatment approaches. As the behavioral guidelines note, both pharmacotherapy and cognitive behavioral therapy tend to target symptom reduction as the major target for treatment outcome. Tinnin, Bills, and Gantt then describe a program of short-term treatment for simple and complex PTSD. Next, Rosenbloom and Williams describe their self-help–oriented workbook treatment of PTSD based on contextualistic self-development theory (McCann and Pearlman, 1990).

In Section III, Turnbull and colleagues present an innovative group treatment approach for PTSD developed at Ticehurst House Hospital in Great Britain. Williams and Gindlesperger Nuss then provide a model for group treatment of survivors of chronic PTSD who have developed a dissociative identity disorder diagnosis or a diagnosis of Disorders of Extreme Stress Not Otherwise Specified (DES-NOS).

Section IV focuses on the treatment of children and families as well as ways to deal with traumatized students and trauma-related topics in the college/university classroom. Lindahl presents a variety of treatment techniques to utilize with traumatized children, and Horenstein presents conclusions from work with school violence and debriefing in French schools. Harris then describes ways to treat traumatic stress in family systems. The final chapter in this section is by Mabe and examines ways to deal with trauma in the college classroom.

Section V of the book looks at competent trauma services with special populations. Lasse Nurmi, of the Police College of Finland, discusses competent hostage negotiations through a case situation. Horn, in his chapter, describes law enforcement and trauma, and looks at the role of critical incident stress management with law enforcement personnel as a healing intervention system. Flora, through narratives and various cases, then examines clinical work with traumatized veterans.

Section VI is designed to provide assistance to traumatologists (both clinicians and researchers) in their work with the media. Ochberg discusses how media could best cover victims in newsworthy, trauma-related stories. Next, Hébert, in a revision of remarks made at the 1997 ISTSS Annual Meeting in Montreal, Canada, discusses how traumatologists can relate to journalists. The final chapter in this section, by Maxson and Simpson, also examines how journalists can work with survivors and how trauma practitioners can work with the media and help survivors.

Section VII, the final chapter of the book, utilizes, in part, the conclusions of the authors of the previous chapters, as well as some comments by trauma survivors, and conclusions by the editors as to what constitutes competency by a clinician. Although healing is a personal journey, survivors can give a perspective to the clinician as to what has assisted them. Not only can they provide personal definitions of healing, but also describe strategies and techniques that helped them most. As one survivor has stated, facing trauma "in the eye" and surviving it has left him forever changed. "He will never be the same again." He no longer sees the world as safe. He knows that human beings can kill, seemingly without cause. Yet he also knows that somehow, somewhere, something good will come out of the horror through which he lived. What that "good" will be remains a mystery; still, the journey to find that "good" drives him forward and "keeps him going." It is our hope that this book will help him and those who work with survivors who are facing similar situations to find meaning in their lives.

Mary Beth Williams
John F. Sommer

REFERENCES

International Society for Traumatic Stress Studies (2001). *Practice Guidelines.* Northbrook, IL: Author.

McCann, I. L. and Pearlman, L. A. (1990). *Psychological trauma and the adult survivor: Theory, therapy, and transformation.* New York: Brunner/Mazel.

Terr, L. C. (1994). *Unchained memories: True stories of traumatic memories lost and found.* New York: Basic Books.

Williams, M. B. and Sommer, J. F. (1994). *Handbook of post-traumatic therapy.* Westport, CT: Greenwood Press.

SECTION I:
INTRODUCTION

Chapter 1

A Short History of PTSD from the Military Perspective

Charles M. Flora

Prior to 1979, Vietnam war veterans who developed troubling psychological symptoms arising from their combat experiences (six months to several years after their return home) were rarely provided treatments that were clinically effective or acceptable to them (Gelsomino and Mackey, 1988; Scurfield, 1985). Traditional military and psychiatric ideologies suggested that adverse reactions to combat were the result of character defects residing within the soldier's personality. These traditional perspectives implied that basically healthy individuals would be relatively impervious to the severe stresses of war (Scurfield, 1985). Thus, the veteran experiencing painful wartime memories—often privately fearful of going crazy—was usually advised that he either had a preexisting pathology or that his experience in Vietnam was not a factor influencing his current postwar civilian adjustment problems. With the advent of the formulation of the post-traumatic stress disorder (PTSD) diagnosis in the American Psychiatric Association's (APA) *Diagnostic and Statistical Manual of Mental Disorders* (DSM-III) in 1980, there was a shift in clinical thinking from predisposing or preexisting psychological factors to the objective elements and psychological aftermath of the veteran's stressful wartime experiences (American Psychiatric Association, 1980). The actual experience of traumatic events became the single most significant factor associated with the emergence of PTSD.

As formulated in the DSM-III, the stressor criterion required the existence of a recognizable stressor that would evoke significant symptoms of distress in almost everyone (American Psychiatric Association, 1980). As revised in 1987, in DSM-III-R, the stressor criterion was elaborated to note that the person experienced an event outside the range of usual experience that was noticeably distressing to almost anyone (American Psychiatric Association, 1987). The stressor criterion as currently formulated in the DSM-IV specifies that the person has experienced, witnessed, or been confronted with an event or events that involve actual or threatened death or serious injury, or a threat to the physical integrity of oneself or others, and that the person's response involved intense fear, helplessness, or horror. In adults, traumatic events that are experienced directly and may lead to PTSD include, but are not limited to, military combat, violent personal assault, being kidnapped, being taken hostage, terrorist attack, torture, incarceration as a prisoner of war or in a concentration camp, natural or manmade disasters, and/or severe automobile or other vehicular accidents. The diagnosis of PTSD requires a determination that the person has been exposed to one of these circumstances (American Psychiatric Association, 1994).

The psychological efficacy of traumatic experiences in precipitating post-traumatic reactions was well understood by the end of the twentieth century. However, these gains in knowledge were subsequently lost until recent decades as a result of conflicting cultural values, confusion, and forgetfulness. As Judith Herman (1992, p. 7) wrote in her book *Trauma and Recovery,* "The study of psychological trauma has a curious history—one of episodic amnesia." Two of the more important historical precursors to the contemporary understanding of PTSD include Pierre Janet's discoveries about trauma and dissociation, and Freud's early clinical work showing a causal relationship between childhood sexual trauma and the adult symptoms of hysteria (Herman, 1992; van der Kolk and van der Hart, 1989; van der Kolk, Brown, and van der Hart, 1989a).

Both Janet and Freud were students of hysteria at the end of the last century under Jean-Martin Charcot at the Salpêtrière in Paris (Gay, 1988; Herman, 1992; Horowitz, 1986; van der Kolk and van der Hart, 1989; van der Kolk, Brown and van der Hart, 1989b). Both clinicians independently developed their theories of psychological trauma to explain hysteria. Janet believed that intense emotional reactivity in response to overwhelmingly stressful life events interrupted the individual's adaptive capacities and the synthesizing functions of the mind (van der Kolk and van der Hart, 1989; van der Kolk, Brown and van der Hart, 1989a). Traumatic memories were "dissociated" and preserved in an altered state apart from the ordinary narrative flow of conscious experience. Dissociated traumatic memories remained highly emotionally charged and continued to disrupt the individual's life functioning. By the time of Janet's death in 1947, however, he and his work had become obscure. His ideas were forgotten, replaced by psychoanalysis as the dominant psychological paradigm of the time (van der Kolk and van der Hart, 1989; van der Kolk, Brown and van der Hart, 1989b).

In 1895, Freud published his theory that childhood sexual trauma causes hysteria and characterized it as a disease of traumatic reminiscences (Herman, 1992; Horowitz, 1986). Similar to Janet, he believed that traumatic memories were the internal impression of traumatic events sealed off in the unconscious mind from the rest of the personality (Horowitz, 1986). However, Freud subsequently abandoned this theory that the actual sexual seduction of a child by an adult caused hysteria, replacing it with his new belief that hysteria was caused by childhood sexual wishes (Herman, 1992; van der Kolk and van der Hart, 1989; van der Kolk, Brown and van der Hart, 1989a). Freud's reasons for reversing his decision on this matter were undoubtedly complicated but included professional and cultural tensions and sensitivities regarding incest and the sexual abuse of children (Gay, 1988; Herman, 1992). In taking this position, Freud set the course for future psychoanalytic investigation: a focus primarily on the vicissitudes of subjective experience and intrapsychic conflict. This either/or thinking away from external trauma to inner conflict relegated traumatic experiences to an ignored and insignificant role in the subsequent history of psychoanalysis.

Given the shift in psychoanalytic thinking away from traumatic experiences, it is paradoxical that the first formulation of the traumatic war neurosis consistent with the modern characterization of PTSD came from within that tradition. Abram Kardiner, MD, returned to New York in the early 1920s following a year-long sabbatical in Vienna where he underwent an analysis with Freud (Kardiner, 1977). In addition to establishing a private practice, Dr. Kardiner accepted a position on the psychiatry staff at the VA Medical Center in Bronx, New York. The latter afforded him the opportunity to work with World War I survivors suffering with combat neurosis. Although deeply interested and intrigued by his veteran patients and their clinical problems, his work proved frustrating because his efforts to relieve their symptoms were to little or no avail. The psychological tools he had acquired through his psychoanalytic training were of little practical use with war-traumatized veterans:

> My efforts to create a theory for the war neurosis proved impossible. Working with the concepts of the libido theory, which are based on instinctual energies, phylogenetically programmed stages of development, and a predetermined Oedipus complex, left little room to explain the response to traumatic experiences. (Kardiner, 1977, p. 121)

In 1936, Dr. Kardiner initiated a series of multidisciplinary seminars in psychology and the social sciences (Kardiner, 1977). Following a fruitful collaboration between himself and a group of cultural anthropologists from Columbia University, Dr. Kardiner became a leading figure in psychological anthropology (Harris, 1968). In 1939, he published *The Individual and His Society,* which concerned itself with the problems of adaptation in primitive society (Kardiner, 1939). By liberating his thinking from much of the theoretical superstructure of psychoanalysis, he developed a theory for integrating personality and culture, as well as a method for identifying the reactions of men to the realities of life (Harris, 1968). Only after he had published his work in anthropology was he able to return with new understanding to the study of war trauma (Herman, 1992; Kardiner, 1977). His study of the relationship between cultural institutions and human adaptation provided him with a perspective that reinforced the reality of the environment and the influence of actual life experiences for understanding human functioning.

Dr. Kardiner's ideas about war trauma were initially published in his 1941 book *The Traumatic Neurosis of War* and revised in 1947 in *War Stress and Neurotic Illness* (Kardiner, 1941; Kardiner and Spiegel, 1947). The latter work was completed in collaboration with Herbert Spiegel, MD, and contained clinical information derived from treating World War II veterans, in addition to the original clinical material on World War I veterans. Kardiner was quite clear in his conception of trauma as an external event: "Trauma . . . is an external factor that initiates an abrupt change in previous adaptation," and as an external event that overwhelms the individual's capacity to function, "the whole apparatus for concerted, coordinated, and purposeful activity is smashed" (Kardiner and Spiegel, 1947, pp. 178, 186). As constant features of the traumatic neurosis, he identified

1. Fixation on the trauma
2. Typical dream life
3. Irritability and startle pattern
4. Tendency to explosive aggressive actions
5. Contraction of the general level of functioning (Kardiner and Spiegel, 1947, p. 200)

Kardiner also classified the trauma neurosis as a physioneurosis, by which he meant that the sufferer remains in a state of physiological preparedness for the return of the trauma (Kardiner and Spiegel, 1947). "A traumatic neurosis is therefore a type of adaptation which follows a break in a previously well integrated pattern of adaptation" (Kardiner and Spiegel, 1947, p. 179).

Kardiner's sense of frustration with trying to use existing psychologies to understand and treat war trauma would find parallels in the experience of clinicians twenty years later treating returning Vietnam veterans. APA deleted any reference to environmental stress reactions, i.e., gross stress reaction, from its DSM-II in 1968, thereby depriving clinicians of an official diagnostic category for making sense of their observations (Gelsomino and Mackey, 1988). This situation resulted in many war veterans being misdiagnosed and provided with ineffective treatments. The Lockean empirical theory of the mind as a tabula rasa was necessary before the impact of traumatic experiences could be fully appreciated. In the face of catastrophic events, the mind is best conceived as a blank tablet upon which traumatic experiences make lasting impressions. By contrast, Freudian thinking had taken on more of the trappings of philosophical rationalism, viewing the mind as a self-contained unfolding of innate tendencies (Allport, 1955; Boring, 1950).

In addition to the primacy of an external traumatic event that overwhelms the individual's adaptive capacities and shatters his or her sense of understanding about self and the world, the contemporary understanding of PTSD includes a series of post-traumatic symptoms that fall into one of three categories (Herman, 1992; Horowitz, 1986). Intrusive symptoms represent the indelible mark of the traumatic event. As both Janet and Kardiner observed, intrusive memories are fragmentary pieces of the traumatic moment dissociated from the normal narrative flow of ordinary memory (van der Kolk and van der Hart, 1989; van der Kolk, Brown and van der Hart, 1989b). Emotional constriction represents the resulting collapse and surrender of the survivor's adaptive behaviors, and hyperarousal reflects the survivor's persistent expectation of danger.

The core psychological phenomenon of delayed traumatic stress reactions consists of the repetitious cycling of intrusive recollections with denial and psychic numbing (Horowitz, 1986). The intrusive symptoms press for recovery via progressive psychological mastery of the trauma, while the defensive avoidance symptoms operate to protect the individual from overstimulation or the fear of retraumatization. By dissociating and denying the traumatic war memories, the veteran can facilitate a partial return to normal functioning. Environmental triggering events, however, can result in periodic intrusions of unintegrated traumatic experiences in the form of recurrent thoughts, images, and distressing dreams. Triggering events in the case of war veterans include any sensory or ideational content that is reminiscent of their war-related experiences.

REFERENCES

Allport, G. W. (1955). *Becoming: Basic considerations for a psychology of personality.* New Haven: Yale University Press.

American Psychiatric Association (APA) (1968). *Diagnostic and statistical manual,* Second edition. Washington, DC: American Psychiatric Association.

___ (1980). *Diagnostic and statistical manual,* Third edition. Washington, DC: American Psychiatric Association.

___ (1987). *Diagnostic and statistical manual,* Third edition, Revised. Washington, DC: American Psychiatric Association.

___ (1994). *Diagnostic and statistical manual,* Fourth edition. Washington, DC: American Psychiatric Association.

Boring, E. G. (1950). *A history of experimental psychology.* New York: Appleton Century-Crofts.

Gay, P. (1988). *Freud: A life for our time.* New York: Norton.

Gelsomino, J. and D. W. Mackey (1988). Clinical interventions in emergencies: War-related events. In M. Lystad (ed.), *Mental health responses to mass emergencies.* New York: Brunner/Mazel, pp. 211-238.

Harris, M. (1968). *The rise of anthropological theory: A history of theories of culture.* New York: Thomas Y. Crowell.

Herman, J. L. (1992). *Trauma and recovery.* New York: Basic Books.

Horowitz, M. J. (1986). *Stress response syndromes.* New York: Jason Aronson.

Kardiner, A. (1939). *The individual and his society.* New York: Columbia University Press.

Kardiner, A. (1941). *The traumatic neurosis of war.* New York: Hoeber.

Kardiner, A. (1977). *My analysis with Freud.* New York: Norton.

Kardiner, A. and H. Spiegel (1947). *War stress and neurotic illness.* New York: Hoeber.

Scurfield, R. M. (1985). Post-traumatic stress assessment and treatment: Overview and formulations. In C. R. Figely (ed.), *Trauma and its wake: The study and treatment of PTSD* (pp. 219-256). New York: Brunner/Mazel.

van der Kolk, B. A., P. Brown, and O. van der Hart (1989a). Pierre Janet on post-traumatic stress. *Journal of Traumatic Stress,* 2(4), 365-378.

van der Kolk, B. A., P. Brown, and O. van der Hart (1989b). Pierre Janet's treatment on post-traumatic stress. *Journal of Traumatic Stress,* 2(4), 379-395.

van der Kolk, B. A. and O. van der Hart (1989). Pierre Janet and the breakdown of adaptation in psychological trauma. *American Journal of Psychiatry,* 146(12), 1530-1540.

Chapter 2

Assessment and Diagnosis of PTSD in Adults: A Comprehensive Psychological Approach

William F. Flack Jr.
Brett T. Litz
Frank W. Weathers
Sherry A. Beaudreau

INTRODUCTION

The assessment of post-traumatic stress disorder (PTSD) is the focus of an increasingly large body of literature. At least four books (Briere, 1997; Carlson, 1997; Stamm, 1996; Wilson and Keane, 1997) and numerous chapters and journal articles have been devoted to various aspects of the subject appearing within the past few years alone. The aim of this chapter is to give an overview of a comprehensive psychological approach to the assessment and diagnosis of PTSD in adults. In the first section, we begin with a discussion of the distinction between the limited goal of establishing a diagnosis and the aim of assessing PTSD from the standpoint of a functional approach to clinical evaluation. We believe that the latter yields a more useful account, in that patients' interpretations of, and adaptations to, a traumatic event are explored within the context of their psychosocial development across the life span. Valid clinical assessment also requires a sensitivity to the possibility of temporal instability in PTSD symptoms and the current level of functioning at which patients present for evaluation since this disorder, similar to other forms of severe psychopathology, has variable manifestations over time.

The next two sections of this chapter contain descriptions of some specific methods that the clinician can use to evaluate PTSD within the life span, contextualized manner that we advocate. These include a trauma-focused psychosocial history, as well as the structured clinical interviews and psychometric instruments that have been developed specifically for assessing PTSD and commonly associated conditions. In addition, we provide suggestions about screening for PTSD in situations in which limitations of time and resources preclude a more comprehensive evaluation.

In the third section, we describe how the results of such an evaluation can be used in planning for treatments. Here we discuss the controversial issue of when, or even whether, treatment should be focused on memories of traumatic events and the symptoms associated with those memories.

DIAGNOSIS VERSUS ASSESSMENT

Unfortunately, simply making a diagnosis of PTSD yields incomplete information to the clinician. There are a number of reasons why this is the case. First, a diagnosis of PTSD alone does not lead to straightforward decisions about treatment. Second, PTSD is a complex condition that typically has a deleterious impact on multiple areas of psychosocial functioning. Therefore, the information conveyed by a diagnosis of PTSD says little about the other areas of patients' lives that may be adversely affected by, or interact with, the condition. Third, the criteria for making a diagnosis of PTSD have changed over the relatively brief period of time during which it has been included in the standard nosology (American Psychiatric Association, 1980; 1994). The results of at least one recent empirical investigation (e.g., King et al., in press) even call into question whether PTSD is a single, coherent disorder or, alternatively, a superordinate category subsuming two or more distinct clinical conditions. Thus, the diagnosis by itself may mask important distinctions that, when taken into account, make possible a more comprehensive, detailed, and idiographic understanding of the disorder as it is manifested by different patients. In short, a diagnosis of PTSD, important though it may be, cannot stand alone. In our view, post-traumatic adjustment must be understood with respect to the development of the afflicted patient over his or her life course. This entails a comprehensive assessment, in which the diagnosis of the disorder is but one part of the process of clinical evaluation.

We recommend that traumatized individuals be evaluated within a life span, contextual approach to clinical assessment. Although beyond the scope of this chapter, such evaluations should be conducted with sensitivity toward a number of patient characteristics, especially differences in age (Nader, 1997; Ruskin and Talbott, 1996), gender (Wolfe and Kimerling, 1997), ethnicity (Manson, 1997; Marsella et al., 1996), and individual differences in the response to traumatic events (Bowman, 1997).

In our approach, we emphasize from the outset the building of a relationship with patients that can both withstand the inevitable difficulties associated with reporting about traumatic events and lead to the development of a positive alliance with the clinician. This is made possible primarily by an accepting and empathic stance on the part of the evaluator, one which is characterized by a capacity to tolerate one's own painful reactions while listening to patients' descriptions of horrific events (Pearlman and Saakvitne, 1995) and by a sensitivity to patients' initial capacity to tolerate discussion of their trauma. Clinicians should assess regularly their own reactions to the traumatic material reported by patients, and seek consultation with colleagues who are experienced in dealing with traumatized individuals if those reactions begin to interfere with the work at hand.

Clinical evaluators of traumatized individuals need to be aware of the cycle of violence and victimization and the significant association between a history of trauma, on the one hand, and self-destructive behavior, aggressive behavior, and risk for subsequent victimization on the other (e.g., Breslau and Davis, 1992). Thus, the clinician should always be ready to assess issues regarding patients' safety early on in an evaluation. For example, patients can be asked direct, specific questions about current and historical tendencies toward self-destructive behavior.

TAKING A PSYCHOSOCIAL HISTORY

In the initial encounter with traumatized patients, after establishing the boundaries regarding safety and confidentiality, we begin with a brief discussion about the current presenting problem(s), then take a psychosocial history which is centered on the traumatic event. While taking this overview of a patient's history, we ask about a wide range of trauma across the life span, knowing that the index event may often be only one instance in an extensive history of traumatization. Such information is rarely taken into account in a standard psychosocial history.

Our approach has several advantages. First, patients are given the opportunity to report briefly about their post-traumatic adjustment, but not to the point of becoming overwhelmed prematurely. Second, starting with general developmental topics that are (presumably, although not inevitably) less affect-laden enables patients to experience themselves as competent autobiographers who are capable of taking an active role in the clinical evaluation. Third, the trauma, once it is broached in detail, is situated within the developmental context of the person' s life.

In taking a general psychosocial history, we recommend that the clinician ask questions in chronological order. It is vital to place equal emphasis on both strengths and weaknesses in patients' histories and current functioning, in order to construct a balanced account that has practical utility in the context of treatment. This part of the assessment interview begins with questions about childhood, early relationships with parents and other significant caregivers, and siblings. Next comes discussion of experiences in school, including academic performance, interpersonal relationships with peers (including intimate ones), and extracurricular activities. Problematic childhood events are then broached, with an emphasis on alcohol and drug use, any antisocial behavior or legal problems, and particularly stressful incidents. The latter may require careful probing about the possibility of abuse, as well as significant losses, during the childhood and adolescent years.

Late adolescence and early adulthood come next, with questions about adjustment to further schooling and work, as well as interpersonal functioning and intimate relationships. Any problematic issues reported to have occurred during childhood should be followed up with specific questions about their development or resolution. This part of the interview should segue naturally into topics relating to patients' current functioning. The major bases to be covered here include psychosocial functioning in the areas of intimate relationships, family relationships (including the extended family), work, and leisure activities.

Once this general contextual information has been gathered, the clinician can then begin narrowing the focus of the assessment toward psychopathology. Patients should be asked about changes they want to make currently, and about factors that may make these changes difficult. Finally, the focus of the assessment is directed toward the target trauma and post-traumatic adjustment.

Caveats in Interviewing

Traumatic events and their psychosocial sequelae are most usefully examined by means of multiple, converging methods of clinical evaluation. However, the clinician is well advised to begin discussion of this material in the context of an interview. In addition, patients should be forewarned that talking about their trauma may well lead to a temporary increase in symptoms, such as intrusive thoughts and nightmares. Again, this material must be handled with caution and with an empathic sensitivity toward patients' capacities to tolerate the memories of the event(s) and associated emotional reactions. Patients may be unable to talk about their trauma, or they may be unable to give complete information, for a variety of reasons, including the forgetting of details, extreme sensitivity to even broaching the topic of trauma, and/or severe numbing, avoidance, and withdrawal. Patients should be informed that they are the sole arbiters regarding what information they divulge and the pace at which they do so. This overt sharing of power and control reinforces the collaborative character of the clinical relationship, and often helps to decrease the anxiety that is almost always associated with direct discussion of traumatic events. Suggested questions for inquiring about traumatic experiences and post-traumatic adjustment are listed in Table 2.1.

METHODS OF ASSESSMENT

Recognizing the inherent limitations of relying on one source of information, we advocate gathering information by means of different types of clinical instruments. This begins with the use of a trauma-focused clinical interview, as outlined earlier. Once information has been gathered from the general interview, additional methods can be brought to bear in the evaluation of specific aspects of PTSD. These methods include structured diagnostic interviews and various psychometric instruments. Although the use of all of these methods are recommended for the purpose of conducting a comprehensive evaluation of PTSD, limitations of time and resources may make such an assessment impossible. Thus, we end this section of the chapter with suggestions for the diagnostic screening for PTSD.

The definition of PTSD contained in the current nosology used in the United States (American Psychiatric Association, 1994) breaks the disorder down into three sets of symptoms: reexperiencing, avoidance and numbing,

TABLE 2.1. Content Areas to Cover When Interviewing Traumatized Individuals

---

A. Pretrauma
1. Developmental (life course) context
2. Life context at the time of the traumatic event(s)
3. Events just prior to the trauma
4. Patient's state of mind just prior to the trauma

B. Trauma
1. What happened (e.g., sights, sounds, thoughts, feelings, actions, meanings)
2. What happened afterward (e.g., others' responses)
3. Unclear or forgotten elements of memories
4. Feelings about recounting trauma during the interview

C. Posttrauma
1. PTSD symptoms
2. Situational cues that trigger reactions
3. Changes in psychosocial functioning
4. Changes in belief system about the self and the world
5. Changes in alcohol and drug use
6. Treatment history and response
7. Current environment and resources

---

and hyperarousal. In addition, symptoms must last for at least one month and must lead to impairment in social or occupational functioning. According to Criterion A, exposure to a traumatic event is defined as the experience (direct or indirect) of an event (or events) that constitutes a threat to the life or limb of self or other, accompanied by extreme fear, horror, or helplessness. A number of instruments are available for assessing such events (see reviews by Briere, 1997; Norris and Riad, 1997). For example, the Evaluation of Lifetime Stressors Questionnaire and Interview (Krinsley et al., 1994) is a comprehensive protocol for assessing a wide range of stressful events across the life span. Another example is the recent Traumatic Life Events Questionnaire (TLEQ) (Kubany, 1995), which is also designed to be consistent with the current DSM-based definition of a Criterion A event. The TLEQ makes possible the subjective evaluation of seventeen traumatic events and associated emotional responses within two and twelve months of the assessment. In addition, instruments such as the Clinician-Administered PTSD Scale (CAPS-DX; Blake et al., 1996) and the Posttraumatic Stress Diagnostic Scale (PDS; Foa et al., 1993) contain checklists to assess the occurrence of Criterion A (traumatic) events.

In the DSM-IV, criterion sets B, C, and D contain the specific symptoms of PTSD, grouped according to their designation as symptoms of reexperiencing (B), avoidance and numbing (C), and hyperarousal (D). Although reexperiencing, avoidance and numbing, and hyperarousal must be present in order to make a diagnosis of PTSD, the specific symptoms required within each criterion set are variable in number, ranging from one (B) to three (C). Since only a subset of symptoms is required from each cluster, and there are no necessary or sufficient symptoms within each cluster, there are quite a few potential combinations of symptoms that may qualify a patient for a diagnosis of PTSD. In other words, patients with a diagnosis of PTSD may present very differently, making an idiographic analysis of patients' constellation of symptoms essential in terms of their frequency of occurrence, intensity of experience, and degree of functional impairment.

A number of methods are available for the assessment of PTSD symptoms. These include structured clinical interviews, self-report scales dedicated to PTSD, and broad spectrum instruments that contain PTSD subscales. At least six structured interviews are available for the assessment of PTSD (see reviews by Briere, 1997; Weathers and Keane, 1998; Weiss, 1997). We recommend the use of the Clinician-Administered PTSD Scale for the DSM-IV (CAPS-DX; Blake et al., 1996). The CAPS-DX allows the clinician to evaluate up to three Criterion A events, as well as each of the seventeen symptoms of PTSD contained in the DSM-IV and five additional symptoms commonly associated with PTSD. Each symptom and associated feature can be characterized on the dimensions of time (current, lifetime), frequency, and intensity. Another example of this kind of assessment instrument is the Structured Interview for PTSD (Davidson, Smith, and Kudler, 1989). Other PTSD interviews include the PTSD module of the Structured Clinical Interview for DSM-IV (First et al., 1996), the Structured Interview for DSM III-R/PTSD (Spitzer et al., 1990), and the interview version of the PTSD Symptom Scale (PSS-I Foa et al., 1993).

In addition to structured interviews, more than a dozen paper-and-pencil measures have been validated for the assessment of PTSD. These can be divided into those that correspond directly to the DSM diagnostic criteria for PTSD, those designed specifically to assess PTSD but that do not correspond exactly to the DSM criteria, and those empirically derived from existing questionnaires (Weathers and Keane, 1998). An example of DSM-correspondent measures is the PTSD checklist (PCL) (Weathers et al., 1993). The PCL consists of seventeen items that correspond to the seventeen PTSD symptoms in the DSM-IV. Each item is rated on a five-point scale, indicating the severity of a symptom over the past month. Similar measures include the PTSD Symptom Scale–Self-Report (PSS-SR) (Foa et al., 1993), which is the paper and-pencil version of the PSS-I, and the recently published Posttraumatic Stress Diagnostic Scale (PDS) (Davidson, Smith, and Kudler, 1989). The PDS is unique among (paper-and-pencil, self-report) measures of PTSD in that it assesses all six (A-F) of the DSM-IV diagnostic criteria for PTSD.

Some of the most widely used measures of PTSD do not conform strictly to the criteria contained in the DSM. Among these are the Mississippi Scale for Combat-Related PTSD (Keane, 1988) and the Impact of Event Scale (IES) (Horowitz, Wilner, and Alvarez, 1979). The Mississippi Scale consists of thirty-five items, rated on a five-point scale, that tap the DSM-III PTSD criteria and a variety of associated features. The civilian version of the Mississippi Scale includes four additional items intended to ensure adequate coverage of DSM-III-R criteria. Also, items on the original Mississippi Scale referring to the military were rephrased for the civilian version. The original IES consisted of fifteen items, with seven items assessing intrusion symptoms and eight items assessing avoidance symptoms. Respondents specify a traumatic event, then rate the frequency of each symptom over the past week, using a four-point scale. The IES was recently updated to bring it more into line with DSM-IV PTSD criteria (Weiss and Marmar, 1997). Seven items were added, primarily tapping hyperarousal symptoms, and the response format was changed to a five-point scale, indicating degree of distress caused by each symptom.

Another instrument in this category is the Penn Inventory (Hammarberg, 1992), a twenty-six–item scale that assesses many, but not all, of the DSM PTSD criteria, as well as a number of associated problems. Similar to the Beck Depression Inventory (BDI-I) (Beck, Steer, and Brown, 1996), items on the Penn consist of four statements graded to reflect increasing symptom severity.

The final category of self-report PTSD measures are PTSD scales derived from existing instruments such as the MMPI and the Symptom Checklist-90-R (SCL-90-R). The most widely used of these is the PK scale of the MMPI and MMPI-2 (Keane, Malloy, and Fairbank, 1984; Lyons and Keane, 1992). The original PK consists of forty-nine MMPI items found to distinguish between combat veterans with and without PTSD. Three repeated items were dropped when the MMPI-2 was published. The PK scale can be used effectively when administered either in the context of the full MMPI-2 or as a stand-alone instrument (Herman et al., 1996; Lyons and Scotti, 1994). Other examples are the PTSD scales of the SCL-90-R. The Crime-Related PTSD Scale (CR-PTSD) (Saunders, Arrate, and Kilpatrick, 1990) consists of twenty-eight SCL-90-R items that discriminate female crime victims with and without PTSD. The War-Zone-Related PTSD Scale (WZ-PTSD) (Weathers et al., 1996) consists of twenty-five SCL-90-R items that discriminate male combat veterans with and without PTSD. Interestingly, these two scales, derived through similar methods but on very different trauma populations, share only eleven items. Subscales have also been developed from some standard psychometric instruments that are typically used to assess a broad range of psychopathological conditions. The PK Scale (Lyons and Keane, 1992) from the Minnesota Multiphasic Personality Inventory-2 (MMPI-2) (Graham, 1993) is one example.

Other instruments are available for the evaluation of specific conditions that are commonly associated with PTSD. The clinician interested in diagnosing other Axis I disorders based on the criteria contained in the DSM-IV can employ the *Structured Clinical Interview for the DSM-IV (Patient Edition)* (SCID-IIP) (First et al., 1996). This may be particularly helpful in identifying depression, substance use disorders, and anxiety disorders that often occur with PTSD. Also useful in evaluating the severity of depression and anxiety are the Beck Depression Inventory (BDI) (Beck, Steer, and Brown, 1996) and the Beck Anxiety Inventory (BAI) (Beck et al., 1988), both of which are brief, self-report scales. Certain disorders of personality, especially borderline personality disorder, are also commonly seen in patients with PTSD. These can be evaluated by means of the *Structured Clinical Interview for the DSM-III-R Axis II* (SCID-II; Spitzer et al., 1990). More broad-based instruments for assessing personality characteristics are also available and some (e.g., MMPI-2) have the added benefit of containing imbedded scales for PTSD.

Although not yet widely used for this purpose, the evaluation of some symptoms of PTSD, especially physiological reactivity and exaggerated startle response, are evaluated most directly by means of psychophysiological measurement (see review by Orr and Kaloupek, 1997). Physiological reactivity can be assessed with measurements of heart rate, skin conductance, and blood pressure in response to a trauma-related "challenge" (e.g., script-driven imagery of an index trauma).

A Brief Screening

The comprehensive assessment of PTSD that we recommend clearly requires considerable resources of personnel and time. Certainly the average clinician working within the current confines of most managed care systems is unlikely to be given the amount of time necessary to administer a battery of structured clinical interviews and psychometric instruments. Although a comprehensive assessment is impossible to perform within a single session, the busy clinician can still conduct a screening for the presence of PTSD within such limits. In this context, we suggest a brief clinical interview combined with either the PCL-C or the PSS-SR. We suggest the use of a more thorough assessment tool (the CAPS, for example) at the beginning of therapy as a means of identifying and clarifying further the targets for intervention.

USING ASSESSMENT RESULTS IN MAKING CLINICAL RECOMMENDATIONS

The final section of this chapter is devoted to the link between the results of a comprehensive assessment of PTSD and the clinician's recommendations for treatment. Whichever methods the clinician uses to perform the assessment, the results must be brought together into a coherent whole that can be used to guide deliberation about specific forms of treatment or clinical management. Such recommendations are informed primarily by two factors. One is the current condition of the patient with PTSD. Flack and colleagues (Flack, Litz, and Keane, 1998; Keane, 1995) recommend tailoring psychotherapeutic treatment to the current presentation of the patient. For example, many patients will present for evaluation and treatment during periods of acute crisis. Clearly, acutely and severely disturbed patients are not good candidates for therapy that is focused on their memories of trauma and associated emotions. Rather, they should be referred for supportive work that is aimed at behavioral and emotional stabilization. Medications may prove helpful in this regard, and those designed for the treatment of anxiety and depression are often favored for patients with PTSD (Friedman, 1991). Once stabilized, such patients may benefit from therapeutic approaches that include stress management, psychoeducation about PTSD, trauma focus, and aftercare.

An important goal in the assessment of PTSD is to prioritize targets for change since experiences of trauma and subsequent posttraumatic pathology are associated with comorbid psychiatric conditions and numerous problems in living (see Keane and Kaloupek, 1998). Comprehensive treatments of PTSD usually entail multiple techniques and strategies that target specific clusters of symptoms and comorbid conditions; reexperiencing symptoms may be treated with exposure therapy of one type or another; symptoms of avoidance may be treated by gradually encouraging the person to increase the range of their interpersonal contacts and activities, coupled with the application of coping skills; hyperarousal symptoms can be addressed by training in stress management.

Exposure Treatments

The emotional processing of trauma-related memories, including various types of direct therapeutic exposure, is usually considered central to the treatment of posttraumatic pathology (Fairbank and Brown, 1987; Flack, Litz, and Keane, 1998; Keane, Zimering, and Caddell, 1985; Keane et al., 1989). Direct therapeutic exposure has the most empirical support in the treatment outcome literature (Solomon, Gerrity, and Muff, 1992). Exposure treatments, however, require considerable resources on the part of both patients and therapists. Deciding whether exposure treatment is indicated for a given combination of patient and therapist is a critical task in the assessment of PTSD.

Several conditions must be met before a therapist should recommend exposure treatments. First, patients must be able to meet the boundary conditions of the technique, such as the ability to form images about traumatic events (see Boudewyns and Shipley, 1980; Levis, 1980). For example, candidates for exposure therapies should report reexperiencing symptoms and exhibit some level of anxious arousal in response to reminders of their trauma. Furthermore, they should be able to follow the therapist's instructions and to imagine various stimuli clearly. A second requirement of exposure techniques is patients' capacities to tolerate the intense levels of arousal associated with the treatment, as well as the increase in PTSD symptoms that often occurs at the beginning of treatment.

The therapist should be especially observant about the potential for therapy dropout when making a decision about recommending exposure treatment. Critical to this decision is patients' abilities to tolerate the intense levels of arousal generated during exposure therapies. Thus, patients should be in relatively good health (moderate to severe heart conditions, for example, are rule-out conditions), have a stable living environment (or some consistent social supports), and not be abusing drugs or alcohol. These decision rules regarding the use of exposure therapies are conventions derived from clinical experience (Litz et al., 1990); specific conditions for positive responses to such treatments have not yet been demonstrated empirically.

SUMMARY

In this chapter, we outlined one approach to the comprehensive assessment of PTSD in adults. The approach is one in which information about exposure to traumatic events and their psychosocial consequences is made meaningful by being embedded within the development of the individual patient across his or her life span. Numerous techniques are available for the elicitation of this information, and recommendations for treatment are based on the current needs of the patient and phase of disorder.

REFERENCES

American Psychiatric Association (1980). *Diagnostic and statistical manual of mental disorders,* Third edition. Washington, DC: Author.

American Psychiatric Association (1994). *Diagnostic and statistical manual of mental disorders,* Fourth edition. Washington, DC: Author.

Beck, A.T., Epstein, N., Brown, G., and Steer, R.A. (1988). An inventory for measuring clinical anxiety: Psychometric properties. *Journal of Consulting and Clinical Psychology, 56,* 893-897.

Beck, A.T., Steer, R.A., and Brown, G.K. (1996). *Beck Depression Inventory-II.* San Antonio, TX: The Psychological Corporation.

Blake, D.D., Weathers, F.W., Nagy, L.M., Kaloupek, D.G., Gusman, F.D., Charney, D.S., and Keane, T.M. (1996). The Clinician-Administered PTSD Scale for DSM-IV: Current and Lifetime Diagnostic Version (CAPS-DX). Unpublished scale. (Available from the Behavioral Science Division, National Center for PTSD, Boston DVAMC, Boston, MA.)

Boudewyns, P.A. and Shipley, R.H. (1980). *Flooding and implosive therapy.* New York: Plenum Press.

Bowman, M. (1997). *Individual differences in posttraumatic response: Problems with the adversity-distress connection.* Mahwah, NJ: Lawrence Erlbaum Associates.

Breslau, N. and Davis, G. (1992). Posttraumatic stress disorder in an urban population of young adults: Risk factors for chronicity. *American Journal of Psychiatry, 149*(5), 671-675.

Briere, J. (1997). *Psychological assessment of adult posttraumatic states.* Washington, DC: American Psychological Association.

Carlson, B. (1997). *Trauma assessments: A clinician's guide.* New York: Guilford Press.

Davidson, J., Smith, R., and Kudler, H. (1989). Validity and reliability of the DSM-III criteria for posttraumatic stress disorder: Experience with a structured interview. *Journal of Nervous and Mental Disease, 177,* 336-341.

Fairbank, J.A. and Brown, T.A. (1987). Current behavioral approaches to the treatment of post-traumatic stress disorder. *The Behavior Therapist. 10,* 57-64.

First, M.B., Gibbon, M., Spitzer, R.L., and Williams, J.B.W. (1996). *User's guide for the SCID-I: Structured clinical interview for DSM-IV Axis I disorders (SCID-L Research version).* New York: Biometrics Research Department, New York State Psychiatric Institute.

Flack, W.F. Jr., Litz, B.T., and Keane, T.M. (1998). Cognitive-behavioral treatment of war-zone-related PTSD: A flexible, hierarchical approach. In V.W. Follette, F.R. Abueg, and J.I. Ruzek (Eds.), *Cognitive-behavioral therapies for trauma* (pp. 77-99). New York: Guilford Press.

Foa, B., Riggs, D., Dancu, D., and Rothbaum, B. (1993). Reliability and validity of a brief instrument for assessing post-traumatic stress disorder. *Journal of Traumatic Stress, 6,* 459-474.

Friedman, M.J. (1991). Biological approaches to the diagnosis and treatment of post-traumatic stress disorder. *Journal of Traumatic Stress, 4,* 67-91.

Graham, J.R. (1993). *MMPI-2: Assessing personality and psychopathology.* New York: Oxford University Press.

Hammarberg, M. (1992). Penn Inventory for Posttraumatic Stress Disorder: Psychometric properties. *Psychological Assessment, 4,* 67-76.

Herman, D.S., Weathers, F.W., Litz, B.T., and Keane, T.M. (1996). Psychometric properties of the embedded and stand-alone versions of the MMPI-2 Keane PTSD scale. *Assessment, 3,* 437-442.

Horowitz, M.J., Wilner, N., and Alvarez, W. (1979). Impact of Event Scale: A measure of subjective stress. *Psychosomatic Medicine, 41,* 209-218.

Keane, T.M. (1988). The Mississippi scale for combat-related PTSD: Three studies in reliability and validity. *Journal of Consulting and Clinical Psychology, 56,* 85-90.

Keane, T.M. (1995). The role of exposure therapy in the psychological treatment of PTSD. *National Center for PTSD (NCP) Quarterly, 5,* 1-6.

Keane, T.M., Fairbank, J.A., Caddell, J.M., and Zimering, R.T. (1989). Clinical evaluation of a measure to assess combat exposure. *Psychological Assessment, 1,* 53-55.

Keane, T.M. and Kaloupek, D.G. (1998). Cormorbid psychiatric disorders in PTSD: Implications for research. In R. Yehuda and A. McFarlane (Eds.), *Psychobiology of posttraumatic stress disorder.* New York: Annals of the New York Academy of Science.

Keane, T.M., Malloy, P.F., and Fairbank, J.A. (1984). Empirical development of an MMPI subscale for the assessment of combat-related posttraumatic stress disorder. *Journal of Consulting and Clinical Psychology, 52,* 888-891.

Keane, T.M., Zimering, R.T., and Caddell, J.M. (1985). A behavioral formulation of posttraumatic stress disorder in Vietnam veterans. *Behavior Therapist, 8,* 9-12.

King, D.W., Leskin, G.A., King, L.A., and Weathers, F.W. (in press). Confirmatory factor analysis of the Clinician-Administered PTSD Scale. *Psychological Assessment.*

Krinsley, K., Weathers, F.W., Vielhauer, M., Newman, E., Walker, E., Young, L., and Kimerling, R. (1994). Evaluation of Lifetime Stressors Questionnaire and Interview. Unpublished scale. (Available from the first author, Behavioral Science Division, National Center for PTSD, Boston DVAMC, Boston, MA.)

Kubany, E. (1995). The Traumatic Life Events Questionnaire (TLEQ): A brief measure of prior traumatic exposure. Unpublished scale. (Available from the author, Pacific Center for PTSD, Honolulu, Hawaii.)

Levis, D.J. (1980). The learned helplessness effect: An expectancy, discrimination deficit, or motivational-induced persistence? *Journal of Research in Personality, 14,* 158-169.

Litz, B.T., Blake, D.D., Gerardi, R.G., and Keane, T.M. (1990). Decision making guidelines for the use of direct therapeutic exposure in the treatment of post-traumatic stress disorder. *The Behavior Therapist, 13,* 91-93

Lyons, J.A. and Keane, T.M. (1992). Keane PTSD scale: MMPI and MMPI-2 update. *Journal of Traumatic Stress, 5,* 111-117.

Lyons, J.A. and Scotti, J.R. (1994). Comparability of two administration formats of the Keane Posttraumatic Stress Disorder Scale. *Psychological Assessment, 6,* 209-211.

Manson, S.M. (1997). Cross-cultural and multiethnic assessment of trauma. In J.P. Wilson and T.M. Keane (Eds.), *Assessing psychological trauma and PTSD* (pp. 239-266). New York: Guilford Press.

Marsella, A.J., Friedman, M.J., Gerrity, E.T., and Scurfield, R.M. (Eds.) (1996). *Ethnocultural aspects of posttraumatic stress disorder: Issues, research, and clinical applications.* Washington, DC: American Psychological Association.

Nader, K.O. (1997). Assessing traumatic experiences in children. In J.P. Wilson and T.M. Keane (Eds.), *Assessing psychological trauma and PTSD* (pp. 291-348). New York: Guilford Press.

Norris, F.H. and Riad, J.K. (1997). Standardized self-report measures of civilian trauma and posttraumatic stress disorder. In J.P. Wilson and T.M. Keane (Eds.), *Assessing psychological trauma and PTSD* (pp. 7-42). New York: Guilford Press.

Orr, S.P. and Kaloupek, D.G. (1997). Psychophysiological assessment of posttraumatic stress disorder. In J.P. Wilson and T.M. Keane (Eds.), *Assessing psychological trauma and PTSD* (pp. 69-97). New York: Guilford Press.

Pearlman, L.A. and Saakvitne, K.W. (1995). *Trauma and the therapist: Countertransference and vicarious traumatization in psychotherapy with incest survivors.* New York: Norton.

Ruskin, P.E. and Talbott, J.A. (Eds.) (1996). *Aging and posttraumatic stress disorder*. Washington, DC: American Psychiatric Press.

Saunders, B.E., Arrate, C.M., and Kilpatrick, D.G. (1990). Development of a crime-related posttraumatic stress disorder scale for women within the Symptom Checklist-90-Revised. *Journal of Traumatic Stress, 3,* 439-448.

Solomon, S.D., Gerrity, E.T., and Muff, A.M. (1992). Efficacy of treatments for post-traumatic stress disorder: An empirical review. *Journal of the American Medical Association, 268,* 633-638.

Spitzer, R.L., Williams, J.B.W., Gibbon, M., and First, M.B. (1990). *Structured clinical interview for DSM III-R/PTSD Personality disorders (SCID-II; Version 1.0).* Washington, DC: American Psychiatric Press.

Stamm, B.H. (Ed.) (1996). *Measurement of stress, trauma, and adaptation*. Lutherville, MD: The Sidran Press.

Weathers, F.W. and Keane, T.M. (1998). Psychological assessment. In P.A. Saigh and J.D. Bremmer (Eds.), *Posttraumatic stress disorder: A comprehensive approach to research and treatment* (pp. 24-34). New York: Allyn & Bacon.

Weathers, F.W., Litz, B.T., Herman, D.S., Huska, J.A., and Keane, T.M. (1993, October). "The PTSD Checklist (PCL): Reliability, validity, and diagnostic utility." Paper presented at the annual meeting of the International Society for Traumatic Stress Studies, San Antonio, TX. (Unpublished scale available from the Behavioral Science Division, National Center for PTSD, Boston DVAMC, Boston, MA.)

Weathers, F.W., Litz, B.T., Herman, D.S., Keane, T.M., Steinberg, H.R., Huska, J.A., and Kraemer, H.C. (1996). The utility of the SCL-90-R for the diagnosis of war-zone-related PTSD. *Journal of Traumatic Stress, 9,* 111-128.

Weiss, D.S. (1997). Structured clinical interview techniques. In J.P. Wilson and T.M. Keane (Eds.), *Assessing psychological trauma and PTSD* (pp. 493-511). New York: Guilford Press.

Weiss, D.S. and Marmar, C.R. (1997). The Impact of Event Scale—Revised. In J.P. Wilson and T.M. Keane (Eds.), *Assessing psychological trauma and PTSD* (pp. 399-411). New York: Guilford Press.

Wilson, J.P. and Keane, T.M. (Eds.) (1997). *Assessing psychological trauma and PTSD*. New York: Guilford Press.

Wolfe, J. and Kimerling, R. (1997). Gender issues in the assessment of posttraumatic stress disorder. In J.P. Wilson and T.M. Keane (Eds.), *Assessing psychological trauma and PTSD* (pp. 192-238). New York: Guilford Press.

Chapter 3

Approaches to the Treatment of PTSD

Bessel A. van der Kolk
Onno van der Hart
Jennifer Burbridge

INTRODUCTION

Terrifying experiences that rupture people's sense of predictability and invulnerability can profoundly alter the ways in which they subsequently deal with their emotions and with their environment. The syndrome of post-traumatic stress disorder (PTSD) can follow such widely different stressors as war trauma, physical and sexual assaults, accidents, and other natural and man-made disasters. Mirroring the confusion and disbelief of people whose basic assumptions are shattered by traumatic experiences, the psychiatric profession periodically has been fascinated by trauma, followed by sudden disbelief in the importance of trauma in the genesis of psychopathology. Over the past decade our profession has experienced the third intense wave of efforts to grasp the reality of trauma on body and soul. The first wave occurred at the Salpêtrière during the closing decades of the nineteenth century, and the second wave, spearheaded by Abram Kardiner (1941), occurred in the 1940s. The findings about the consequences of trauma and what constitutes effective treatment have been extraordinarily consistent over these 120 years.

Several studies in recent years have shown that post-traumatic stress disorder (PTSD) is among the most common of psychiatric disorders. The National Vietnam Veterans Readjustment Study (Kulka, Schlenger, and Fairbank, 1990) found that approximately twenty years after the end of the Vietnam war, 15.2 percent of Vietnam theater veterans continued to suffer from PTSD. However, PTSD is not confined to combat soldiers, but is quite common in the general population, particularly among psychiatric patients. Various studies have demonstrated a lifetime prevalence of between 1.3 percent (Helzer, Robins, and McEvoy, 1987) and 9 percent (Breslau, Davis, and Andreski, 1991) in the general population and at least 15 percent in psychiatric inpatients (Saxe et al., 1993). Although PTSD is associated with high levels of chronicity, comorbidity, and functional impairment, the general level of functioning varies a great deal between affected individuals.

Lack of predictability and controllability are the central issues for the development and maintenance of PTSD. The combination of intrusive and numbing symptoms has been consistently noted over the past century (e.g., Janet, 1904; Kardiner, 1941), and forms the basis of our understanding of the nature of PTSD. What distinguishes people who develop PTSD from people who are merely temporarily overwhelmed is that people who develop PTSD become "stuck" on the trauma and keep reliving it in thoughts, feelings, or images. Evidence during the 1990s supports the notion that it is the intrusive reliving, rather than the traumatic event itself, that is responsible for the complex biobehavioral change that we call PTSD (McFarlane, 1988). Once they become dominated by intrusions of the trauma, traumatized individuals begin organizing their lives around avoiding having them (van der Kolk and Ducey, 1984). Avoidance may take many different forms: keeping away from reminders, ingesting drugs or alcohol that numb awareness of distressing emotional states, or utilizing dissociating to keep unpleasant experiences from conscious awareness. The helplessness, conditioned hyperarousal, and other trauma-related changes may permanently change how a person deals with stress, alter his or her self-concept, and interfere with the view of the world as a basically safe and predictable place.

A relative sense of safety and predictability are preconditions for effective planning and personal action. Freud (1911/1959) described how, in order to function properly, people need to be able to define their needs, anticipate how to meet them, and plan for appropriate action. In order to do this, people need to be able to mentally entertain a range of options, without resorting to action. He called this capacity "thought as experimental action." Traumatized people seem to lose this essential capacity and have difficulty turning inward to utilize their emotions as guides for action (van der Kolk and Ducey, 1984). Instead, their internal world becomes a danger zone and they seem to spend their energies on *not* thinking and planning.

The therapeutic relationship with these patients tends to be extraordinarily complex. It confronts all participants with intense emotional experiences, forcing them to explore the darkest corners of their mind, and to face the entire spectrum of human glory and degradation. The devastating effects of trauma on affect modulation, attention, perception, and the giving and taking of pleasure bring us face to face with the full destructive impact of traumatic stress to dominate, use, and control others.

The Role of Memory and Dissociation

Pierre Janet (1889) first described how the central issue in trauma is dissociation: memories of what has happened cannot be integrated into one's general experiential schemes and are split off from the rest of personal experience. Physiological hyperarousal seems to be a central precondition for dissociation to occur. Lack of integration on a schematic level causes the experience to be stored as affect states or as somatosensory elements of the trauma (van der Kolk and Fisler, 1994), which return into consciousness when reminders activate customary response patterns: physical sensations (such as panic attacks), visual images (such as flashbacks and nightmares), obsessive ruminations, or behavioral reenactments of elements of the trauma.

Most studies of people who develop PTSD find significant dissociative symptomatology (Bremner et al., 1993; Marmar et al., 1994). The most extreme form of posttraumatic dissociation is seen in patients who suffer from dissociative identity disorder. Janet (1889) first described how traumatized people become "attached" (Freud [1959] would later use the term "fixated") to the trauma:

> unable to integrate traumatic memories, they seem to have lost their capacity to assimilate new experiences as well. It is as if their personality definitely stopped at a certain point and cannot enlarge any more by the addition or assimilation of new elements. (p. 532)

This suggests that traumatized people are prone to revert to earlier modes of cognitive processing of information when faced with new stresses.

Because the core problem in PTSD consists of a failure to integrate an upsetting experience into autobiographical memory, the goal of treatment is to find a way in which people can acknowledge the reality of what has happened without having to reexperience the trauma all over again. For this to occur, merely uncovering memories is not enough: they need to be modified and transformed, i.e., placed in their proper context and reconstructed into neutral or meaningful narratives. Thus, in therapy, memory paradoxically becomes an act of creation, rather than the static recording of events that is characteristic of trauma-based memories.

PTSD As a Biologically Based Disorder

Abram Kardiner (1941) introduced the notion that "traumatic neuroses" are "physioneuroses" and that patients with PTSD remain on constant alert for environmental threat: "[t]he subject acts as if the original traumatic situation were still in existence and engages in protective devices which failed on the original occasion" (p. 82). In PTSD, the physiological state of chronic overarousal is accompanied by difficulties in attention and concentration, as well as distortions in information processing, including narrowing of attention onto sources of potential challenge or threat. It appears that for traumatized people, all emotions become dangerous. Although the function of their hyperarousal is to prepare them for some form of action in the face of threat, it does not build up specific skills and feelings of mastery and control, because the anticipated action is not specific.

Over the past few years, it has become increasingly evident that the intensity of the initial somatic response to a potentially traumatic experience is the most significant predictor of long-term outcome. If the stress is sufficiently overwhelming, the resulting trauma sets up a conditional emotional response in which the body continues to go into a fight, flight, or freeze response at the least provocation: traumatized people keep experiencing life as a continuation of the trauma and remain in a state of constant alert for its return. Many traumatized people who have consciously put the trauma behind them continue to experience anxiety and increased physical arousal when exposed to situations that remind them of the trauma, or even to unexpected events such as loud noises, and go into fight/flight reactions, without necessarily being aware of the origin of these extreme behaviors.

Though the biological underpinnings of response to trauma are extremely complex, forty years of research on humans and other mammals have demonstrated that trauma (particularly trauma early in the life cycle) has long-term effects on the neurochemical response to stress. This includes the magnitude of the catecholamine response, the duration and extent of the cortisol response, as well as a number of other biological systems, such as the serotonin and endogenous opioid system (for an extensive review on the psychobiology of trauma, see van der Kolk, 1994).

THE SYMPTOMATOLOGY OF PTSD

Although posttraumatic stress has been recognized in the poetry of Homer, Shakespeare, and Goethe, psychiatry has consistently recognized its existence only since 1980 when PTSD was introduced into the DSM-III. Table 3.1 shows the diagnostic criteria for simple PTSD. Since 1980, there has been a growing body of literature documenting the posttraumatic symptoms of hyperarousal, hyperreactivity to stimuli reminiscent of the trauma, avoidance and emotional numbing in a large variety of traumatized populations, including war veterans, children who have experienced physical or sexual assaults, women who have been battered and raped, people exposed to natural disasters, refugees, and political prisoners. Regardless of the origin of the terror, the central nervous system (CNS) reacts consistently to

TABLE 3.1. Simple PTSD (DSM-IV)

A. Exposure to life-threatening events
   1. Intense subjective distress upon exposure
B. Reexperiencing the trauma
   1. Recurrent intrusive memories or repetitive play
   2. Recurrent dreams
   3. Suddenly acting or feeling as if the traumatic event were happening again
   4. Intense distress upon reexposure to events similar to or referring back to the trauma
   5. Physiological reactions after reexposure
C. Persistent avoidance or numbing of responsiveness
   1. Efforts to avoid thoughts or feelings associated with trauma
   2. Efforts to avoid activities
   3. Inability to remember all or part of the trauma
   4. Less interest in activities
   5. Feelings of detachment, estrangement, lack of connection
   6. Sense of future that is shortened
D. Persistent symptoms of increased arousal
   1. Problems falling or staying asleep
   2. Irritability, outbursts of anger
   3. Problems concentrating
   4. Overawareness of surroundings
   5. Exaggerated startle reaction

---

overwhelming, threatening, and uncontrollable experiences with conditioned emotional responses. For example, rape victims may respond to conditioned stimuli, such as the approach by an unknown man, as if they were about to be raped again, and experience panic.

Intrusive Reexperiencing

Remembrance and intrusion of the trauma is expressed on many different levels, ranging from flashbacks, affective states, somatic sensations, nightmares, interpersonal reenactments, including transference repetitions, character styles, and pervasive life themes. Laub and Auerhahn (1993) organized the different forms of knowing along a continuum according to the distance from the traumatic experience. Each form also progressively represents a consciously deeper and more integrated "level of knowing." The different forms of remembering trauma include

1. not knowing;
2. fugue states (in which events are relived in an altered state of consciousness);
3. retention of the experience as compartmentalized, undigested fragments of perceptions that break into consciousness (with no conscious meaning or relation to oneself);
4. transference phenomena (wherein the traumatic legacy is lived out as one's inevitable fate);
5. its partial, hesitant expression as an overpowering narrative;
6. the experience of compelling, identity-defining and pervasive life themes (both conscious and unconscious); and
7. its organization as a witnessed narrative.

These various forms of knowing are not mutually exclusive.

Autonomic Hyperarousal

Although people with PTSD tend to deal with their environment by emotional constriction, their bodies continue to react to certain physical and emotional stimuli as if there were a continuing threat of annihilation. Conditioned autonomic arousal to trauma-related stimuli has consistently been shown to occur in a variety of traumatized populations. Autonomic arousal, which serves the essential function of alerting the organism to potential danger, seems to lose that function in traumatized people: the easy triggering of somatic stress reactions causes people with PTSD to be unable to rely on bodily sensations to warn them against impending threat. Instead, the persistent warning signals lose their function as signals of impending danger and cease to alert the organism to take appropriate action.

Numbing of Responsiveness

Aware of their difficulties in controlling their emotions, traumatized people seem to spend their energies on avoiding distressing internal sensations, instead of attending to the demands of the environment. In addition, they lose satisfaction in matters that previously gave them a sense of satisfaction and may feel "dead to the world." This emotional numbing may be expressed as depression, anhedonia and lack of motivation, psychosomatic reactions, or as dissociative states. In contrast with the intrusive PTSD symptoms, which occur in response to outside stimuli, numbing is part of these patients' baseline functioning. In children, numbing has been observed among elementary school children who have been attacked by a sniper, among witnesses to parental assault or murder, and among victims of physical or sexual abuse. They become less involved in playful social interactions, and often are withdrawn and isolated. After being traumatized, many people stop feeling pleasure from exploration and involvement in activities, and they feel that they just "go through the motions" of everyday living. Emotional numbness also gets in the way of resolving the trauma in psychotherapy: they give up on recovery and it keeps them from being able to imagine a future for themselves.

Intense Emotional Reactions and Sleep Problems

The loss of neuromodulation that is at the core of PTSD leads to a loss of affect regulation. Traumatized people go immediately from stimulus to response without being able to first figure out what makes them so upset. They tend to experience intense fear, anxiety, anger, and panic in response to even minor stimuli. This makes them either overreact and intimidate others, or shut down and freeze. Both adults and children with such hyperarousal will experience sleep problems, both because they are unable to still themselves sufficiently to go to sleep, and because they are fearful of having traumatic nightmares. Many traumatized people report dream-interruption insomnia: they wake themselves up as soon as they start having a dream, for fear that this dream will turn into a trauma-related nightmare. They also are liable to exhibit hypervigilance, exaggerated startle response, and restlessness.

Learning Difficulties

Physiological hyperarousal interferes with the capacity to concentrate and to learn from experience. Aside from amnesias about aspects of the trauma, traumatized people often have trouble remembering ordinary events, as well. Easily triggered into hyperarousal by trauma—related stimuli, and beset with difficulties paying attention, they may display symptoms of attention deficit disorder. After a traumatic experience, people often lose some maturational achievements and regress to earlier modes of coping with stress. In children, this may show up as an inability to take care of themselves in such areas as feeding and toilet training; in adults, it is expressed in excessive dependence and in a loss of capacity to make thoughtful, autonomous decisions.

Memory Disturbances and Dissociation

Increased autonomic arousal not only interferes with psychological comfort, anxiety itself also may trigger memories of previous traumatic experiences. The administration of a salt or ester of lactic acid, which stimulates the physiological arousal system, elicits flashbacks and panic attacks in people with PTSD. Yohimbine injections (which stimulate norepinephrine

[NE] release from the locus coeruleus) are able to induce flashbacks in Vietnam veterans with PTSD. Any arousing situation may trigger memories of long-ago traumatic experiences and precipitate reactions that are irrelevant to present demands (see van der Kolk and Fisler, 1994).

In addition to intrusive memories, chronically traumatized people, particularly children, may develop amnestic syndromes related to the traumatic event. During the stage of life that children, in a stage-appropriate way, try on different identities in their daily play activities, children who are exposed to prolonged and severe trauma may be capable of organizing whole personality fragments in order to cope with traumatic experiences. In the long-term, this may give rise to the syndrome of dissociative identity disorder, which occurs in about 4 percent of psychiatric inpatients in the United States (Saxe et al., 1993).

Patients who have learned to dissociate in response to trauma are likely to continue to utilize dissociative defenses when exposed to new stresses. They develop amnesia for some experiences, and tend to react with fight or flight responses to feeling threatened, neither of which may be consciously remembered afterward. People who suffer from dissociative disorders are a clinical challenge, including helping them acquire a sense of personal responsibility for both their actions and reactions, while forensically, they are a nightmare.

Aggression Against Self and Others

Numerous studies have demonstrated that both adults and children who have been traumatized are likely to turn their aggression against others or themselves. Being abused as a child sharply increases the risk for later delinquency and violent criminal behavior. In one study of eighty-seven psychiatric outpatients (van der Kolk, Perry, and Herman, 1991) self-mutilators invariably had severe childhood histories of abuse and/or neglect. Evidence suggests that self-mutilative behavior is related to endogenous opioid changes in the CNS secondary to early traumatization. Problems with aggression against others have been particularly well documented in war veterans, traumatized children, and prisoners with histories of early trauma.

Psychosomatic Reactions

Chronic anxiety and emotional numbing also get in the way of learning to identify and articulate internal states and wishes (Pennebaker, 1993).

People traumatized as children frequently suffer from alexithymia—an inability to translate somatic sensations into basic feelings, such as anger, happiness, or fear. This failure to translate somatic states into words and symbols causes them to experience emotions simply as physical problems. This naturally plays havoc with intimate and trusting interpersonal communications. These people have somatization disorders and relate to the world through their bodies. They experience distress in terms of physical organs, rather than as psychological states (Saxe et al., 1994).

Developmental Level Affects and the Behavioral and Biological Concomitants of Trauma

Over the past thirty years, the differential effects of trauma at various age levels have been unravelled. Modern psychiatry has begun to reconsider the ways in which failure of attachment and traumatic separation affect the developing organism. Bowlby (1969) has emphasized that attachment behavior is first of all a vital biological function, indispensable for both reproduction and survival. A rapidly expanding body of research has shown that disturbances of childhood attachment bonds can have long-term neurobiological consequences. In addition to the disturbances in affect regulation, a large variety of studies, both in animals and in humans, have shown that childhood abuse, neglect, and separation have far-reaching biopsychosocial effects, including lasting biological changes which affect the capacity to modulate emotions, difficulty in learning new coping skills, alterations in immune competency, and impairment in the capacity to engage in meaningful social affiliation. Aided by work on other animal species, a voluminous research literature on the effects of childhood physical and sexual abuse, and the field trials for the DSM-IV, it has become understood that there are critical stages in the development of the CNS that make children particularly vulnerable to developing lasting disturbances secondary to abuse, neglect, and separation. Because of the awareness of the fact that trauma at an early age has profound effects on affect regulation, levels of consciousness, the tendency to organize experience on a somatic level, and characterological adaptations to chronic exposure to danger and fear, the DSM-IV PTSD committee recommended an expanded definition of PTSD for inclusion in the DSM-IV. The DSM-IV classification system now recognizes the pervasive effects of trauma on the totality of personality functioning in its new section on "associated features." Table 3.2 gives the associated features of PTSD in the DSM-IV.

TABLE 3.2. Complicated PTSD

A. Alteration in regulation of affect and impulses
  1. Affect regulation
  2. Modulation of anger
  3. Self-destructive
  4. Suidical preoccupation
  5. Difficulty modulating sexual involvement
  6. Excessive risk taking
B. Alterations in attention or consciousness
  1. Amnesia
  2. Transient dissociative episodes and depersonalization
C. Somatization
  1. Digestive system
  2. Chronic pain
  3. Cardiopulmonary symptoms
  4. Conversion symptoms
  5. Sexual symptoms
D. Alterations in self-perception
  1. Ineffectiveness
  2. Permanent damage
  3. Guilt and responsibility
  4. Shame
  5. Nobody can understand
  6. Minimizing
E. Alterations in perception of the perpetrator
  1. Adopting distorted beliefs
  2. Idealization of the perpetrator
  3. Preoccupation with hurting perpetrator
F. Alterations in relations with others
  1. Inability to trust
  2. Revictimization
  3. Victimizing others
G. Alterations in systems of meaning
  1. Despair and hopelessness
  2. Loss of previously sustaining beliefs

PRINCIPLES OF TREATMENT

The treatment of PTSD has three principal components:

1. Processing and coming to terms with the horrifying, overwhelming experience
2. Controlling and mastering physiological and biological stress reactions
3. Reestablishing secure social connections and interpersonal efficacy

The aim of these therapies is to help the traumatized individual to move from being dominated and haunted by the past to being present in the here and now, capable of responding to current exigencies with his or her fullest potential. Thus, the trauma needs to be placed in the larger perspective of a person's life, as a relatively isolated historical event, or series of events, that occurred at a particular time, and in a particular place, and that can be expected not to recur if the traumatized individual takes charge of his or her life. Tragically, many traumatized people are involved in situations of ongoing trauma, in which they have little or no personal control over what happens to them. However, even under those circumstances, learning how to properly assess what is going on and planning one's responses, possibly in collaboration with other people, still can be expected to have significant psychological benefits.

Acute Trauma

Immediately after the trauma, emphasis needs to be placed on self-regulation and on rebuilding. This means the reestablishment of a sense of security and predictability, and active engagement in adaptive action. Only a limited proportion of people who are traumatized develop PTSD. Most traumatized people seem to be able to successfully negotiate these initial adaptive phases without succumbing to the long-term progression of their acute stress reaction into PTSD. For them, the trauma becomes merely a terrible experience that happened to them some time in their past. It is quite unclear whether talking about what has happened is always useful in preventing the development of PTSD. Some surprising findings have come out of careful Critical Incidence Stress Debriefing research: the few controlled studies that have examined the preventative effect of debriefing immediately following exposure to a traumatic event have suggested a poorer outcome following debriefing as compared with no intervention (McFarlane, 1994). Given the paucity of controlled studies, we are left with the clinical impression that the initial response to trauma consists of reconnecting with ordinary supportive networks, and of engaging in activities that reestablish a sense of mastery. It is obvious that the role of mental health professionals in these initial recuperative efforts is quite limited.

The Need for Phase-Oriented Treatment

Trauma needs to be treated differently at different phases of people's lives following the trauma, and at the different stages of the PTSD disorder. Treatments that may be effective at some stages of treatment might not be effective at others. For example, on a pharmacological level, initial management with drugs that decrease autonomic arousal will decrease nightmares and flashback, promote sleep, and are likely to prevent the kindling effects that are thought to underlie the long-term establishment of PTSD symptomatology. These same drugs, once the disorder has been established, have, at best, a palliative function. Serotonin reuptake blockers, which seem to have little immediate benefit, can be immensely helpful in allowing people to attend to current tasks, and not to dwell on past fears, interpretations, and fixations. In this context, Foa et al. (1991) found that in the initial stages of treatment of rape victims, stress inoculation training turned out to be as effective a treatment of PTSD as was prolonged imaginal exposure. However, on follow-up, imaginal flooding had superior results to stress inoculation. If there are differential effects of therapeutic modalities within a four-month time frame, it is likely that there would be differential effects over longer time spans. It is likely that some forms of therapy might be effective at some stages, but have negative outcomes at other phases of the illness. Another example is abreaction. Abreaction as a treatment is most effective early in the course of the illness, and its effectiveness decreases over time. For example, exposure therapy using "flooding" techniques have been found to worsen the symptoms of some patients, particularly in those in whom the focal trauma was decades earlier (Pitman et al., 1991). When intrusions of fragments of the trauma are the predominant symptom, exposure and desensitization may be what is most required. At a later stage of the progression of the disorder, when people have organized their entire lives around avoidance of triggers of the trauma, and approach other people as potential triggers of traumatic intrusions, helplessness, suspicion, anger, and interpersonal problems may dominate the symptom picture. When that is the case, primary attention needs to be paid to stabilization in the social realm.

Psychotherapeutic Interventions

The key element of the psychotherapy of people with PTSD—as perhaps for all psychotherapy—is the integration of the alien, the unacceptable, the terrifying, the incomprehensible. Life events initially experienced as alien, as if imposed from outside upon passive victims, must come to be "personalized" affectively as integrated aspects of one's history and life experiences (van der Kolk and Ducey, 1989). The massive defenses, initially established as emergency protective measures, must gradually relax their grip upon the psyche, so that dissociated aspects of experience do not continue to intrude into one's life experience and thereby threaten to retraumatize an already traumatized victim.

Psychotherapy must address two fundamental aspects of PTSD: the deconditioning of anxiety, and the pervasive effects that trauma has on the way victims view themselves and the world. In only the simplest cases will it be sufficient to decondition the anxiety associated with the trauma. In the vast majority of patients, both aspects will have to be treated, which means the use of a combination of procedures for reconditioning anxiety, for changing beliefs, and for developing a cognitive system that somehow allows a person to continue to cope effectively in a world that now is known to be capable of great destructiveness (Epstein, 1991).

Stabilization

In the treatment of simple cases of PTSD, it is perhaps possible to move quickly to activating the traumatic memory. In more complex cases, it should be part of a more encompassing treatment model, which must include careful preparation, with an eye on providing the patient with a capacity to feel safe while accessing traumatic material (e.g., Brown and Fromm, 1986). In the twentieth century, psychotherapeutic clinicians basically adopted a phase-oriented model that consists of reintegration and rehabilitation (cf. van der Hart, Brown, and van der Kolk, 1989; Herman, 1992). In the first phase, the foundation is laid that enables the patient to deal with the challenge of confronting the trauma. The patient is helped with establishing more stability and safety in daily life, including social support, stress inoculation, ways of controlling symptoms, and ways of containing intrusive memories (e.g., van der Hart et al., 1993). Psychopharmacological management often is an integral part of stabilization.

The Identification of Feelings by Verbalizing Somatic States

The function of emotions is to alert people to the occurrence, significance, and nature of subjectively significant events (Krystal, 1978). Ordinarily, emotions are deactivated when schemas and situations have been realigned (e.g., by taking action that conforms situations to schemas, or by amending schemas to better fit situations) (Horowitz, 1986). Thus, emotions function as signals to readjust one's expectations of the world and to take adaptive action. Krystal (1978) first noted that, in people with PTSD, emotions seem to lose much of their alerting function: a dissociation is set up between emotional arousal and goal-directed action. Traumatized people lose their capacity to interpret the meaning of their emotional arousal, which thus becomes irrelevant as a current signal. Unable to interpret the meaning of their emotional arousal, feelings themselves become endowed with a negative valence. Because no release can be found in adaptive action, emotions merely become reminders of one's inability to affect the outcome of one's life. Hence, aside from the concrete, usually visual, reminders of the trauma, feelings in general come to be experienced as traumatic reminders, and are to be avoided (van der Kolk and Ducey, 1989).

Unable to neutralize affects with adaptive action, traumatized people tend to experience their affects as somatic states: either through their smooth or striated musculature. Thus, people with PTSD tend to somatize (Saxe et al., 1994), or to discharge their emotions with actions that are irrelevant to the stimulus that precipitated the emotion: with aggressive actions against self or others (van der Kolk, Perry, and Herman, 1991). When the disorganizing intrusions can be understood as failures of integration of traumatic experiences into the totality of one's life, the psychotherapist is in a position to recognize seemingly overwhelming affective experiences as actual reliving of past terror. The natural proclivity in psychotherapy is to help the patient avoid experiencing undue pain; yet the patient's affective experiences are part and parcel of healing and integration. The psychotherapist who understands the nature of trauma can aid the process of integration by staying with the patient through his suffering, by providing a perspective that the suffering is meaningful and bearable, and by helping in the mastery of trauma through putting the experience into symbolic, communicable form, such as words, thoughts, and feelings. The patient's "repeating" the trauma in action is the forerunner to his "remembering" and symbolizing it in words, which in turn is the precursor accompaniment to his "working it through" in emotional experience.

Deconditioning of Traumatic Memories and Responses

This consists of (1) controlled activation of the traumatic memories, and (2) corrections of faulty traumatic beliefs. The critical issue is to introduce the capacity to flexibly remember the trauma. For this to occur, some new information that is incompatible to the traumatic memory must be introduced (Foa, Steketee, and Olasov, 1989). The most important new information is probably that the patient is able to confront the traumatic memory with a trusted therapist in a safe environment (van der Hart and Spiegel, 1993). To help the patient regulate emotional arousal, secure attachment may be even more important than evoking the traumatic memories. Therefore, it is important for the patient to establish and maintain an emotional connection with the therapist. Although behavioral therapists speak about exposure procedures, which are either systematic desensitization procedures, or implosive therapy or flooding procedures, they neglect to write about the intensely personal element in all psychotherapeutic procedures, which is a critical element in the success of effective treatment. So, while these clinicians and researchers almost exclusively present their data about decreases of fear or anxiety through controlled exposure to (1) the stimulus components (environmental cues), (2) the response components (e.g., motoric actions, heart pounding), and (3) the meaning elements (e.g., cues regarding morality and guilt) of the traumatic memory (Foa and Kozak, 1986; Foa, Steketee, and Olasov, 1989; Litz and Keane, 1989), their results are most likely heavily affected by their personal investment in the well-being of their patients, which is communicated and translated into a subjective sense of safety.

According to Foa and Kozak (1985) two conditions are required for anxiety reduction in the treatment of PTSD: (1) A person must attend to fear-relevant information in a manner that will activate his or her own fear memory. As long as the fear is not experienced, the fear structure cannot be modified. (2) In order to form a new, nonfear structure, some of the information that evoked the fear must be absent in the new context in which the fear is being provoked. Exposure to information consistent with a fear memory would be expected to strengthen the fear (i.e., sensitize and thereby increase the likelihood of developing PTSD). Hence, the critical issue in treatment is to expose the patient to an experience that contains elements that are sufficiently similar to an existing traumatic memory in order to activate it, and at the same time, be an experience that contains aspects that are incompatible enough to change it (for example, experiencing a traumatic memory in a safe and controllable environment, being able to evoke a traumatic image, without feeling overwhelmed by the associated emotions).

There are at least two significant problems with this exposure technique: (1) Because excessive arousal interferes with the acquisition of new information, excessive arousal impedes habituation (Strian and Klicpera, 1978). When that occurs, the fear structure will not be corrected, but instead, will be confirmed: instead of promoting habituation, it accidentally fosters sensitization. (2) An additional serious obstacle to effective treatment is that the strong response elements in the PTSD structure may promote avoidance: strong fear and discomfort motivates people who suffer from PTSD to avoid or escape confrontation with situations that remind them of the trauma. To overcome the intrusive, sensorimotor elements of the trauma, a person must transform the traumatic (nonverbal) memory into a personal narrative, in which the trauma is experienced as a historical event that is part of their autobiography. This entails being able to tell the story of the shocking event without reexperiencing it. It is generally assumed that once all relevant elements of the total traumatic experience have been identified and thoroughly and deeply examined and experienced in the therapy, successful synthesis will take place. The work by Resick and Schnicke (1992) supports the notion that exposure of all elements of the trauma, and their associated shifts in perception of self and others does lead to successful resolution of trauma-related symptomatology.

Restructuring of Trauma-Related Schemas of Internal and External Reality

Apart from the treatment that is needed to address specific trauma—related memories, and fostering deconditioning—treatment needs to address the effects of the trauma on people's perceptions of themselves, and the world around them. People are meaning-making creatures. As we develop, we organize our world according to a personal theory of reality, some of which may be conscious, but much of which is an unconscious integration of accumulated experience. These mental schemas organize psychological experience via the process of assimilation and accommodation and assure the continuity of one's identity (Horowitz, 1991). Although most people cannot clearly articulate the content of their mental schemes, they nonetheless determine what sensory input is selected for further coding and categorization. Adaptive resolution to a stressful experience consists of the modification, or accommodation of one's view of self and others that permits adaptive action and continued attention to the exigencies of daily life. To successfully deal with a distressing experience, it is necessary to not generalize from that experience to the totality of existence, but to view it merely as one terrible event that has taken place at a particular place at a particular time (Epstein, 1991).

Traumatic experiences, i.e., experiences that do not fit into people's personal schemes, may be assimilated (directly taken in) ("That never happened"; "I caused it to happen"), or people may accommodate to the experience by altering their conceptions of the world ("There is no safe place"; "This happened because people are out to hurt me") (Resick and Schnicke, 1992; Hollon and Garber, 1988).

Traumatic experiences are not only processed by means of currently existing mental schemas, but they may also activate latent self-concepts and views of relationships that were formed earlier in life. This activation of latent schemes is particularly relevant for people with prior histories of trauma, even in those who subsequently have been able to make a successful adaptation. When trauma activates these earlier self-schemas, these will compete and coexist with more mature schemas in explaining cause and effect relationships in regard to the trauma. These different, and often competing mental schemas then will determine the psychological organization of the traumatic experience.

Psychotherapy needs to specifically address how the trauma has affected a person's sense of self—efficacy, capacity for trust and intimacy, ability to negotiate personal needs, and the ability to feel empathy for other people (McCann and Pearlman, 1990).

Exposure to Restitutive Experiences

Considering that the central psychological preoccupation of traumatized people is either the reliving or the warding off of the memory of the trauma, there is little room for new, gratifying experiences which might allow for reparation of past injuries to the self. Patients need to actively expose themselves to experiences that provide them with feelings of mastery and pleasure. Engagement in physical activities, such as sports or wilderness ventures, gratifying physical experiences, such as massages, or artistic accomplishments may be experiences that patients have that are not contaminated by the trauma, and which may serve as a core of new gratifying experiences.

GROUP PSYCHOTHERAPY

Emotional attachment is the primary protection against being traumatized. People have always gathered in communities and organizations to deal with outside challenges, and to seek close, emotional relationships with others to help anticipate, meet, and integrate difficult experiences. Contemporary research (e.g., Quanterelli, 1985; Holen, 1990) has shown that as long as the social support network remains intact, people are relatively well protected against even catastrophic stresses. For young children, the family usually is a very effective source of protection against traumatization, and most children are amazingly resilient as long as they have a caregiver who is emotionally and physically available (van der Kolk, Perry, and Herman, 1991, McFarlane, 1988). Adults also rely on their families, colleagues, and friends to provide such a trauma membrane. In recognition of this need for affiliation as a protection against trauma, it has become widely accepted that the central issue in acute crisis intervention is the provision and restoration of social support (Lystad, 1988; Raphael, 1986; Mitchell, 1983). However, curiously, research has not supported the efficacy of standardized stress debriefing interventions following trauma.

The task of group therapy and community interventions is to help victims regain a sense of safety and of mastery. After an acute trauma, fellow victims often provide the most effective short-term bond because the shared history of trauma can form the nucleus of retrieving a sense of communality.

Regardless of the nature of the trauma, or the structure of the group, the aim of group therapy is to help people actively attend to the requirements of the moment, without undue intrusions from past perceptions and experiences. Group therapy is widely regarded as a treatment of choice for patients with trauma histories. It has been used for victims of interpersonal violence (Mitchell, 1983), natural disasters (Lystad, 1988; Raphael, 1986), childhood sexual abuse (Herman and Schatzow, 1987; Ganzarain and Buchele, 1987; Schacht, Kerlinsky, and Carldon, 1990), rape (Yassen and Glass, 1984), spouse battering (Rounsaville, Lifton, and Bieber, 1979), concentration camps (Danieli, 1985) and war trauma (Parson, 1988). In a group of individuals who have gone through similar experiences, most traumatized people eventually are able to find the appropriate words to express what has happened to them. As was observed over fifty years ago, if people work out their problems in a small group, are they better able to face the larger group, i.e., their world, in an easier manner (Grinker and Spiegel, 1946)?

Many levels of trauma-related group psychotherapies exist, with different degrees of emphasis on stabilization, memory retrieval, bonding, negotiation of interpersonal differences, and support. However, to varying degrees, the purpose of all trauma related groups is to

1. stabilize psychological and physiological reactions to the trauma,
2. explore and validate perceptions and emotions,
3. retrieve memories,
4. understand the effects of past experience on current affects and behaviors, and
5. learn new ways of coping with interpersonal stress (see van der Kolk, 1992).

CONCLUDING REMARKS

After a trauma which fully confronts a person with existential helplessness and vulnerability, life can never be exactly the same. The traumatic experience will somehow become part of a person's life. Sorting out exactly what happened and sharing one's reactions with others can make a great deal of difference in one's eventual adaptation. Putting the feelings and cognitions related to the trauma into words is essential in the treatment of posttraumatic reactions. After intense efforts to ward off reliving the trauma, therapists cannot expect that the resistances to remember will suddenly melt away under their empathic efforts. The trauma can only be worked through when a secure bond is established with another person; this then can be utilized to hold the psyche together when the threat of physical disintegration is reexperienced.

Failure to approach trauma-related material gradually is likely to lead to intensification of posttraumatic symptomatology, leading to increased somatic, visual, or behavioral reexperiences. Once the traumatic experiences have been located in time and place, a person can start making distinctions between current life stresses and past trauma, and decrease the impact of the trauma on present experience. Talking about the trauma is not enough. Trauma survivors need to take some action that symbolizes triumph over helplessness and despair. The Holocaust Memorial in Yad Vashem in Jerusalem, and the Vietnam Veterans Memorial in Washington, DC, are good examples of symbols for survivors to mourn the dead and establish the historical and cultural meaning of the traumatic events. Most of all, they serve to remind survivors of the ongoing potential for communality and sharing. This also applies to other survivors who may have to build less visible memorials and common symbols around which they can gather to mourn and express their shame about their own vulnerability. This may take the form of writing a book, taking political action, helping other victims, or any of the myriad of creative solutions that human beings can find to defy even the most desperate plight.

BIBLIOGRAPHY

Bowlby, J. (1969). *Attachment and loss:* Volume 1, *Attachment.* New York: Basic Books.

Bremner, J.D., Steinberg, M., Southwick, S.M., et al. (1993). Use of the structured clinical interview for DSM-IV dissociative disorders for systematic assessment of dissociative symptoms in post-traumatic stress disorder. *American Journal of Psychiatry, 150,* 1011-1014.

Breslau, N., Davis, G.C., and Andreski, P. (1991). Traumatic events and post traumatic stress disorder in an urban population of young adults. *Archives of General Psychiatry, 48,* 216-222.

Brown, M. and Fromm, E. (1986). *Hypnoanalysis and hypnotherapy.* Hillsdale, NY: Lawrence Erlbaum Associates.

Danieli, Y. (1985). The treatment and prevention of long-term effects and inter-generational transmission of victimization: A lesson from holocaust survivors and their children. In C.R. Figley (Ed.), *Trauma and its wake* (Volume 1, pp. 295-313). New York: Brunner/Mazel.

Davidson, J.R.T. (1992). Drug therapy of post traumatic stress disorder. *British Journal of Psychiatry, 160,* 309-314.

Davidson, J.R.T., Kudler, H., Smith, R., Mahorney, S., Lipper, S., Hammett, E., Saunders, W., and Cavenar, J.O. (1990). Treatment of post-traumatic stress disorder with amitriptylene and placebo. *Archives of General Psychiatry, 47,* 259-266.

Davidson, J.R.T. and Nemeroff, C.B. (1989). Pharmacotherapy in PTSD: Historical and clinical considerations and future directions. *Psychopharmacology Bulletin,* 422-425.

Davidson, J.R.T., Roth, S., and Newman, E. (1991). Treatment of post-traumatic stress disorder with fluoxetine. *Journal of Traumatic Stress, 3,* 419-423.

Epstein, S. (1991). The self-concept, the traumatic neurosis, and the structure of personality. In D. Ozer, J.M. Healy Jr., and A.J. Stewart (Eds.), *Perspectives in personality* (Volume 3, Part A, pp. 63-98). London: Jessica Kingsley.

Foa, E.B. and Kozak, M.J. (1985). Treatment of anxiety disorders: Implications for psychopathology. In A. H. Tuma and J. D. Maser (Eds.), *Anxiety and anxiety disorders.* Hillsdale, NY: Lawrence Erlbaum Associates.

Foa, E.B. and Kozak, M.J. (1986). Emotional processing of fear: Exposure to corrective information. *Psychological Bulletin, 99,* 20-35.

Foa, E., Rothbaum, B.O., Riggs, D.S., and Murdock, G.B. (1991). Treatment of post-traumatic stress disorder in rape victims: Comparison between cognitive behavioral procedures and counseling. *Journal of Consulting and Clinical Psychology, 59,* 715-725.

Foa, E.B., Steketee, G., and Olasov, B.R. (1989). Behavioral/cognitive conceptualizations of post-traumatic stress disorder. *Behavior Therapy, 20,* 155-176.

Frank, J.B., Kosten, T.R., Giller, E.L., and Dan, E. (1988). A preliminary study of pheneizine and imipramine for post-traumatic stress disorder. *American Journal of Psychiatry, 145,* 1289-1291.

Freud, S. (1959). Formulations on the two principles of mental functioning. In J. Strachey (Ed. and Trans.), *Complete psychological works* (Standard edition, Volume 12, pp. 9-82). London: Hogarth Press. (Original work published 1911.)

Friedman, M. (1988). Toward rational pharmacotherapy of post traumatic stress disorder. *American Journal of Psychiatry, 145,* 281-285.

Ganzarain, R. and Buchele, B. (1987). Acting out during group psychotherapy for incest. *International Journal of Group Psychotherapy, 37,* 185-200.

Gray, J. (1988). *The psychology of fear and stress* (Second edition). Cambridge: Cambridge University Press.

Grinker, R. and Spiegel, H. (1946). *Men under stress.* New York: Basic Books.

Helzer, J.E., Robins, L.N., and McEvoy, L. (1987). Post-traumatic stress disorder in the general population. *New England Journal of Medicine, 317*(26), 1630-1634.

Herman, J.L. (1992). *Trauma and recovery.* New York: Basic Books.

Herman, J.L. and Schatzow, E. (1987). Recovery and verification of memories of childhood sexual trauma. *Psychoanalytic Psychology, 3*(1), 1-14.

Holen, A. (1990). *A long-term study of survivors from a disaster.* Oslo: University of Oslo Press.

Hollon, S.D. and Garber, J. (1988). Cognitive therapy. In L.Y. Abrahamson (Ed.), *Social cognition and clinical psychology: A synthesis* (pp. 204-253). New York: Guilford Press.

Horowitz, M.J. (1986). *Stress response syndromes* (Second edition). Northvale, NJ: Aronson.

Horowitz, M.J. (1991). *Person schemas and maladaptive interpersonal patterns.* Chicago: University of Chicago Press.

Janet, P. (1889). *L'Automatisme Psychologie.* Paris: Alcan.

Janet, P. (1904). L'amnesie at la dissociation des souvenirs par emotion. *Journal de Psychologie, 1,* 417-453.

Kardiner, A. (1941). *The traumatic neuroses of war.* New York: Hoeber.

Kosten, T.R., Frank, J.B., Dan, E., McDougle, C.J., and Giller, E.L. (1991). Pharmacotherapy for post traumatic stress disorder using pheneizine and imipramine. *Journal of Nervous and Mental Disorders, 179,* 366-370.

Krystal, H. (1978). Trauma and affects. *Psychoanalytic Study of Children, 33,* 81-116.

Kulka, R.A., Schlenger, W., and Fairbank, J. (1990). *Trauma and the Vietnam War generation.* New York: Brunner/Mazel.

Laub, D. and Auerhahn, N.C. (1993). Knowing and not knowing massive psychic trauma: Forms of traumatic memory. *International Journal of Psychoanalysis, 74,* 287-301.

Litz, B.T. and Keane, T.M. (1989). Information processing in anxiety disorders: Application to the understanding of post-traumatic stress disorder. *Clinical Psychology Review, 9,* 243-257.

Lystad, M. (1988). *Mental health response to mass emergencies.* New York: Brunner/Mazel.

March, J. (1992). Fluoxetine and flovoxamine in PTSD [Letter to the editor] *American Journal of Psychiatry, 149,* 413.

Marmar, C.R., Weiss, D.S., Schlenger, W.E., Fairbank, J.A., Jordan, K., Kulka, R.A., and Hough, R.L. (1994). Peritraumatic dissociation and posttraumatic stress in male Vietnam theater veterans. *American Journal of Psychiatry, 151,* 902-907.

McCann, I.L. and Pearlman, L.A. (1990). *Psychological trauma and the adult survivor: Theory, therapy and transformation.* New York: Brunner/Mazel.

McFarlane, A.C. (1988). Recent life events and psychiatric disorder in children: The interaction with preceding extreme adversity. *Journal of Clinical Psychiatry, 29*(5), 677-690.

McFarlane, A.C. (1994). Individual psychotherapy for post-traumatic stress disorder. *Psychiatric Clinics of North America, 17*(2), 393-408.

Mitchell, J. (1983). The critical incident stress debriefing. *Journal of Emergency Medical Services, 8,* 36-39.

Nagy, L.M., Morgan, C.A., Southwick, S.M., and Charney, D.S. (1993). Open prospective trial of fluoxetine for post traumatic stress disorder. *Journal of Clinical Psychopharmacology, 13,* 107-114.

Parson, E.R. (1988). Post-traumatic accelerated cohesion: Its recognition and management in group treatment of Vietnam veterans. *Group, 9*(4), 10-23.

Pennebaker, J.W. (1993). Putting stress into words: Health, linguistic, and therapeutic implications. *Behavioral Residental Therapy, 31*(6), 539-548.

Pitman, R.K., Altman, B., Greenwald, E., Longpre, R.E., Macklin, M.L., Poire, R.E., and Steketee, G.S. (1991). Psychiatric complications during flooding therapy for posttraumatic stress disorder. *Journal of Clinical Psychiatry, 52*(1), 17-20.

Quanterelli, E.L. (1985). An assessment of conflicting views on mental health: The consequences of traumatic events. In C.R. Figley (Ed.), *Trauma and its wake* (Volume 1). New York: Brunner/Mazel.

Raphael, B. (1986). *When disaster strikes: How individuals and communities cope with catastrophe.* New York: Basic Books.

Rauch, S., van der Kolk, B.A., Fisler, R., Alpert, N., Orr, S., Savage, C., Jenike, M., and Pitman, R. (in press). A symptom provocation study using positron emission tomography and script driven imagery. *Archives of General Psychiatry.*

Reist, C., Kaufman, C.D., and Haier, R.J. (1989). A controlled trial of desipramine in 18 men with PTSD. *American Journal of Psychiatry, 146,* 513-516.

Resick, P.A., and Schnicke, M.K. (1992). Cognitive processing therapy for sexual assault victims. *Journal of Consulting and Clinical Psychology, 60*(5), 748-756.

Rounsaville, B., Lifton, N., and Bieber, M. (1979). The natural history of a psychotherapy group for battered women. *Psychiatry, 42,* 63-78.

Saxe, G.N., Chinman, G., Berkowitz, R., Hall, K., Lieberg, G., Schwartz, J., and van der Kolk, B.A. (1994). Somatization in patients with dissociative disorders. *American Journal of Psychiatry, 151,* 1329-1335.

Saxe, G., van der Kolk, B.A., Hall, K., Schwartz, J., Chinman, G., Hall, M.D., Lieberg, G., and Berkowitz, R. (1993). Dissociative disorders in psychiatric inpatients. *American Journal of Psychiatry, 150*(7), 1037-1042.

Schacht, A., Kerlinsky, D., and Carldon, C. (1990). Group therapy with sexually abused boys: Leadership, projective identification, and countertransference issues. *International Journal of Group Psychotherapy, 40*(4), 401-417.

Shetatsky, M., Greenberg, D., and Lerer, B. (1988). A controlled trial of pheneizine in posttraumatic stress disorder. *Psychiatry Research, 24,* 149-155.

Strian, F. and Klicpera, C. (1978). Die bedeuting psychoautotonomische reaktionen im entstehung und persistenz von angstzustanden. *Nervenartzt, 49,* 576-583.

van der Hart, O., Brown, P., and van der Kolk, B.A. (1989). Pierre Janet's treatment of posttraumatic stress. *Journal of Traumatic Stress, 2*(4), 379-395.

van der Hart, O. and Spiegel, D. (1993). Hypnotic assessment and treatment of trauma induced psychoses: The early psychotherapy of H. Breukink and modern views. *International Journal of Clinical and Experimental Hypnosis, 41,* 191-209.

van der Hart, O., Steele, K., Boon, S., and Brown, P. (1993). The treatment of traumatic memories: Synthesis, realization, and integration. *Dissociation, 6,* 162-180.

van der Kolk, B.A. (1987). The drug treatment of post-traumatic stress disorder. *Journal of Affective Disorders, 13,* 203-213.

van der Kolk, B.A. (1992). Group psychotherapy with post traumatic stress disorders. In H. Kaplan and B. Sadock (Eds.), *Comprehensive group psychotherapy* (pp. 550-560). Philadelphia: Williams and Wilkins.

van der Kolk, B.A. (1994). The body keeps the score: Memory and the evolving psychobiology of post traumatic stress. *Harvard Review of Psychiatry, 1,* 253-265.

van der Kolk, B.A., Dreyfuss, D., Berkowitz, R., Saxe, G., and Michaels, M. (1994, December). Fluoxetine in post traumatic stress. *Journal of Clinical Psychiatry.*

van der Kolk, B.A. and Ducey, C. (1984). Clinical implications of the Rorschach in post-traumatic stress disorder. In B.A. van der Kolk (Ed.), *Post traumatic stress disorder: Psychological and biological sequelae,* (pp. 30-42). Washington, DC: American Psychiatric Press.

van der Kolk, B.A. and Ducey, C. (1989). The psychological processing of traumatic experience: Rorschach patterns in PTSD. *Journal of Traumatic Stress, 2*(2), 259-274.

van der Kolk, B.A., and Fisler, R. (1994). Childhood abuse and neglect and loss of self-regulation. *Bulletin of Menninger Clinic 58,* 145-168.

van der Kolk, B.A. and Fisler, R. (1995). Dissociation and the fragmentary nature of traumatic memories: Background and experimental evidence. *Journal of Traumatic Stress, 8*(4), 505-525.

van der Kolk, B.A., Perry, J.C., and Herman, J.L. (1991). Childhood origins of self-destructive behavior. *American Journal of Psychiatry, 148,* 1665-1671.

Yassen, J. and Glass, L. (1984). Sexual assault survivor groups. *Social Work, 37,* 252-257.

Chapter 4

Psychopharmacological Treatment in PTSD

Ronald Albucher
Michelle Van Etten-Lee
Israel Liberzon

INTRODUCTION

Originally, psychological mechanisms alone were presumed to play a central role in the etiology and pathophysiology of post-traumatic stress disorder (PTSD) (Kinzie and Goetz, 1996). In its earliest conceptualization, the symptoms that appeared after a traumatic experience were presumed to be a short-lived, "normal response," even classified as an adjustment reaction. Long-term symptoms were presumed to reflect unresolved neurotic conflict or character pathology. Not surprisingly, medication treatment for PTSD may have been perceived as unnecessary or contraindicated, either because it interfered with needed psychotherapeutic intervention or, at best, because it sedated overexcited patients so that they could proceed with therapy. Although this view has dominated the fields of psychiatry and clinical psychology for almost 100 years, biological theories on "traumatic neurosis" were also developed during this time.

Beginning with Da Costa's description of "irritable heart" during the American Civil War, then as memory "disruption" by Janet, and later as "physioneurosis" around World War II by Abram Kardiner, researchers integrated empirical observations of psychopathology and physiology with known neurobiology to develop an evidence-based, scientific approach to the field of trauma (Da Costa, 1871; Janet, 1889; Kardiner, 1941). This created the necessary background for the development of both neurobiological research in PTSD, and the development of rational and informed pharmacological treatment strategies.

In the last twenty years, the fields of psychology and neuroscience have come to appreciate the intricate interplay between the underlying biological substrate of the individual and the complex human experience of trauma. This more recent progress also allowed the delineation of a biological diathesis for several psychiatric disorders, including PTSD, and clarified the potential importance of psychopharmacological interventions to these syndromes (Davidson, 1997; Friedman, Charney, and Deutch, 1995; Grillon, Southwick, and Charney, 1996). In the majority of conditions, psychology and biology are extensively intertwined. In this emerging view, PTSD is not just an abnormal "psychological" response to an extraordinary stressor; rather, the traumatic experience alters the patient's neurophysiology, which may initiate or maintain the symptoms (Heim et al., 1997; Hockings et al., 1993; Kosten et al., 1987). Because the interaction between biology and experiences is important, individual differences in neurophysiology might result in some individuals being more susceptible to the effects of trauma than others. Recent evidence indicating a genetic predisposition to the development of PTSD further supports this assertion (True et al., 1993).

These recent manifestations offer a new conceptual frame for the development of pharmacological treatments for trauma survivors, while maintaining the importance of psychotherapy in the treatment of PTSD. Evidence suggests that psychotherapeutic interventions affect both biology (regional cerebral blood flow) and improve mental functioning similar to pharmacological interventions (Baxter et al., 1992). Consistent with this new information, treatment approaches have become more comprehensive, combining both psychotherapeutic and pharmacological interventions and tailoring them more specifically to the symptom profiles of specific patients.

In view of the complex interaction between biology and individual experience, it is not surprising that the development of pharmacological treatments for PTSD is quite challenging. PTSD is a heterogeneous illness and its symptoms vary in intensity from patient to patient. Patients may manifest intrusive memories of the original trauma, flashbacks, or nightmares, hyperarousal symptoms, avoidance, numbing, anxiety, anger, impulsivity, or aggression. In addition, the disorder has a high degree of comorbidity with other psychiatric disorders such as depression, substance abuse, and panic disorder. It is therefore not surprising that a single medication has not been found to alleviate the diverse symptoms clustered within the PTSD syndrome. Yet despite the complexity of PTSD, advances in neurobiology have shed light on its clinical features, as well as the neurobiologic systems that have been permanently altered by exposure to extreme stress.

The neurobiological findings implicate a number of neurotransmitters, neuronal mechanisms, and neuroendocrine systems in PTSD pathophysiology. Of greatest interest are the noradrenergic and serotonergic portions of the central nervous system, the hypothalamic-pituitary-adrenal axis, and concepts such as sensitization and kindling. These same systems and theoretical mechanisms are involved in the mediation of stress response, fear conditioning, and in memory and arousal regulation.

The noradrenergic abnormalities reported in this disorder can be linked in the most obvious way to PTSD symptoms. Considerable similarity exists between the behavioral and physiologic manifestations of anxiety seen in PTSD and increased catecholaminergic functioning, such as tachycardia, flushing, tremor, and sweating. Thus, PTSD symptoms such as increased arousal, overactive startle response, tension, and abnormalities in heart rate and blood pressure responses to traumatic reminders might involve abnormalities in the noradrenergic system (Bremner et al., 1996; Yatham, Sacamano, and Kusumakar, 1996). Other reported neurotransmitter abnormalities that might play a role in the pathophysiology of PTSD symptoms include serotonin, which may be linked to anger, violence, numbing, and depression (Arora et al., 1993; Davis et al., 1997; van der Kolk, 1994); endogenous opioids, which may be connected to pain, substance abuse, and dissociation (Hockings et al., 1993; Pitman et al., 1990; van der Kolk et al., 1989); gamma-aminobutyric acid (GABA) and cholecystokinin, which are possibly related to anxiety (Adamec, 1997; Adamec, Shallow, and Budgell, 1997; Friedman et al., 1995); and dopamine, which may be linked to intrusive symptoms (Yehuda et al., 1992).

Abnormalities in neuroendocrine systems such as the hypothalamic-pituitary-adrenal axis (HPA) (Friedman et al., 1995; Henry et al., 1992; Hockings et al., 1993; Kosten et al., 1990; Yehuda et al., 1992), and the thyroid axis (Mason et al., 1996) are very interesting and appear to be PTSD specific; however, their link to symptom production or pharmacological treatment is less obvious. Kindling of the limbic system has been proposed as a model for some PTSD symptoms, as has the *N*-methyl-D-aspartate (NMDA)-mediated potentiation of anxietylike behaviors in other species (Adamec, Shallow, and Budgell, 1997; Grillon, Southwick, and Charney, 1996). Although the empirical data to support the validity of these PTSD models is still missing, they provide insight into PTSD symptoms such as rage and anger outbursts, enhanced startle response, and sensitivity to specific reminders of the original trauma. They also offer a scientific rational for the use of antikindling (anticonvulsant) agents such as mood stabilizers to treat PTSD.

Problems in each of these systems might explain some PTSD symptoms, but a single abnormality in one system cannot explain them all. Therefore, a number of different pharmacological agents have been used effectively in the treatment of PTSD, as a single agent, or combined with other medications. This chapter reviews the existing literature on medications that impact the biological systems listed above.

Despite the prevalence of PTSD in the general population, the amount of research conducted in this area is relatively small. The treatment outcome literature for several different classes of medications that have been used in the treatment of PTSD is presented as follows. Where possible, the authors have emphasized results from randomized, controlled trials and augmented this information with less controlled research clarifying the limitations along the way. In the descriptions that follow, drug doses in parentheses refer to mean daily maximum doses used in that study.

Finally, it is suggested that the pharmacological treatment of PTSD can have at least four different goals. The first is to provide immediate relief to patients for overt symptoms such as sleep disturbance, intrusive memories, impulsivity, or hypervigilance. Second, by reducing the core symptoms, the patient will be more able to participate in psychotherapy, an essential part of healing and recovery (Bleich et al., 1986). Learning and working through issues in psychotherapy is more difficult, if not impossible, in the context of severe symptoms (Foy, 1992) . Third, it is often necessary to treat comorbid symptoms and syndromes, such as depression or panic attacks. Fourth, medication may correct alterations of the neurobiologic systems caused by the trauma itself, thereby restoring these systems to their premorbid state or tempering the degree of dysfunction.

ANTIDEPRESSANTS

Originally developed to treat depression, this class of medications is effective in a range of psychiatric disorders, including panic disorder, obsessive-compulsive disorder, chronic pain problems, and eating disorders. Given the high degree of comorbidity between PTSD and depression and the similar symptoms present in PTSD and other anxiety disorders (anxiety, agoraphobia, panic attacks), it is not surprising that the majority of research studies have focused on the efficacy of antidepressants for PTSD. As a group, antidepressants increase the amount of synaptic neurotransmitters available by increasing secretion, decreasing the uptake, or preventing the breakdown of monoaminergic neurotransmitters such as norepinephrine, serotonin, and dopamine.

Tricyclic Antidepressants (TCAs)

Most TCAs block the reuptake of norepinephrine and serotonin to varying degrees. For instance, desipramine is a potent norepinephrine reuptake inhibitor with relatively little effect on serotonin. Conversely, clomipramine has less effect on norepinephrine, but is a more effective serotonin reuptake inhibitor. In general, side effects from this group are more extensive than with the newer antidepressants (e.g., the selective serotonin reuptake inhibitors) and tend to appear early in the treatment course, while the therapeutic effects accrue after several weeks. Side effects are due to the blockade of nontherapeutic receptor sites, such as the muscarinic system (dry mouth, sedation, constipation, and blurred vision), histamine (sedation and weight gain), and adrenergic blockade (hypotension and the slowing of atrioventricular node depolarization).

TCAs are among the most extensively researched medications for the treatment of PTSD. Three controlled trials and several uncontrolled studies have been reported to date, including studies of imipramine, desipramine, and amitriptyline. In one of the larger TCA studies, imipramine (225 mg) was compared to phenelzine (68 mg) in a placebo-controlled, eight-week trial with sixty combat veterans (Kosten et al., 1991). Treatment retention to eight weeks was relatively low (52 percent), and end-point analysis was utilized in this study. Here, posttreatment time points varied across subjects (i.e., for subjects that dropped out prior to week eight, scores from their last week in treatment were carried forward). Although intrusive symptoms decreased on imipramine relative to placebo, no imipramine benefit was observed for avoidance or depressive symptoms.

Another large, double-blind, placebo-controlled, eight-week trial compared amitriptyline (200-300 mg) and placebo in forty-six combat veterans (Davidson et al., 1990). Treatment retention was considerably better in this study (72 percent). Improvement was noted for amitriptyline relative to placebo for depression, anxiety, and both intrusive and avoidance symptoms on self-reported, but not observer-rated measures. Avoidance symptoms were more markedly improved than intrusions.

An earlier trial by Reist and colleagues examined the efficacy of desipramine (165 mg) in a placebo-controlled, crossover design in eighteen inpatients with combat-related PTSD (Reist et al., 1989). Each arm of the study was four weeks in duration with a two-week wash-out period between phases. In this brief trial, desipramine was superior to placebo for improving depressive, but not anxiety- or PTSD-specific symptoms.

A number of uncontrolled trials have also examined the efficacy of TCAs for PTSD. In a two- to three-week open trial of imipramine (260 mg) in fifteen patients with noncombat PTSD, imipramine improved intrusive, but not avoidance, symptoms (Burstein, 1984). A four-week, open trial with desipramine (200 mg) in eight inpatients with combat-related PTSD demonstrated decreased intrusions, avoidance, and depression (Kauffman et al., 1987). Finally, a retrospective chart review of seventeen combat veterans treated with various TCAs reported that 82 percent were "much improved" on medication, with sleep and mood being the most reliably improved symptoms, followed by benefit to intrusive symptoms and general anxiety (Falcon et al., 1985).

In sum, available data suggest that TCAs can be effective in treating PTSD spectrum symptoms, with the most convincing evidence coming from two large placebo-controlled trials by Davidson (Davidson et al., 1990) and Kosten (Kosten et al., 1991). Their third controlled trial had less promising results, but the brevity of treatment duration could have contributed to negative findings. Most of the studies report improvement of depression and intrusive symptoms, and some reported overall improvement in PTSD and general anxiety levels. Although one study by Davidson and colleagues reported greater improvement of avoidance symptoms than intrusive symptoms (Davidson et al., 1990), other studies suggest that intrusive symptoms are more reliably impacted with TCAs than are avoidance symptoms. Finally, none of the TCA medications stand out as more effective than the others, though the two studies using desipramine had split results, whereas imipramine and amitriptyline reports were all positive.

Not surprisingly, given the broad side effect profiles of these drugs, dropout rates with TCAs tend to be high (28 to 48 percent), suggesting that these medications are often difficult for PTSD patients to tolerate. It should also be kept in mind that all of the controlled trials, and all but one of the uncontrolled trials of TCAs, were completed with combat veterans with chronic PTSD, who are known to be a particularly treatment-refractory population. Thus, the evidence of moderate efficacy obtained in these studies should be accepted with greater enthusiasm. In general, it appears that for those patients who are able to tolerate TCAs, these medications are likely to offer some improvement to their PTSD symptoms.

Monoamine Oxidase Inhibitors (MAOIs)

MAOI antidepressants increase synaptic monoamine levels by inhibiting neurotransmitter breakdown and metabolism. These medications are especially effective in the treatment of depression and some anxiety disorders, such as social phobia. However, their clinical utility is limited by the need for patients to follow a low-tyramine diet. Foods such as aged meats, cheeses, and wines must be avoided, as they contain high levels of tyramine that interact with this class of medication leading to a potentially life-threatening hypertensive crisis. MAOIs that reversibly bind to the MAO enzyme are not currently available in the United States, but may represent a safer way to use this class of medication in the future. The most frequent side effects in this group are insomnia, weight gain, and orthostatic hypotension.

Four controlled trials and at least six uncontrolled reports examined the efficacy of MAOIs for the treatment of PTSD, including trials with phenelzine, brofaromine, and moclobemide. Kosten and colleagues compared phenelzine (68 mg) and imipramine (225 mg) in a double-blind, placebo-controlled trial in combat veterans with PTSD (see the previous section on TCAs) (Kosten et al., 1991). Drop-out rates were high, with only 52 percent of the original sixty patients completing the full eight weeks of treatment. Phenelzine decreased intrusive but not avoidance or depressive symptoms relative to placebo, and symptom reduction was slightly greater for phenelzine than imipramine. Shestatzky and colleagues similarly studied phenelzine (60 mg) using a within-subject, placebo-controlled crossover design, in patients with noncombat PTSD (Shestatzky, Greenberg, and Lerer, 1988). The dropout rate was very high, the number of subjects was small, and the trial duration was brief in this study. Although designed as a five-week crossover trial, only six (46 percent) of the original thirteen patients completed the full five weeks, so results were reported for the ten patients completing at least four weeks on each arm. In contrast to Kosten's promising results, Shestatzky and colleagues found that phenelzine was not superior to placebo in reducing PTSD, depression, or anxiety symptoms.

More recently, two large, placebo-controlled trials for PTSD have been published. These trials used brofaromine, a combined MAO-Alserotonin reuptake inhibitor that has not been available in the United States since 1993, but is currently available in Europe. In one report, Baker and colleagues studied brofaromine (150 mg) versus placebo over twelve weeks in 113 patients with PTSD due to various traumas (Baker et al., 1995). The drop-out rate was fairly low (30 percent), considering the relatively long duration of the study. Brofaromine was not superior to placebo in reducing any PTSD symptoms; however, the placebo response in this study was notably greater than that in other reported medication trials for PTSD, thus potentially obscuring positive results. This was attributed to potentially therapeutic patient-interviewer attention received in repeated interview assessments.

In the other brofaromine report, Katz and colleagues similarly compared brofaromine (up to 150 mg) to placebo in sixty-eight diverse-trauma patients participating in a fourteen-week, multisite, multicountry trial (Katz et al., 1994). The drop-out rate was 34 percent, quite similar to the one reported by Baker and colleagues. Katz and colleagues reported that brofaromine was not superior to placebo in treating PTSD symptoms among the total sample of PTSD patients, but that it did significantly reduce PTSD symptoms relative to placebo among those patients with chronic PTSD (symptoms present for at least one year). Findings for specific PTSD symptom clusters were not reported. Although some patients improved notably, nearly half of brofaromine-treated patients continued to meet criteria for PTSD at the end of the trial.

In addition, several open trials have been published examining the efficacy of MAOIs in PTSD. In one of the earlier open trials, phenelzine (1 mg/kg) was administered to eleven combat veterans with PTSD over eight weeks (Milanes et al., 1984). The drop-out rate was 40 percent; but among the six completers, four reported improvements in depression, overall PTSD symptoms, and global level of distress. Davidson and colleagues also conducted an open trial with phenelzine (45-60 mg) in eleven combat veterans treated for four to six weeks (Davidson, Walker, and Kilts, 1987). The drop-out rate to week six was 36 percent, but ten of the eleven patients completed at least the minimum four weeks of the trial. Among these completers, phenelzine resulted in rapid improvements in intrusions, estrangement, sleep disturbance, and startle response on observer-rated measures. No improvement was noted on self-reported outcomes, but this may have been the result of difficulty in interpreting the questionnaires, or of secondary gain issues (e.g., concern of losing disability compensation).

Lerer and colleagues used phenelzine (60 mg) in twenty-two combat veterans who completed a four- to eighteen-week trial (Lerer et al., 1987). The drop-out rate prior to week four was not reported. Among those completing at least four weeks of treatment, six patients were treated for four to eight weeks, seven for nine to thirteen weeks, and nine for fourteen to eighteen weeks. Although a few patients in the nine- to thirteen-week treatment group experienced improved PTSD symptoms on phenelzine, the level of symptom reduction was minimal and was not as evident for the two other groups. The only clinically significant improvement on phenelzine was for sleep. More recently, Neal and colleagues reported results from a twelve-week open trial of moclobemide (600 mg), a reversible inhibitor of MAO-A (Neal, Shapland, and Fox, 1997). Among their twenty patients with PTSD from diverse traumas, dropout was 10 percent to week four, and 20 percent to week twelve, which is much lower than in trials with traditional MAOIs. Moclobemide significantly reduced intrusions, avoidance, and hyperarousal symptoms of PTSD as well as depression relative to placebo, with improvement being most marked for avoidance/numbing symptoms.

Finally, at least two case reports have commented on the efficacy of MAOIs in treating PTSD. In one report, various MAOIs reduced intrusions, hyperarousal, and depression symptoms in five Indochinese survivors of trauma; avoidance symptoms, however, were not affected (DeMartino, Mollica, and Wilk, 1995). Another case report described five treatment-resistant combat veterans who experienced elimination of nightmares, flashbacks, and startle response following treatment with phenelzine (45-75 mg) (Hogben and Cornfield, 1981). Again, avoidance symptoms did not improve.

In summary, the controlled research examining the efficacy of MAOIs in the treatment of PTSD revealed some mixed findings; however, PTSD patients using this class of medication showed greater global improvement than those treated with TCAs. Of the four placebo-controlled trials conducted with MAOIs, there was one positive and one negative phenelzine report and one positive and one negative brofaromine report. The uncontrolled reports were more promising, with three of four open trials and several case reports demonstrating positive results with MAOIs. These medications appeared to be helpful for at least some PTSD patients, but the difficulty in using the MAOIs currently available in the United States may prohibit their future use, especially in an impulsive patient population. As with TCAs,

presynaptic alpha-2 autoreceptor. Pilot data from an open-label study of mirtazapine up to 45 mg/day for eight weeks in six civilian outpatients with severe, chronic PTSD demonstrated a 50 percent or more improvement in both PTSD and depression symptoms in three of the six patients (Connor, Davidson, and Weisler, 1998).

Bupropion is a unique antidepressant and has a chemical structure similar to amphetamines and other central nervous system stimulants. No reports could be found in the literature relating the efficacy of this medication to PTSD symptoms.

Venlafaxine is another structurally novel antidepressant which inhibits serotonin and norepinephrine reuptake and weak inhibition of dopamine reuptake. There are no studies indicating its potential use for PTSD patients.

BUSPIRONE

Buspirone is an anxiolytic that is unrelated to either the barbiturates or the benzodiazepines. Its mechanism of action is unknown, but it binds at the serotonin (5-HT_{1A} and 5-HT_2), as well as the dopamine (D_2) receptor binding sites. A major drawback of this medication, especially when compared to the benzodiazepines, is the three to four week delay until symptom relief appears. The most common side effects include dizziness, nausea, headache, nervousness, dry mouth, and diarrhea. In one open trial, three patients with PTSD were successfully treated with buspirone in final maximum dosages ranging from 35-60 mg daily. Symptoms that improved included anxiety, insomnia, flashbacks, and depressed mood, and the patients experienced no side effects (Wells et al., 1991). In another open trial, Duffy and Malloy examined eight patients with PTSD. Seven out of eight patients exhibited a significant reduction in symptoms, with a dose ranging from 5 to 30 mg per day (Duffy and Malloy, 1994).

LITHIUM

Originally introduced for the treatment of manic-depressive illness, lithium has now been used effectively in the augmentation of antidepressants and in patients with impulse control problems and aggression. The precise mechanism of action of lithium is still not understood; however, "stabilization" of cell membranes and modulation of the inositol phosphate secondary messenger system have been discussed in the literature. Lithium is effective within a narrow range of serum blood levels, above which toxicity prevails. Thus kidney, thyroid, and cardiac functions have to be monitored regularly during lithium treatment. The literature on lithium's effectiveness in PTSD is limited. In one open trial, lithium (300-600 mg) improved anxiety, anger, irritability, and insomnia in five treatment-resistant combat veterans with PTSD, with one case responding best to combined lithium and 10 mg of propranolol (Kitchner and Greenstein, 1985).

ANTICONVULSANTS

As their name suggests, these medications were originally developed to treat seizure disorders. They later became useful in the treatment of manic-depressive illness (as a mood stabilizer) and to decrease the frequency of impulsive or violent behaviors. With the development of the kindling model as a possible pathophysiological abnormality underlying mood oscillations, these medications were found to have antikindling properties, offering a possible explanation for their pharmacological effects. The best studied medications in this category are carbamazepine and valproic acid. Both have side effects such as gastrointestinal disturbance, possible bone marrow suppression, or hepatitis, and require periodic laboratory tests.

Although no controlled trials have been published on the use of anticonvulsants in the treatment of PTSD, four open trials and several case reports have suggested efficacy of these agents in treating some PTSD symptoms. Lipper and colleagues observed improved intrusive symptoms, depression, anxiety, and sleep in seven out of ten combat veterans with PTSD who were treated in an open trial with carbamazepine (Lipper et al., 1986). Wolf and colleagues reported a notable decrease in angry outbursts in ten combat veterans treated with carbamazepine (Wolf, Alavi, and Mosnaim, 1988). In a third open trial, carbamazepine eliminated core aspects of PTSD symptoms in twenty-two of twenty-eight sexually abused children and decreased symptoms in the remaining six patients (Looff et al., 1995). Finally, an open trial of valproic acid led to improvement in PTSD symptoms, particularly hyperarousal symptoms, in ten of sixteen combat veterans with PTSD (Fesler, 1991). Several case reports have also supported the efficacy of carbamazepine (Ford, 1996), valproate (Berigan and Holzgang, 1995), and vigabatrin (Macleod, 1996) in the management of nightmares, flashbacks, sleep disturbances, and startle response, with the latter being most frequently reported as successfully treated. Doses of carbamazepine in these reports were generally between 800-1000 mg. Valproic acid doses ranged from 1000-1500 mg and vigabatrin from 250-500 mg. In sum, anticonvulsants may improve intrusive symptoms and probably reduce hypervigilance and startle response.

BENZODIAZEPINES

In the last thirty years, benzodiazepines have replaced barbiturates as first line sedative (sleep inducing) and anxiolytic (antianxiety) agents. They are safer, especially if one overdoses and, although they can be addictive, they have less abuse potential than barbiturates. They are active in the widely distributed GABAergic system, which is a major inhibitory system in the brain. These medications are not effective in the treatment of depressive disorders, but their antianxiety effect has a more rapid onset of action than any of the antidepressants. Dependence can develop in some patients, especially when the medication is used chronically to treat sleep disturbances. This can lead to a withdrawal syndrome, which may be indistinguishable from the original symptoms, if the medication is abruptly discontinued. Benzodiazepine use in patients with past histories of substance abuse problems must be weighed against the potential benefit of the treatment.

Only one controlled trial has been conducted using benzodiazepines in the treatment of PTSD. In that study, alprazolam (3.75 mg) was compared to placebo in a five-week, crossover design, with a two-week washout between drug and placebo phases (Braun et al., 1990). Although overall anxiety ratings decreased on the drug relative to placebo, no changes in core PTSD symptoms were observed. Shalev and colleagues have also reported a failure of clonazepam and alprazolam to suppress auditory startle responses in PTSD patients (Shalev et al., 1998; Shalev and Rogel-Fuchs, 1992), as well as a failure of early administration of these drugs (two to eighteen days posttrauma) to alter the course of PTSD symptoms over six months (Gelpin et al., 1996). Clonazepam may be useful in the treatment of the severe dissociative symptoms, often present in refractory PTSD, as suggested by an open trial of this medication in five patients diagnosed with multiple personality disorder (Lowenstein, Hornstein, and Farber, 1988). However, no other reports provided further support for this specific area of efficacy.

In sum, although these drugs may seem to be a logical choice for the treatment of pervasive anxiety syndromes, there is little empirical support for their efficacy in PTSD. Furthermore, several factors suggest that initiation of benzodiazepine treatment in PTSD might require careful consideration. Because it is known that PTSD patients frequently have comorbid substance dependence, there is a potential for the development of benzodiazepine abuse and dependence as well. In addition, withdrawal from benzodiazepines can exacerbate PTSD symptoms (Risse et al., 1990). On the other hand, the abuse potential in other anxiety disorders has been overstated in the past (Shader and Greenblatt, 1993), and should not constitute an exclusive consideration, thus depriving PTSD patients of a potentially helpful pharmacological agent. Clinically, benzodiazepines are used regularly to treat symptoms such as sleep disturbance, the persistence of general anxiety symptoms, anger, irritability, and agoraphobia. Because they are relatively ineffective at treating core PTSD symptoms and have higher risks as previously described, practitioners should have clear indications in mind when prescribing these agents. Illicit substance use should be monitored during the medication trial and a gradual taper should be the method of discontinuing a benzodiazepine trial.

NEUROLEPTICS OR ANTIPSYCHOTIC AGENTS ("MAJOR TRANQUILIZERS")

In the last two decades, neuroleptics or antipsychotic agents have been less frequently prescribed for PTSD patients; however, they were extensively used in the 1960s and 1970s. Prior to the official recognition of PTSD as a unique diagnostic entity in DSM-III, patients presenting with severe agitation, explosive behavior, rage, and flashbacks were prescribed antipsychotic agents for symptoms that appeared psychotic. Since that time, however, PTSD has been reconceptualized as an anxiety disorder rather than a psychotic disorder and there has been little support for the use of these medications as first-line treatments for PTSD. There is no theoretical or empirical evidence to suggest that antipsychotic agents (blocking dopaminergic transmission) have PTSD-specific activity. When sedation is necessary, other medications are available that do not have the same risk factors and have overall fewer side effects.

Nonetheless, there have been isolated reports of benefit for some PTSD patients using neuroleptics. For example, PTSD patients with extreme suspiciousness or aggressive paranoia, intense anger, self-destructive behavior, and frequent hallucinatory flashbacks may respond to a neuroleptic trial (Dillard, Bendfeldt, and Jernigan, 1993; Walker, 1982). Mueser and Butler reported on five Vietnam veterans with PTSD and auditory hallucinations whose symptoms improved on antipsychotics (Mueser and Butler, 1987). Similarly, Hamner reported on a Vietnam veteran with both PTSD and Psychotic Disorder NOS whose psychotic and PTSD symptoms improved on 600 mg per day of clozapine (Hamner, 1996). The atypical neuroleptic, risperidone, has been used to successfully treat four male patients with vivid flashbacks and nightmares, allowing them to participate in psychotherapeutic treatment (Leyba and Wampler, 1998).

Thus, neuroleptics have been readily used in the past for PTSD, but should not be considered a first-line treatment, given the lack of solid data on their efficacy and their potentially severe side effects, especially tardive dyskinesia. On the other hand, these agents might be helpful for a particular symptom profile or patient subtype. Their use may become more acceptable with the advent of the new atypical neuroleptics, such as olanzapine, clozapine, or risperidone, which have more favorable side effect profiles than the traditional antipsychotics.

ADRENERGIC AGENTS

The principle pharmacological action of adrenergic agents used in psychiatry is decreasing catecholaminergic (adrenergic and noradrenergic) tone associated with arousal, anxiety, and panic symptoms. Adrenergic blockers such as propranolol directly block the postsynaptic adrenergic receptor sites, while adrenergic agonists such as clonidine achieve similar goals by acting on presynaptic adrenergic autoreceptors and decreasing neurotransmitter release. Originally, these medications were used for the management of hypertension and cardiac arrhythmias; however, psychiatrists began using them to treat psychiatric symptoms such as performance anxiety, aggressive or impulsive behavior, alcohol withdrawal, medication-induced tremor, and akathisia. Although often not a primary psychopharmacological treatment or "first line" medication, these agents can often supplement and augment other psychiatric medications. Potential side effects for this group include sedation, hypotension, bradycardia, exacerbation of asthma or diabetes, impotence, and possibly depression.

No placebo-controlled trials have been conducted using adrenergic agents in PTSD patients. One multiple-baseline case report on eleven sexually or physically abused children with PTSD found that propranolol (up to 2.5 mg/kg) was effective in decreasing PTSD symptoms (Famularo, Kinscherff, and Fenton, 1988). Similarly, van der Kolk reported that propranolol (120-160 mg) improved PTSD symptoms in eleven of twelve combat veterans, and clonidine (0.2-0.4 mg), an alpha-2 agonist, improved PTSD symptoms in eight of nine combat veterans (van der Kolk, 1983). Two other reports indicated similarly positive results with clonidine. In the first, clonidine (0.2 mg, up to 0.6 mg) combined with imipramine (150 mg) decreased both depressive and PTSD symptoms (especially sleep problems and nightmares) beyond the improvement observed for imipramine alone, in Cambodian refugees with PTSD (Kinzie and Leung, 1989). In the second report, clonidine (up to 0.2 mg patch) used with seven preschool children with PTSD due to severe abuse and neglect, improved aggression, hyperarousal, and sleep difficulties (Harmon and Riggs, 1996). Two other case reports note suppression of nightmares on clonidine, with reemergence of the nightmares in the early morning hours after several weeks on the medication (Horrigan, 1996; Horrigan and Barnhill, 1996). Sustained suppression of nightmares was achieved when guanfacine, a longer-acting alpha-2 agonist, was tried.

In sum, several reports suggest efficacy of adrenergic agents in treating some PTSD symptoms, particularly nightmares and hyperarousal symptoms. Double-blind, controlled studies are needed to confirm these findings and to further explore the efficacy of these agents in PTSD specific symptomatology.

OPIATE ANTAGONISTS

Originally used to treat opioid addiction or overdose, these medications may have some role in treating a wide variety of psychiatric disorders, including PTSD. Two reports have commented on the use of opiate antagonists in the treatment of PTSD symptoms. Based on the hypothesis that emotional numbing of PTSD patients is an opiate-mediated phenomenon, 400 mg of nalmefene, an oral opiate antagonist (not available in the United States), was administered to eighteen combat veterans with PTSD in an open trial. Eight of the eighteen patients reported decreased numbing, intrusive symptoms, and startle response (Glover, 1993). In the second report, naltrexone (50 mg) was administered to two patients with noncombat PTSD, in a multiple-baseline, on-off-on design. In both cases, flashbacks decreased significantly on the drug and returned when drug use was discontinued (Bills and Kreisler, 1993). Flashbacks may represent a form of self-injurious behavior, mediated by recurrent endogenous endorphin release that can be treated with naloxone.

CONCLUSION

Clinical experience and research have demonstrated the complexity of the PTSD syndrome, as well as the need for continued research to integrate effective treatments and to improve outcomes. Although achieving a "cure" from PTSD through pharmacotherapy is out of reach, numerous medications are clearly effective in alleviating symptoms and facilitating recovery.

In general, antidepressants appear effective for the treatment of PTSD, especially in patients with depression, sleep disturbance, or intrusive and hyperarousal symptoms. They might be less effective in the treatment of avoidance behavior; however, this has to be further studied. Data do not seem to show clear differential efficacy between the SSRIs, MAOIs, or TCAs. It is reasonable, therefore, to advocate the use of the SSRIs as a first-line treatment, given their greater ease of use, lower risk of harm in overdose, and, perhaps, fewer side effects. The mood stabilizers also show significant promise, especially for the treatment of impulsivity, irritability, and mood fluctuation. Benzodiazepines were not studied enough to draw any conclusions regarding their efficacy. In the little research available, they have not been shown to be effective. Clinically, though, they are used quite extensively for sleep problems, panic symptoms, and residual anxiety in PTSD patients. Similarly, there is insufficient data demonstrating efficacy of the neuroleptics in the treatment of PTSD. Given the potential serious side effects of classical neuroleptics, their use should be carefully considered. Some adrenergic agents might hold promise for the treatment of hyperarousal symptoms, in combination with other agents. The other agents mentioned in this chapter should still be considered "experimental."

A number of particular methodological issues make the interpretation and the integration of the existing data, from the PTSD treatment studies a particularly complex task. Symptom profiles can differ among patients meeting PTSD diagnostic criteria (e.g., the relative predominance of numbing, avoidance, anger, or intrusive symptoms). Significant variation exists among the studies with regard to comorbidities, type of trauma leading to PTSD, degrees of severity, chronicity, litigation, and secondary gain. For instance, we know that combat veterans in general, and those with chronic PTSD in particular, are more treatment-refractory than other patient populations. Studies done exclusively with these groups may miss potentially effective treatments for other cohorts. Numerous outcome measures are also used across different studies. Both the sensitivity and the specificity can vary across these instruments, as well, whether they are self- or clinician-administered, as the latter will often provide larger effect sizes (Lambert et al., 1986; Taylor, 1995). Finally, the study design and the controls used vary significantly in these studies, making generalization possible from some of the studies, but not others. Randomization, use of appropriate control groups, adequate duration of treatment trials, blinding procedures, assessment of drug concentration in blood samples, and other research design elements contribute to the scientific rigor and confidence in the outcomes.

The future of psychopharmacology for PTSD holds much hope. Research will further clarify the efficacy and the utility of medications such as mood stabilizers, atypical neuroleptics, and newer antidepressants. Meanwhile, innovative treatments, for example, inositol and cyproheptadine (a serotonin/histamine antagonist), are already being tested (Gupta et al., 1998; Kaplan et al., 1996). Finally, with the better understanding of the pathophysiology of PTSD, anxiety, and depression, more specific pharmacological agents (such as CRF antagonists) are expected to become available in the near future. A deeper understanding of the risk factors and the pathophysiology of PTSD (i.e., the effects of early trauma on corticotrophin releasing factor [CRF] containing neural circuits) will ultimately allow the development of early intervention and prevention strategies (Heim et al., 1997).

REFERENCES

Adamec, R. (1997). Transmitter systems involved in neural plasticity underlying increased anxiety and defense—Implications for understanding anxiety following traumatic stress. *Neuroscience and Biobehavioral Reviews, 21,* 755-765.

Adamec, R. E., Shallow, T., and Budgell, J. (1997). Blockade of CCK(B) but not CCK(A) receptors before and after the stress of predator exposure prevents lasting increases in anxiety-like behavior: Implications for anxiety associated with posttraumatic stress disorder. *Behavioral Neuroscience, 111,* 435-449.

Arora, R. C., Fichtner, C. G., O'Connor, F., and Crayton, J. W. (1993). Paroxetine binding in the blood platelets of post-traumatic stress disorder patients. *Life Sciences, 53,* 919-928.

Baker, D. G., Diamond, B. I., Gillette, G., Hanmer, M., Katzelnick, D., Keller, T., Mellman, T. A., Pontius, E., Rosenthal, M., Tucker, P., et al. (1995). A double-blind, randomized, placebo-controlled, multi-center study of brofaromine in the treatment of post-traumatic stress disorder. *Psychopharmacology, 122,* 386-389.

Baxter, L. R. Jr., Schwartz, J. M., Bergman, K. S., Szuba, M. P., Guze, B. H., Mazziotta, J. C., Alazraki, A., Selin, C. E., Ferng, H. K., Munford, P., et al. (1992). Caudate glucose metabolic rate changes with both drug and behavior therapy for obsessive-compulsive disorder. *Archives of General Psychiatry, 49,* 681-689.

Berigan, T. R. and Holzgang, A. (1995). Valproate as an alternative in post-traumatic stress disorder: A case report. *Military Medicine, 160,* 318.

Bills, L. J. and Kreisler, K. (1993). Treatment of flashbacks with naltrexone [letter]. *American Journal of Psychiatry, 150,* 1430.

Bleich, A., Siegel, B., Garb, R., and Lerer, B. (1986). Post-traumatic stress disorder following combat exposure: Clinical features and psychopharmacological treatment. *British Journal of Psychiatry 149*(September), 365-369.

Brady, K., Farfel, G., and SPS, G. A. (1998). "Double-blind multicenter comparison of sertraline and placebo in PTSD." Paper presented at the American College of Neuropsychopharmacology, 37th Annual Meeting, Las Croabas, Puerto Rico, December.

Brady, K. T., Sonne, S. C., and Roberts, J. M. (1995). Sertraline treatment of comorbid posttraumatic stress disorder and alcohol dependence. *Journal of Clinical Psychiatry, 56,* 502-505.

Braun, P., Greenberg, D., Dasberg, H., and Lerer, B. (1990). Core symptoms of posttraumatic stress disorder unimproved by alprazolam treatment. *Journal of Clinical Psychiatry, 51,* 236-238.

Bremner, J. D., Krystal, J. H., Southwick, S. M., and Charney, D. (1996). Noradrenergic mechanisms in stress and anxiety: II. Clinical studies. *Synapse, 23,* 39-51.

Burdon, A. P., Sutker, P. B., Foulks, E. F., Crane, M. U., and Thompson, K. E. (1991). Pilot program of treatment for PTSD [letter]. *American Journal of Psychiatry, 148,* 1269-1270.

Burstein, A. (1984). Treatment of post-traumatic stress disorder with imipramine. *Psychosomatics, 25,* 681-687.

Connor, K., Davidson, J., and Weisler, R. (1998). "A pilot study of mirtazapine in posttraumatic stress disorder." Paper presented at the American College of Neuropsychopharmacology, 37th Annual Meeting, Las Croabas, Puerto Rico, December.

Da Costa, J. (1871). On irritable heart: A clinical study of a form of functional cardiac disorder and its consequence. *American Journal of Medical Science, 16,* 17-52.

Davidson, J. R. (1997). Biological therapies for posttraumatic stress disorder: An overview. *Journal of Clinical Psychiatry, 58,* 29-32.

Davidson, J., Kudler, H., Smith, R., Mahorney, S. L., Lipper, S., Hammett, E., Saunders, W. B., and Cavenar, J. O. Jr. (1990). Treatment of posttraumatic stress disorder with amitriptyline and placebo. *Archives of General Psychiatry, 47,* 259-266.

Davidson, J., Roth, S., and Newman, E. (1991). Fluoxetine in post-traumatic stress disorder. *Journal of Traumatic Stress, 4,* 419-423.

Davidson, J., Walker, J. I., and Kilts, C. (1987). A pilot study of phenelzine in the treatment of post-traumatic stress disorder. *British Journal of Psychiatry, 150* (February), 252-255.

Davidson, J. R., Weisler, R. H., Malik, M. L., and Connor, K. M. (1998). Treatment of posttraumatic stress disorder with nefazodone. *International Clinical Psychopharmacology, 13,* 111-113.

Davidson, J. R., Weisler, R. H., Malik, M., and Tupler, L. A. (1998). Fluvoxamine in civilians with posttraumatic stress disorder [letter]. *Journal of Clinical Psychopharmacology, 18,* 93-95.

Davis, L. L., Suns, A., Lambert, M. T., Heimberg, C., and Petty, F. (1997). Posttraumatic stress disorder and serotonin: New directions for research and treatment. *Journal of Psychiatry and Neuroscience, 22,* 318-326.

De Boer, M., Op den Velde, W., Falger, P. J., Hovens, J. E., De Groen, J. H., and Van Duijn, H. (1992). Fluvoxamine treatment for chronic PTSD: A pilot study. *Psychotherapy and Psychosomatics, 57,* 158-163.

DeMartino, R., Mollica, R. F., and Wilk, V. (1995). Monoamine oxidase inhibitors in posttraumatic stress disorder. Promise and problems in Indochinese survivors of trauma. *Journal of Nervous and Mental Disease, 183,* 510-515.

Dillard, M. L., Bendfeldt, F., and Jernigan, P. (1993). Use of thioridazine in post-traumatic stress disorder. *Southern Medical Journal, 86,* 1276-1278.

Duffy, J. D. and Malloy, P. F. (1994). Efficacy of buspirone in the treatment of post-traumatic stress disorder: An open trial. *Annals of Clinical Psychiatry, 6,* 33-37.

Falcon, S., Ryan, C., Chamberlain, K., and Curtis, G. (1985). Tricyclics: Possible treatment for posttraumatic stress disorder. *Journal of Clinical Psychiatry, 46,* 385-388.

Famularo, R., Kinscherff, R., and Fenton, T. (1988). Propranolol treatment for childhood posttraumatic stress disorder, acute type. A pilot study. *American Journal of Diseases of Children, 142,* 1244-1247.

Fesler, F. A. (1991). Valproate in combat-related posttraumatic stress disorder. *Journal of Clinical Psychiatry, 52,* 361-364.

Ford, N. (1996). The use of anticonvulsants in posttraumatic stress disorder: Case study and overview. *Journal of Traumatic Stress, 9,* 857-863.

Foy, D. (1992). *Treating PTSD: Cognitive-behavioral strategies.* New York: Guilford Press.

Friedman, M., Charney, D., and Deutch, A. (1995). *Neurobiological and clinical consequences of stress.* Philadelphia: Lippincott-Raven.

Gelpin, E., Bonne, O., Pen, T., Brandes, D., and Shalev, A. Y. (1996). *Treatment of recent trauma survivors with benzodiazepines: A prospective study.* Jerusalem, Israel: Hadassah University.

Glover, H. (1993). A preliminary trial of nalmefene for the treatment of emotional numbing in combat veterans with post-traumatic stress disorder. *Israel Journal of Psychiatry and Related Sciences, 30,* 255-263.

Grillon, C., Southwick, S. M., and Charney, D. S. (1996). The psychobiological basis of posttraumatic stress disorder. *Molecular Psychiatry, 1,* 278-297.

Gupta, S., Popli, A., Bathurst, E., Hennig, L., Droney, T., and Keller, P. (1998). Efficacy of cyproheptadine for nightmares associated with posttraumatic stress disorder. *Comprehensive Psychiatry, 39,* 160-164.

Hamner, M. B. (1996). Clozapine treatment for a veteran with comorbid psychosis and PTSD [letter]. *American Journal of Psychiatry, 153,* 841.

Harmon, R. J. and Riggs, P. D. (1996). Clonidine for posttraumatic stress disorder in preschool children. *Journal of the American Academy of Child and Adolescent Psychiatry, 35,* 1247-1249.

Heim, C., Owens, M. J., Plotsky, P. M., and Nemeroff, C. B. (1997). Persistent changes in corticotropin-releasing factor systems due to early life stress: Relationship to the pathophysiology of major depression and post-traumatic stress disorder. *Psychopharmacology Bulletin, 33,* 185-192.

Henry, J. P., Haviland, M. G., Cummings, M. A., Anderson, D. L., Nelson, J. C., MacMurray, J. P., MeGhee, W. H., and Hubbard, R. W. (1992). Shared neuroendocrine patterns of posttraumatic stress disorder and alexithymia. *Psychosomatic Medicine, 54,* 407-415.

Hertzberg, M. A., Feldman, M. E., Beckham, J. C., and Davidson, J. R. (1996). Trial of trazodone for posttraumatic stress disorder using a multiple baseline group design. *Journal of Clinical Psychopharmacology, 16,* 294-298.

Hertzberg, M. A., Feldman, M. E., Beckham, J. C., Moore, S. D., and Davidson, J. R. (1996). Open trial of nefazodone for combat-related posttraumatic stress disorder. *Journal of Clinical Psychiatry, 59,* 460-464.

Hockings, G. I., Grice, J. E., Ward, W. K., Walters, M. M., Jensen, G. R., and Jackson, R. V. (1993). Hypersensitivity of the hypothalamic-pituitary-adrenal axis to naloxone in post-traumatic stress disorder. *Biological Psychiatry, 33,* 585-593.

Hogben, G. L. and Cornfield, R. B. (1981). Treatment of traumatic war neurosis with phenelzine. *Archives of General Psychiatry, 38,* 440-445.

Horrigan, J. P. (1996). Guanfacine for PTSD nightmares [letter]. *Journal of the American Academy of Child and Adolescent Psychiatry, 35,* 975-976.

Horrigan, J. P. and Barnhill, L. J. (1996). The suppression of nightmares with guanfacine [letter]. *Journal of Clinical Psychiatry, 57,* 371.

Janet, P. (1889). *L'automatisme psychologique;essai de psychologie experimentale sur les formes inferieures de l'activite humaine, par Pierre Janet.* Paris: Alcan.

Kaplan, Z., Amir, M., Swartz, M., and Levine, J. (1996). Inositol treatment of post-traumatic stress disorder. *Anxiety, 2,* 51-52.

Kardiner, A. (1941). *The traumatic neurosis of war.* Washington, DC: National Research Council.

Katz, R. J., Lott, M. H., Arbus, P., Crocq, L., Herlobsen, P., Lingjaerde, O., Lopez, G., Loughrey, G. C., MacFarlane, D. J., Melvor, R., et al. (1994). Pharmacotherapy of post-traumatic stress disorder with a novel psychotropic. *Anxiety, 1,* 169-174.

Kauffman, C. D., Reist, C., Djenderedjian, A., Nelson, J. N., and Haier, R. J. (1987). Biological markers of affective disorders and posttraumatic stress disorder: A pilot study with desipramine. *Journal of Clinical Psychiatry, 48,* 366-367.

Kinzie, J. D. and Goetz, R. R. (1996). A century of controversy surrounding post-traumatic stress stress-spectrum syndromes: The impact on DSM-III and DSM-IV. *Journal of Traumatic Stress, 9,* 159-179.

Kinzie, J. D. and Leung, P. (1989). Clonidine in Cambodian patients with post-traumatic stress disorder [see comments]. *Journal of Nervous and Mental Disease, 177,* 546-550.

Kitchner, I. and Greenstein, R. (1985). Low dose lithium carbonate in the treatment of post-traumatic stress disorder: Brief communication. *Military Medicine, 150,* 378-381.

Kline, N. A., Dow, B. M., Brown, S. A., and Matloff, J. L. (1994). Sertraline efficacy in depressed combat veterans with posttraumatic stress disorder [letter]. *American Journal of Psychiatry, 151,* 621.

Kosten, T. R., Frank, J. B., Dan, E., McDougle, C. J., and Giller, E. L. Jr. (1991). Pharmacotherapy for posttraumatic stress disorder using phenelzine or imipramine. *Journal of Nervous and Mental Disease, 179,* 366-370.

Kosten, T. R., Mason, J. W., Giller, E. L., Ostroff, R. B., and Harkness, L. (1987). Sustained urinary norepinephrine and epinephrine elevation in post-traumatic stress disorder. *Psychoneuroendocrinology, 12,* 13-20.

Kosten, T. R., Wahby, V., Giller, E., Jr., and Mason, J. (1990). The dexamethasone suppression test and thyrotropin-releasing hormone stimulation test in post-traumatic stress disorder. *Biological Psychiatry, 28,* 657-664.

Lambert, M., Hatch, D., Kingston, M., and Edwards, B. (1986). Zung, Beck, and Hamilton rating scales as measures of treatment outcome: A meta-analytic comparison. *Journal of Consulting and Clinical Psychology, 54,* 54-59.

Lerer, B., Bleich, A., Kotler, M., Garb, R., Hertzberg, M., and Levin, B. (1987). Posttraumatic stress disorder in Israeli combat veterans. Effect of phenelzine treatment. *Archives of General Psychiatry, 44,* 976-981.

Leyba, C. M. and Wampler, T. P. (1998). Risperidone in PTSD [letter]. *Psychiatric Services, 49,* 245-246.

Lipper, S., Davidson, J. R., Grady, T. A., Edinger, J. D., Hammett, E. B., Mahorney, S. L., and Cavenar, J. O. Jr. (1986). Preliminary study of carbamazepine in posttraumatic stress disorder. *Psychosomatics, 27,* 849-854.

Looff, D., Grimley, P., Kuller, F., Martin, A., and Shonfield, L. (1995). Carbamazepine for PTSD [letter]. *Journal of the American Academy of Child and Adolescent Psychiatry, 34,* 703-704.

Lowenstein, R. J., Hornstein, N., and Farber, B. (1988). Open trial of clonazepam in the treatment of posttraumatic stress symptoms in multiple personality disorder. *Dissociation, 1,* 3-12.

Macleod, A. D. (1996). Vigabatrin and posttraumatic stress disorder [letter]. *Journal of Clinical Psychopharmacology, 16,* 190-191.

March, J. S. (1992). Fluoxetine and fluvoxamine in PTSD [letter]. *American Journal of Psychiatry, 149,* 413.

Marmar, C. R., Schoenfeld, F., Weiss, D. S., Metzler, T., Zatzick, D., Wu, R., Smiga, S., Tecott, L., and Neylan, T. (1996). Open trial of fluvoxamine treatment for combat-related posttraumatic stress disorder. *Journal of Clinical Psychiatry, 57,* 66-70; discussion 71-72.

Marshall, R. D., Schneier, F. R., Fallon, B. A., Knight, C. B., Abbate, L. A., Goetz, D., Campeas, R., and Liebowitz, M. R. (1998). An open trial of paroxetine in patients with noncombat-related, chronic posttraumatic stress disorder. *Journal of Clinical Psychopharmacology, 18,* 10-18.

Mason, J., Weizman, R., Laor, N., Wang, S., Schujovitsky, A., Abramovitz-Schneider, P., Feiler, D., and Charney, D. (1996). Serum triiodothyronine elevation with posttraumatic stress disorder: A cross-cultural study. *Biological Psychiatry, 39,* 835-838.

McDougle, C. J., Southwick, S. M., Charney, D. S., and St. James, R. L. (1991). An open trial of fluoxetine in the treatment of posttraumatic stress disorder [letter]. *Journal of Clinical Psychopharmacology, 11,* 325-327.

Milanes, F., Mack, C. N., Dennison, J., and Slater, V. (1984). Phenelzine treatment of post-Vietnam stress syndrome. *VA Practitioner,* 40-49.

Mueser, K. T. and Butler, R. W. (1987). Auditory hallucinations in combat-related chronic posttraumatic stress disorder. *American Journal of Psychiatry, 144,* 299-302.

Nagy, L. M., Morgan, C. A. D., Southwick, S. M., and Charney, D. S. (1993). Open prospective trial of fluoxetine for posttraumatic stress disorder. *Journal of Clinical Psychopharmacology, 13,* 107-113.

Neal, L. A., Shapland, W., and Fox, C. (1997). An open trial of moclobemide in the treatment of post-traumatic stress disorder. *International Clinical Psychopharmacology, 12,* 231-237.

Pitman, R. K., van der Kolk, B. A., Orr, S. P., and Greenberg, M. (1990). Naloxone-reversible analgesic response to combat-related stimuli in posttraumatic stress disorder. A pilot study. *Archives of General Psychiatry, 47,* 541-544.

Reist, C., Kauffmann, C. D., Haier, R. J., Sangdahl, C., DeMet, E. M., Chicz-DeMet, A., and Nelson, J. N. (1989). A controlled trial of desipramine in 18 men with posttraumatic stress disorder [see comments]. *American Journal of Psychiatry, 146*, 513-516.

Risse, S. C., Whitters, A., Burke, J., Chen, S., Scurfield, R. M., and Raskind, M. A. (1990). Severe withdrawal symptoms after discontinuation of alprazolam in eight patients with combat-induced posttraumatic stress disorder. *Journal of Clinical Psychiatry, 51*, 206-209.

Rothbaum, B. O., Ninan, P. T., and Thomas, L. (1996). Sertraline in the treatment of rape victims with posttraumatic stress disorder. *Journal of Traumatic Stress, 9*, 865-871.

Shader, R. I. and Greenblatt, D. J. (1993). Use of benzodiazepines in anxiety disorders. *NEJM, 328*, 1398-1405.

Shalev, A. Y., Bloch, M., Peri, T., and Bonne, O. (1998). Alprazolam reduces response to loud tones in panic disorder but not in posttraumatic stress disorder. *Biological Psychiatry, 44*, 64-68.

Shalev, A. Y. and Rogel-Fuchs, Y. (1992). Auditory startle reflex in post-traumatic stress disorder patients treated with clonazepam. *Israel Journal of Psychiatry and Related Sciences, 29*, 1-6.

Shay, J. (1992). Fluoxetine reduces explosiveness and elevates mood of Vietnam combat veterans with posttraumatic stress disorder. *Journal of Traumatic Stress, 5*, 97-101.

Shestatzky, M., Greenberg, D., and Lerer, B. (1988). A controlled trial of phenelzine in posttraumatic stress disorder. *Psychiatry Research, 24*, 149-155.

Taylor, S. (1995). Assessment of obsessions and compulsions: Reliability, validity, and sensitivity to treatment effects. *Clinical Psychology Review, 15*, 261-296.

True, W. R., Rice, J., Eisen, S. A., Heath, A. C., Goldberg, J., Lyons, M. J., and Nowak, J. (1993). A twin study of genetic and environmental contributions to liability for posttraumatic stress symptoms. *Archive of General Psychiatry, 50*, 257-264.

van der Kolk, B. A. (1983). Psychopharmacology. Psychopharmacological issues in posttraumatic stress disorder. *Hospital and Community Psychiatry, 34*, 683-684, 691.

van der Kolk, B. A. (1994). The body keeps the score: Memory and the evolving psychobiology of posttraumatic stress. *Harvard Review of Psychiatry, 1*, 253-265.

van der Kolk, B. A., Dreyfuss, D., Michaels, M., Shera, D., Berkowitz, R., Fisler, R., and Saxe, G. (1994). Fluoxetine in posttraumatic stress disorder [see comments]. *Journal of Clinical Psychiatry, 55*, 517-522.

van der Kolk, B. A., Greenberg, M. S., Orr, S. P., and Pitman, R. K. (1989). Endogenous opioids, stress-induced analgesia, and posttraumatic stress disorder. *Psychopharmacology Bulletin, 25*, 417-421.

Walker, J. I. (1982). Chemotherapy of traumatic war stress. *Military Medicine, 147,* 1029-1033.

Wells, B. G., Chu, C. C., Johnson, R., Nasdahl, C., Ayubi, M. A., Sewell, E., and Statham, P. (1991). Buspirone in the treatment of posttraumatic stress disorder. *Pharmacotherapy, 11,* 340-343.

Wolf, M. E., Alavi, A., and Mosnaim, A. D. (1988). Posttraumatic stress disorder in Vietnam veterans clinical and EEG findings; possible therapeutic effects of carbamazepine. *Biological Psychiatry, 23,* 642-644.

Yatham, L. N., Sacamano, J., and Kusumakar, V. (1996). Assessment of noradrenergic functioning in patients with non-combat-related posttraumatic stress disorder: A study with desmethylimipramine and orthostatic challenges. *Psychiatry Research, 63,* 1-6.

Yehuda, R., Southwick, S., Giller, E. L., Ma, X., and Mason, J. W. (1992). Urinary catecholamine excretion and severity of PTSD symptoms in Vietnam combat veterans. *Journal of Nervous and Mental Disease, 180,* 321-325.

SECTION II:
TREATMENT OF PTSD IN GENERAL

Chapter 5

Cognitive-Behavioral Treatment of PTSD

Lori A. Zoellner
Edna B. Foa
Lee A. Fitzgibbons

In the aftermath of a traumatic experience such as an assault, a natural disaster, a tragic accident, or war, the development of post-traumatic stress disorder (PTSD) is a common occurrence. Epidemiological data estimate lifetime prevalence of PTSD from 1.0 percent (Helzer, Robins, and McEvoy, 1987) to 12.3 percent (Resick et al., 1993). However, most epidemiological studies of PTSD have focused on specific types of extreme events and examined the prevalence of PTSD among those subjected to that particular trauma. For example, Resick et al. (1993) found that 32 percent of female robbery victims met criteria for lifetime prevalence of PTSD. For war trauma, the National Vietnam Veterans Readjustment Study (NVVRS) (Kulka et al., 1988) found a 30.9 percent lifetime prevalence of PTSD in male Vietnam veterans. For other traumas such as natural disasters and motor vehicle accidents, similar prevalence rates of PTSD can also be found (e.g., Green et al., 1990; McFarlane and Papay, 1992; Shore, Vollmer, and Tatum, 1989; Taylor and Koch, 1995). Given the high rates of resulting PTSD from a variety of traumatic events, the development of efficacious and cost-effective treatments has become imperative.

Please address all correspondence concerning this manuscript to Dr. Lori A. Zoellner, Center for the Treatment and Study of Anxiety Disorders, MCP University, 3200 Henry Avenue, Philadelphia, PA 19129. Electronic mail may be sent to <zoellner@auhs.edu>. The preparation of this chapter was supported in part by a grant from the National Institute of Mental Health (MH-52272) awarded to Dr. Edna B. Foa.

THE EFFICACY OF PSYCHOSOCIAL TREATMENTS

The most studied psychosocial treatment programs for PTSD have utilized cognitive-behavioral techniques (Foa and Meadows, 1997). These consist of a variety of treatment programs including exposure procedures, cognitive restructuring, and anxiety management.

Prolonged Imaginal and In Vivo Exposure

All exposure programs involve the confrontation of feared stimuli, either in imagination or in vivo. With PTSD, exposure therapy usually involves repeated confrontation with the memories of the trauma (i.e., imaginal exposure) and with trauma-related situations that give rise to extreme fear (i.e., in vivo exposure).

One of the earliest exposure techniques used to treat posttrauma reactions was systematic desensitization (SD) (Wolpe, 1958). In SD, relaxation is paired with short, imaginal exposures to trauma reminders. These stimuli are presented in a hierarchical fashion, beginning with the least anxiety-producing image and gradually moving to the most anxiety-evoking images. Case reports and uncontrolled studies (e.g., Frank and Stewart, 1983, 1984) indicate that SD was somewhat effective in reducing trauma-related symptoms.

More recently, prolonged exposure with or without relaxation has replaced SD as a technique. With respect to war veterans, three controlled studies using imaginal exposure have been conducted (Cooper and Clum, 1989; Keane et al., 1989; Boudewyns and Hyer, 1990; Boudewyns et al., 1990). Imaginal exposure ranged from six to sixteen sessions. Cooper and Clum (1989) compared individual and group counseling with the inclusion of imaginal exposure, to individual and group counseling alone. They found that the imaginal exposure group decreased PTSD symptoms but did not show any benefits on either depression or trait anxiety. Keane et al. (1989) compared imaginal exposure preceded by relaxation with a no-treatment, wait-list condition. Although the numbing and social avoidance components of PTSD did not differ between groups, the imaginal exposure group experienced reduction in reexperiencing, anxiety, and depression. Finally, Boudewyns and colleagues published two reports (Boudewyns and Hyer, 1990; Boudewyns et al., 1990) examining group treatment supplemented with either traditional weekly psychotherapy or weekly imaginal exposure. The group supplemented with imaginal exposure evidenced improvement on self-reported psychological functioning more than the control group, but no group differences in physiological responding were detected.

With female assault victims, two controlled studies have examined the efficacy of nine-session exposure treatment for chronic PTSD in compari-

fronting trauma-related situations that the client fears and avoids, and daily listening to an audiotape of the imaginal exposure. Table 5.1 depicts an outline of the treatment program.

The Educational Component

The education stage consists of discussing the various PTSD symptoms as well as other common reactions to a traumatic event. This presentation takes the form of a dialogue to address the client's unique responses to the trauma. The definition of PTSD, the role of fear and anxiety, and a description of common PTSD symptoms are all discussed. In addition to the PTSD symptoms, other common trauma-related disturbances are also discussed. Depressive symptoms are especially common. Careful attention should be paid to suicidal ideation and appropriate risk assessment conducted. Guilt or shame associated with the assault, a sense of loss of control, and low self-esteem are other issues discussed. Often, trauma survivors also experience disruptions in relationships. Following rape, and to a lesser extent other traumas, the client may experience a significant loss of interest in sexual activity as well as evidencing sexual problems. Such problems are identified

TABLE 5.1. Outline of Treatment Program

Session 1:	Structured interview to discuss trauma and reactions Overview of the program and rationale for techniques Breathing retraining Homework: breathing practice
Session 2:	Common reactions Rationale for in vivo exposure Construction of in vivo hierarchy Homework: breathing and in vivo exposure assignments
Session 3:	Rationale for cognitive restructuring Cognitive restructuring Homework: breathing, in vivo exposure, daily diary (CR)
Session 4:	Rationale of prolonged imaginal exposure Prolonged imaginal exposure—sixty minutes Homework: breathing, in vivo exposure, daily diary, and imaginal exposure via audiotape
Session 5-8 (or 11):	Prolonged imaginal exposure—thirty to forty minutes Cognitive restructuring—thirty minutes Homework: breathing, in vivo exposure, daily diary, and imaginal exposure via audiotape
Final Session:	Prolonged imaginal exposure—twenty to thirty minutes Review of progress Discussion of relapse prevention

and their relationship to the traumatic experience is noted. Following this discussion, the client is provided with a handout that summarizes common reactions to trauma and he or she is instructed to reread the handout and encouraged to share this information with important people in his or her life. An example of the handout is in the Appendix at the end of this chapter.

Breathing Retraining

Breathing skills are taught to help manage anxiety and distress. The therapist briefly explains the relationship of hyperventilation and physical symptoms of anxiety and notes that to reduce anxiety, inhalation should be relatively shallow and exhalation should be slow. The therapist initially models the breathing by taking a normal breath and exhaling very slowly, silently uttering the word *"calm."* After a brief pause, another breath is taken. The sequence is repeated approximately ten to fifteen times. After the therapist's modeling, the therapist and client try the breathing together. Finally, the therapist watches the client practicing on his or her own to monitor for any difficulties. As homework, the skill is practiced three times daily.

Exposure

Exposure to feared but safe situations as well as to imagery of traumatic memory allows activation of the trauma-related fear and subsequent modification of the pathological elements that maintain PTSD. Thus, repeated and prolonged confrontation of feared situations and images allows emotional processing to take place, resulting in amelioration of the psychological difficulties experienced by the client. The goal of therapy is to help the client resume preassault daily functioning and to be able to remember the trauma without undue anxiety and distress.

In Vivo Exposure

Fears associated with the trauma are often unrealistic or excessive. Repeatedly confronting situations that are anxiety provoking, but not objectively dangerous, results in reduction of trauma-related anxiety evoked by these situations. The belief that the situations are unsafe is disconfirmed, as is the belief that anxiety will continue forever unless escape is realized. As a by-product, in vivo exposure enhances self-efficacy and self-esteem. The therapist explains the rationale underlying in vivo exposure and also illustrates the process using a common example for the client:

> Imagine the taxicab driver who lived in New York and developed a fear of driving across bridges. This fear created serious problems in

his work since he was unable to drive customers across bridges. Each time he approached a bridge he pretended that something was mechanically wrong with the taxi and called another cab to take his customers to their destination. The taxicab driver, with the support of a therapist, practiced driving over bridges daily. Within a week he was able to cross a bridge with the therapist following him in another car. By the end of two weeks, with repeated practice, he was able drive over small bridges by himself. (Foa and Rothbaum, 1998, p. 146)

After the rationale, the therapist inquires about a variety of areas in the client's life. Although avoidance is often trauma-specific, typical situations that are avoided include such events as reading about a trauma in the newspaper, seeing an unfamiliar man, walking through a parking garage or parking lot, or going to a crowded store. For every item on the hierarchy, the objective safety of the situation must be assessed. Confrontation with truly dangerous situations will not be helpful in the reduction of anxiety.

Next, a 0 to 100 point scale called the Subjective Units of Discomfort Scale (SUDS) is introduced. Zero indicates "no discomfort at all" and 100 indicates "severe discomfort." A SUDS level is obtained for each item. Initially, the therapist and client choose situations that evoke moderate levels of anxiety (e.g., SUDS = 50) for the first exposure homework. The client is instructed to stay in each situation for thirty to forty-five minutes, or until his or her anxiety drops considerably (at least 50 percent). Eventually, more anxiety-producing items on the hierarchy are assigned, until the client is able to comfortably confront most items. Toward the end of therapy, SUDS scores are reobtained for each situation in order to evaluate progress and assess areas for future intervention.

Imaginal Exposure to Trauma

Trauma survivors often try hard to push intrusive memories of the event out of their minds. However, by engaging in the memory rather than avoiding it, they learn that the memories of the trauma are not intrinsically dangerous. Consequently, the trauma can be remembered without intense or disruptive anxiety. During imaginal exposure, the client recalls the memory as vividly as possible, imagining the trauma as if it is happening at that moment. The client is encouraged to describe the trauma in the present tense and recount as many details as possible, including specific thoughts and feelings. The therapist monitors the SUDS level during the reliving, approximately every five minutes. The therapist also asks for vividness ratings on a scale from 0 to 100, as to how real the image feels. Typical instructions for prolonged imaginal exposure are as follows:

I will ask you to recall the trauma as vividly as possible. We call this reliving. I don't want you to tell the story about the trauma in the past tense. What I would like you to do is to describe it in the present tense, as if it is happening now, right here. I'd like you to close your eyes and tell me what happened during the trauma in as much detail as you can remember. We will work on this together. If you start to feel too uncomfortable and want to run away or avoid it by leaving the image, I will help you to stay with it. When you are finished with the story, I'll ask you to start over again, without pause. It is very important you don't stop in the middle and you don't push the memories away, even if they are painful. Don't stop in the middle to talk about your trauma or about your feelings; we'll have some time afterwards to talk about your experience with the exposure. (Foa and Rothbaum, 1998, p. 162)

Imaginal exposure continues for approximately forty-five to sixty minutes, repeating the story as many times as necessary. The therapist needs to help the client obtain a vivid image of the memory during the exposure. Although details are helpful in enhancing vividness, the goal is not to recall as many details as possible or recover "lost" memories. As therapy proceeds, the imaginal exposure focuses on the most difficult parts of the trauma ("hot spots") to promote anxiety reduction. The therapist's role during the imaginal exposure is to help modulate distress, by either encouraging more detail and affect if the client is not sufficiently engaged emotionally, or by diminishing detail and affect if the client becomes overwhelmed. Following the reliving, time is allotted to discuss the client's reaction to the reliving experiences as well as to the experiences she or he had during the in vivo exposure. The client is instructed to listen to the audiotape of the imaginal exposure daily and to record pre-, post-, and peak SUDS levels. The therapist monitors the imaginal exposure homework to make sure that the client is listening to the tape in a manner that will encourage full engagement with the trauma memory (e.g., the client is not listening to the tape in the car on the way to work).

Cognitive Restructuring

The goal of cognitive restructuring is to reduce dysfunctional thoughts about the world, other people, and themselves by having the clients identify, evaluate, and modify these thoughts and beliefs. After a traumatic experience, a client's appraisal of self and of the world in general often changes dramatically. Initially, an assessment is made of the client's belief in a variety of trauma-related thoughts. Common themes include unrealistic assumptions such as, "I have to be in control at all times"; "I am vulnerable"; "No one is trustworthy"; "The world is dangerous"; and "It's all my fault."

The therapist presents a brief rationale for cognitive restructuring, emphasizing the kinds of unhelpful beliefs that may develop following a trauma. A sample introduction follows:

> Let's discuss what happens to people's thoughts after they experience a trauma. After a traumatic event, thoughts and beliefs about ourselves and the world go through a drastic change. Often survivors believe that the world is entirely dangerous and they are unworthy people who cannot cope with stress. The goal of treatment is to help you evaluate your thoughts and beliefs about safety and about yourself, and to identify unhelpful thoughts that make you feel distressed. In this therapy we will work together as a detective team to identify those thoughts and then we will evaluate together the evidence for and against these beliefs. (Foa et al., 1994, p. 25)

After this introduction, the therapist uses an example to show how the same event (e.g., a crash outside the window) leads to completely different emotional and behavioral responses depending on the interpretation (e.g., "there is a burglar in there" or "the garbage collector is getting the trash"). After this general example, the client describes a recent emotion-evoking situation. The therapist uses a "Daily Diary" to help identify the situation, the feelings and their intensity, and the negative thoughts or images that occurred. The therapist assesses the rationality of the beliefs by challenging them using a series of questions (e.g., "What is the evidence for this idea?", "Is there an alternative explanation?"), and then replacing them with more realistic thoughts. For a more detailed explanation regarding cognitive restructuring with trauma survivors, see Foa and Rothbaum (1998).

CASE ILLUSTRATION

Case Description

The client, Maria, was a twenty-seven-year-old Hispanic woman. Maria was the eldest of three daughters, from a close, Catholic family. Her father was overly controlling and prone to physical and verbal abuse; her mother, passive. Maria stated that it was important to please her parents. She also reported a strong fear and resentment toward her father. At the time Maria presented to our clinic, she was studying business administration at a large metropolitan university. During the previous academic year, Maria had been robbed at gunpoint one evening after leaving her off-campus apartment to meet a friend. Two young, African-American men appeared suddenly, screamed at her, called her names, held a gun to her head, and demanded that she give them all her money.

Maria sought treatment the next school year after summer vacation. She was referred to treatment by one of her professors because she was not attending classes and not completing her schoolwork. Prior to the robbery, Maria had been an "A" student in a demanding academic program. She had led an active social life, liked being at school, and had looked forward to attending graduate school.

At intake, Maria reported disturbances clearly related to the robbery. She had recurrent thoughts and disturbing nightmares about the robbery as well as intense physical responses when reminded of the incident. She consistently tried to avoid situations, thoughts, and feelings related to the robbery and felt detached from others, had difficulty falling asleep, and had difficulty concentrating. Maria was constantly scared, whether at school, in public, or even in her own apartment. She felt she had no place of safety. She had withdrawn nearly completely from all of her friends, no longer enjoyed or took interest in her studies, and had little interest in school. Furthermore, she doubted whether the future she had dreamed of would ever materialize.

Assessment and Case Formulation

Maria was assessed extensively as part of the treatment research project. This included a full diagnostic interview (SCID: Structured Clinical Interview for DSM-IV Axis I Disorders), a structured interview for PTSD (PTSD Symptom Scale-Interview, PSS-I) (Foa et al., 1993), and several self-report measures, including the Posttraumatic Stress Diagnostic Scale (PDS) (Foa, 1995), the Beck Depression Inventory (Beck et al., 1961), and the Beck Anxiety Inventory (Beck et al., 1988). During the first treatment session, additional information was gathered by the therapist. Maria was cooperative throughout the interview and readily gave information about her preassault history. The only previous traumatic incident was the physical punishment inflicted by her father. Based on the SCID and the PDS, Maria had posttraumatic stress disorder in the moderate to severe range, subthreshold social phobia, and subthreshold prior major depression. She also reported current depressive symptoms in the mild range (BDI-17), but did not meet diagnostic criteria for a current depressive disorder.

An assessment of Maria's beliefs about herself, others, and the world revealed that she strongly believed in the following : "I should have been able to tell they were dangerous, I did not do enough to stop it, and I have to be on guard all the time." In addition to these themes of blame and danger, Maria also voiced beliefs that other people should not be trusted: "I can't rely on other people, I feel isolated and set apart from others." It seemed that the cognitions that were maintaining her PTSD, her isolation, and her depression resulted from the excessively high standards which she consistently placed on herself in every domain of her life. In other words, she thought that the assault was her fault and reflected her incompetence. Consequently, she was unwilling to share her experience and thereby obtain support from others.

Course of Treatment

Maria's treatment focused on the reduction of symptoms of PTSD via imaginal exposure, in vivo exposure, and cognitive restructuring, as described previously. Her intense self-blame, dangerousness of the world, and isolation were other targets for intervention. An additional target was to closely monitor her depressive symptoms.

The initial treatment session focused on explaining the rationale and process for treatment during the next nine to twelve weeks. Maria easily grasped the rationale for treatment. However, she expressed some trepidation about the exposure because she was quite convinced that every situation she was currently avoiding was truly highly dangerous. Because some of her avoidance was reasonable as she was living in a neighborhood notorious for its crime, the therapist reassured Maria that each exposure practice would be carefully assessed for realistic risk. Finally, the therapist explained the rationale for breathing retraining and modeled the procedure before Maria attempted it herself. Maria mastered the exercise easily and reported that she felt calmer at its completion.

In the next session, Maria reported that she was able to practice the breathing exercise at home several times and that she found it very helpful. She expressed some skepticism and reserved judgment regarding the remaining treatment components. However, the usefulness of the breathing exercise during the week did fuel some hope in the potential efficacy of the treatment. In the second session, common reactions to trauma were described. Maria actively participated in the discussion, relating the reactions to her own experiences. Her overall response, however, was ambivalent. She indicated that, while she felt less abnormal for having these reactions, she still felt that she should be doing better. Finally, in order to identify her patterns of avoidance, her therapist discussed changes in her daily life and interactions that she had made because of the assault. Together, Maria and her therapist used these situations to create a hierarchy, as seen in Table 5.2.

Her first in vivo homework assignment involved turning the telephone ringer on, since Maria had turned off the phone in order to avoid talking to people and to prevent being startled. She was told that, with repeated exposure to the telephone rings, she would startle less and gradually gain confidence in her ability to deal with callers. She was also instructed to attempt to share and discuss the common reactions handout with friends and family.

TABLE 5.2. In Vivo Hierarchy List

SUDS Session 2	SUDS Session 9	Items on Hierarchy
25	10	Making eye contact with people on the street
40	10	Leaving the phone on, but not answering the phone
30	10	Walking up and down street alone during the day-time
30	10	Going to a movie during the daytime alone
40	15	Reading the school paper
50	15	Talking with a friend about the assault
50	10	Going to the grocery store with a friend
50	10	Sitting on the front steps, telling a security guard she was there
60	15	Riding in a car at dusk with a friend
75	15	Walking up and down her street alone at dusk
75	15	Sitting on the front steps, not telling a security guard she was there
80	15	Driving in a car alone at dusk
80	60	Leaving the lights off after a nightmare
80	50	Going to functions at night alone
80	40	Going to a movie at night alone

Maria agreed to discuss her assault-related difficulties only with friends as she did not feel ready to reveal her assault to her family.

In the third session, Maria reported that she had reviewed the common reactions with a number of friends and was also able to leave the telephone on. Her mood improved considerably and she seemed pleased with the risks she had taken and the progress she had made. She noted that her practice exercises were getting easier and that she found the in vivo exercises to be extremely helpful. The main goal of the third session was to introduce cognitive restructuring. During this session, Maria identified an anxiety-producing situation that had occurred during the week, which seemed appropriate for the exercise. She saw two men, dressed similarly to her assailants, loitering near the door of a local fast-food restaurant in which she was eating. Seeing these men made her moderately scared (SUDS = 50) as she thought: they are going to rob the restaurant and kill us. She rated her belief in the thought at 75 percent (on a scale from 0 to 100 percent). The therapist helped her challenge the negative thought by encouraging her to consider alternative explanations for the behavior of the men and examine the available evidence that they indeed were robbers. Maria realized that her only evidence for their intentions to rob and kill was their vague resemblance to her assailants and her own fear reaction. With prompting from the therapist, Maria recognized that her conclusions were erroneous. She then generated alternative explanations such as: "they were waiting for someone" or "just hanging out." Although she agreed, rationally, that the probability of a robbery occurring in that restaurant was quite low, she still felt that the restaurant was dangerous. For homework, Maria agreed to go shopping alone to a local mall during the daytime and agreed to practice sitting alone on her front steps. She was also given cognitive restructuring worksheets ("Daily Diaries") to complete when she felt upset during the week (see Foa and Rothbaum, 1998).

During the next week, Maria used the cognitive restructuring worksheets to evaluate several instances that caused her to be upset. Yet, she had a great deal of difficulty generating a rational response to these anxiety-producing situations. The therapist found it difficult to understand Maria's difficulties; Maria was bright and possessed an analytical thinking style. However, she was reluctant to dismiss her gut feelings as unacceptable "hard" evidence of danger.

In the fourth session, the imaginal reliving of the trauma began. Although Maria expressed some reluctance, she clearly understood the rationale and willingly complied with the program. The exercise progressed very well. Maria talked in a quiet voice and maintained present tense with little prompting. She generated vivid imagery and emotional engagement. Her initial SUDs was 40 and increased to 80 within the first five minutes. She started with the image of leaving her apartment and ended with the image of being driven home by a victim assistance officer. Her anxiety level fluctuated greatly within this imagery. High points included the moments when the assailants screamed at her as well as when she was questioned by a police officer who reprimanded her for walking alone. After the reliving, Maria appeared exhausted. As is often the case after the first reliving practice, Maria was not sure how helpful it was. However, she did express amazement that she had been able to tell the story, because she had not believed she would be able to do so. Furthermore, she agreed to take the "imaginal tape" home, to listen to it, and to actively imagine the incident daily.

In the following session, Maria reported that she had listened to the tape one time, with minimal discomfort (SUDS = 20), and reported that the exercise was very helpful. The therapist was concerned by her report because a low SUDS level early in treatment is rare and usually signifies cognitive avoidance. Maria explained that she thought the reliving was helpful mostly because she felt more comfortable throughout the day, especially in public places and when alone in her apartment. She attributed her reduced anxiety to the in vivo exercises. She reported that she did the imaginal exercise one time only because it was a difficult academic week, she was feeling better, and she did not want to ruin her week. The therapist congratulated her on her in vivo work and her progress, but reiterated the rationale for further imaginal work and encouraged her to risk possibly exacerbating her symptoms in the short run in favor of fully processing the trauma and achieving long-term symptom relief.

Maria engaged in her second imaginal reliving of the robbery. Unlike the first session, her anxiety level stayed low, between 15 and 25, and the vividness of the image was medium. During the reliving, Maria was instructed to focus on the assault itself rather than the police activity following the assault. Again, the therapist was surprised by the low distress during the imagery and repeatedly prompted Maria to share thoughts and feelings. Maria reported she was feeling numb and frozen. Queries of her thoughts repeatedly elicited judgmental recriminations. In addition, the therapist struggled to keep Maria in the present tense. Following the reliving exercise, Maria admitted that she had not wanted do the exercise and was tearful. She felt depressed and spoke of her belief that she should have stopped the assault.

Maria's self-blame easily led into a continued discussion of how thoughts evoke feelings that can then affect behaviors and avoidance. Maria then admitted that she had not wanted to do the reliving exercise during the week because of feeling ashamed and guilty. As the discussion progressed, Maria adamantly insisted that she should have and could have stopped the assault because she had a "gut feeling" about her assailants. She repeatedly said, "If only I hadn't frozen, it wouldn't have happened." With the therapist's help, Maria calculated the time that she had to react (essentially none) and what actions she might have taken. This careful analysis helped her realize that she had had no options. She realized that she had had insufficient time to run back to her building or to get to the nearest public place; there was no one to call to for help; and if she had fought or even run, the assault might have been worse. She concluded, "There was nothing I could have done, even though I knew they were dangerous." She stated that she believed this rational response 100 percent.

During subsequent sessions, Maria engaged in the imaginal reliving without cognitive avoidance. She easily reported her thoughts and feelings and her vividness was high. Throughout subsequent sessions, her SUDS levels were high until they began to decrease in session six (SUDS = 15). She worked on the reliving exercise at home, practicing four to six times per week. Similarly, Maria made good progress as she exposed herself to fearful situations in real life. She was able to be alone in the dark, to go out during the daytime alone, and to increase her social activities. Yet, she still remained prone to anxiety whenever she encountered young, African-American males, was still afraid of going out of her apartment alone at night, and was reluctant to seek escorts or friends to accompany her. Unfortunately, Maria lived in an urban area where crime was high; yet she also needed to be able to leave her apartment and function during the evening. The therapist addressed this issue carefully, discussing the discrimination between real and exaggerated danger. The therapist reviewed with Maria the recommendations provided by the campus police, and Maria then began utilizing the university escort service and arranging to walk with available friends.

Probably the most difficult aspect of the therapy was the cognitive restructuring surrounding her fear of young African-American males. By the end of treatment, Maria was able to recognize that her beliefs were somewhat exaggerated ("He will rape, rob, or murder me"), but she still maintained a high degree of belief in them. Although she was also able to generate alternative thoughts and more realistic probabilities, she was reluctant to dismiss her "gut feeling." The therapist revisited common reactions in a discussion of how triggers (in her case, young black males) reliably elicit fear in PTSD. The therapist gave an example of how "gut feelings" are similar to a car alarm malfunction. Although the gut feelings may have been accurate before the assault, after the assault, they may be overly sensitive and can usually be ignored. However, Maria believed that her "gut feelings" during the assault had been accurate and that for that reason she should continue to listen to them.

At the end of treatment, Maria and her therapist reviewed her treatment progress. Both were pleased that her symptoms had reduced markedly. In fact, she was doing so well that it was difficult to identify situations that she needed to address via cognitive restructuring. They agreed that the turning point for her had occurred when she was able to let go of her self-blame for the incident because she realized that she had not had time to escape the assault. After that realization, Maria remembered the assault without excessive shame or guilt, which permitted emotional processing to occur. Very quickly, she felt that the memory was no longer dangerous, although it was annoying. Furthermore, Maria felt that she had gained much insight from the imaginal exposure, especially tying together her freezing response to similar experiences that she had had when her father screamed at her during her childhood. This realization prompted her to practice asserting herself in similar situations when she felt unduly criticized. Maria also realized that her avoidance had kept her isolated. She now felt more comfortable reaching out to others, and consequently she became more connected to her friends and became better able to cope with their occasional insensitivity. These results reflected both increased ability to take risks with her friends by sharing her feelings as well as shifts in attitudes toward trusting people.

Outcome

Maria was again evaluated at the end of treatment. Her PTSD symptoms had dropped substantially and she no longer met diagnostic criteria for PTSD (see Table 5.3), although she still reported occasional nightmares that were not explicitly connected to the robbery. Furthermore, her main symptom that persisted was moderate hypervigilance when she was alone. Her depressive symptoms completely disappeared, although she still reported a significant amount of general anxiety. A summary of her pre- and posttreatment scores is presented in Table 5.3.

After a six-month follow-up, Maria reported no symptoms of reexperiencing or avoidance, stating that "it [the robbery] just doesn't come up anymore." Her nightmares and her hypervigilance had completely disappeared and she reported a reduction of general anxiety and depression; however, she continued to report feeling easily started. Since treatment, she had graduated from college, had begun to work at a major corporation, and had moved from the city. She reported no limitations in being able to go out with friends, shopping, or movies.

SUMMARY

Maria's case clearly demonstrates the value of a structured approach to alleviate symptoms of PTSD and related problems following a trauma. Although cognitive restructuring appeared to be an important aspect of Maria's treatment, her shifts in self-blame and dangerousness of the world seem to have been altered largely by imaginal and in vivo exposure. Future research on the treatment of PTSD should help clarify the necessity of cognitive restructuring. At the present time, the addition of cognitive restructuring or other cognitive behavioral procedures has not augmented treatment efficacy over treatment by in vivo and imaginal exposure alone.

TABLE 5.3. Symptom Severity at Pretreatment and Posttreatment

Measure	Pretreatment	Posttreatment
BAI	15	16
BDI	17	0
PSS-I	39	6
PDS	36	6

Note: BAI = Beck Anxiety Inventory; BDI = Beck Depression Inventory; PSS-I = PTSD Symptom Scale Interview; PDS = Post-traumatic Stress Diagnostic Scale.

APPENDIX: COMMON REACTIONS TO ASSAULT HANDOUT

An assault is a traumatic experience that produces emotional shock and causes many emotional problems. This handout describes some of the common reactions people have after a trauma. Because everyone responds differently to traumas, you may have some of these reactions more than others. Please read it carefully, and think about any changes in your feelings, thoughts and behaviors since the assault.

Remember, many changes after a trauma are common. In fact, 95 percent of rape victims have severe problems two weeks after the rape. About half of these women feel much better within three months after the rape, but the other half recovers more slowly, and many do not recover enough without help. Becoming more aware of the changes you've undergone since your assault is the first step toward recovery.

Some of the most common problems after a trauma are described as follows.

1. *Fear and anxiety.* Anxiety is a common and natural response to a dangerous situation. For many it lasts long after the assault ended. This happens when views of the world and a sense of safety have changed. You may become anxious when you remember your assault. But sometimes anxiety may come from out of the blue. *Triggers* or *cues* that can cause anxiety may include places, times of day, certain smells or noises, or any situation that reminds you of the assault. As you begin to pay more attention to the times you feel afraid, you can discover the triggers for your anxiety. In this way, you may learn that some of the out-of-the-blue anxiety is really triggered by things that remind you of your assault.

2. *Reexperiencing the trauma.* Women who have been assaulted often reexperience the trauma. For example, you may have *unwanted thoughts* of the assault, and find yourself unable to get rid of them. Some women have *flashbacks,* or very vivid images as if the assault is occurring again. *Nightmares* are also common. These symptoms occur because a traumatic experience is so shocking and so different from everyday experiences that you cannot fit it into what you know about the world. So in order to understand what happened, your mind keeps bringing the memory back, as if to better digest it and fit it in.

3. *Increased arousal* is also a common response to trauma. This includes feeling jumpy, jittery, shaky, being easily startled, and having trouble concentrating or sleeping. Continuous arousal can lead to *impatience* and *irritability,* especially if you are not getting enough sleep. The arousal reactions are due to the fight or flight response kicking in in your body. The fight or flight response is the way we protect ourselves against danger, and it occurs also in animals. When we protect ourselves from danger by fighting or run-

ning away, we need a lot more energy than usual, so our bodies pump out extra adrenaline to help us get the extra energy we need to survive.

People who have been assaulted often see the world as filled with danger, so, their bodies are on constant alert, always ready to respond immediately to any attack. The problem is that increased arousal is useful in truly dangerous situations, such as if we find ourselves facing a tiger. But, alertness becomes very uncomfortable when it continues for a long time even in safe situations. Another reaction to danger is to *freeze,* like the deer in the headlights, and this reaction can also occur during an assault.

4. *Avoidance* is a common way of managing trauma-related pain. The most common is avoiding situations that remind you of the assault, such as the place where it happened. Often situations that are less directly related to the trauma are also avoided, such as going out in the evening if you were assaulted at night. Another way to reduce discomfort is trying to push away painful thoughts and feelings. This can lead to feelings of *numbness,* in which you find it difficult to have both fearful and pleasant or loving feelings. Sometimes the painful thoughts or feelings may be so intense that your mind just blocks them out altogether, and you may not remember parts of the assault.

5. Many people who have been assaulted feel *angry* not only at the assailant but also with others. If you are not used to feeling angry this may seem scary as well. It may be especially confusing to feel angry at those who are closest to you. Sometimes people feel angry because of feeling irritable so often. Anger can also arise from a feeling that the world is not fair.

6. Trauma often leads to feelings of *guilt* and *shame.* Many people blame themselves for things they did or didn't do to survive. For example, some women believe that they should have fought off an assailant, and blame themselves for the assault. Others feel that if they had not fought back they would not have gotten hurt. You may feel ashamed because during the assault you were forced to do something that you would not otherwise have done. Sometimes, other people may blame you for being assaulted.

Feeling guilty about the assault means that you are taking responsibility for what your assailant did. Although this may make you feel somewhat more in control, it can also lead to feelings of helplessness and depression.

7. *Depression* is also a common reaction to assault. It can include feeling down, sad, hopeless, or despairing. You may cry more often. You may lose interest in people and activities you used to enjoy. You may also feel that plans you had for the future do not seem to matter anymore, or that life is not worth living. These feelings can lead to thoughts of wishing you were dead, or doing something to hurt or kill yourself. Because the assault has changed so much of how you see the world and yourself, it makes sense to feel sad and to grieve for what you lost because of the assault.

8. *Self-image* and *views of the world* often become more negative after an assault. You may tell yourself, "If I hadn't been so weak or stupid this wouldn't have happened to me." Many women see themselves as more negative overall after the assault ("I am a bad person and deserved this").

It is also very common to see others more negatively, and to feel that you cannot *trust* anyone. If you used to think about the world as a safe place, the assault suddenly makes you think that the world is dangerous. If you had previous bad experiences, the assault convinces you that the world is dangerous and others are not to be trusted. These negative thoughts often make women feel that they have been changed completely by the assault. Relationships with others can become tense and it is difficult to become intimate with people as your trust decreases.

9. *Sexual relationships* may also suffer after a traumatic experience. Many women find it difficult to feel sexual or to have sexual relationships. This is especially true for women who have been sexually assaulted, since in addition to the lack of trust, sex itself is a reminder of the assault.

Many of the reactions to trauma are connected to one another. For example, a flashback may make you feel out of control, and will therefore produce fear and arousal. Many women think that their common reactions to the trauma mean that they are "going crazy" or "losing it." These thoughts can make them even more fearful. Again, as you become aware of the changes you have gone through since the assault, and as you process these experiences during treatment, the symptoms should become less distressing.

REFERENCES

Beck, A.T., Epstein, N., Brown, G., and Steer, R.A. (1988). An inventory for measuring clinical anxiety: The Beck Anxiety Inventory. *Journal of Consulting and Clinical Psychology, 56,* 893-897.

Beck, A.T., Ward, C.H., Mendelsohn, M., Mock, J., and Erbaugh, J. (1961). An inventory for measuring depression. *Archives of General Psychiatry, 4,* 561-571.

Boudewyns, P.A. and Hyer, L. (1990). Physiological response to combat memories and preliminary treatment outcome in Vietnam veterans: PTSD patients treated with direct therapeutic exposure. *Behavior Therapy, 21,* 63-87.

Boudewyns, P.A., Hyer, L., Woods, M.G., Harrison, W.R., and McCranie, E. (1990). PTSD among Vietnam veterans: An early look at treatment outcome using direct therapeutic exposure. *Journal of Traumatic Stress, 3,* 359-368.

Cooper, N.A. and Clum, G.A. (1989). Imaginal flooding as a supplementary treatment for PTSD in combat veterans: A controlled study. *Behavior Therapy, 3,* 381-391.

Foa, E.B. (1995). *PDS (Posttraumatic Stress Diagnostic Scale) manual.* Minneapolis, MN: National Computer Systems, Inc.

Foa, E.B. (1997). Psychopathology of PTSD and its treatment: New findings. Keynote lecture in the Conference of the European Association for Cognitive and Behavioral Therapies. Venice, Italy.

Foa, E.B., Dancu, C., Hembree, E., Jaycox, L., and Meadows, E. (1997). Cognitive behavior therapy for chronic PTSD in female assault victims: Comparison of exposure therapy, stress inoculation training and their combination. Manuscript in preparation.

Foa, E.B., Hearst-Ikeda, D.E., Dancu, C., Hembree. F., and Jaycox, L. (1994). Cognitive therapy and prolonged exposure (CT/PE) manual.

Foa, E.B. and Jaycox, L.H. (2000). Cognitive-behavioral treatment of post-traumatic stress disorder. In D. Spiegel (Ed.), *Psychotherapeutic frontiers: New principles and practices.* Washington, DC: American Psychiatric Press.

Foa, E.B. and Kozak, M.J. (1985). Treatment of anxiety disorder: Implications for psychopathology. In A.H. Tuma and J.D. Maser (Eds.), *Anxiety and the anxiety disorders* (pp. 451-452). Hillsdale, NJ: Erlbaum.

Foa, E.B. and Kozak, M.J. (1986). Emotional processing of fear: Exposure to corrective information. *Psychological Bulletin 99,* 20-35.

Foa, E.B. and Meadows, E.A. (1997). Psychosocial treatment for post-traumatic stress disorder: A critical review. In J. Spence (Ed.), *Annual Review of Psychology, 48,* 449-480.

Foa, E.B. and Riggs, D.S. (1993). Post-traumatic stress disorder in rape victims. In J. Oldham, M.B. Riba, and A. Tasman (Eds.), *American Psychiatric Press review of psychiatry.* Volume 12 (pp. 273-303). Washington, DC: American Psychiatric Press.

Foa, E.B., Riggs, D.S., Dancu, C.V., and Rothbaum, B.O. (1993). Reliability and validity of a brief instrument for assessing post-traumatic stress disorder. *Journal of Traumatic Stress, 6,* 459-473.

Foa, E.B. and Rothbaum, B.O. (1998). *Treating the trauma of rape.* New York: Guilford Publications.

Foa, E.B., Rothbaum, B.O., Riggs, D., and Murdock, T. (1991). Treatment of post-traumatic stress disorder in rape victims: A comparison between cognitive-behavioral procedures and counseling. *Journal of Consulting and Clinical Psychology, 59,* 715-723.

Foa, E.B., Steketee, G., and Rothbaum, B. (1989). Behavioral/cognitive conceptualizations of post-traumatic stress disorder. *Behavior Therapy, 20,* 155-176.

Frank, E., and Stewart, B.D. (1983). Physical aggression: Treating the victims. In E.A. Bleckman (Ed.), *Behavior modification with women* (pp. 245-272). New York: Guilford Press.

Frank, E. and Stewart, B.D. (1984). Depressive symptoms in rape victims. *Journal of Affective Disorders, 1,* 269-277.

Green, B.L., Grace, M.C., Lindy, J.D., Gleser, G.C., and Lonard, A. (1990). Risk factors for PTSD and other diagnoses in a general sample of Vietnam veterans. *American Journal of Psychiatry, 147,* 729-733.

Helzer, J.E., Robins, L., and McEvoy, L. (1987). Post-traumatic stress disorder in the general population. *New England Journal of Medicine, 317,* 1630-1634.

Keane, T.M., Fairbank, J.A., Caddell, J.M., and Zimering, R.T. (1989). Implosive (flooding) therapy reduces symptoms of PTSD in Vietnam combat veterans. *Behavior Therapy, 20,* 245-260.

Kessler, R.C., Sonnega, A., Bromet, E. Hughes, M., and Nelson, C.B. (1995). Posttraumatic stress disorder in the National Comorbidity Survey. *Archives of General Psychiatry, 52,* 1048-1060.

Kilpatrick, D.G., Veronen, L.F., and Resick, P.A. (1982). Psychological sequelae to rape: Assessment and treatment strategies. In D.M. Dolay and R.L. Meredith (Eds.), *Behavioral medicine: Assessment and treatment strategies* (pp. 473-497). New York: Plenum Press.

Kulka, R.A., Schelenger, W.E., Fairbank, J.A., Jough, R.L., Jordan, B.K. (1988). *Contractional report of the finding from the National Vietnam Veterans Readjustment Study.* Research Triangle Park, NC: Research Triangle Institute.

Lohr, J.M., Tolin, D.F., and Lilienfeld, S.O. (1998). Efficacy of eye movement desensitization and reprocessing: Implications for behavior therapy. *Behavior Therapy, 29,* 123-156.

Marks, I., Lovell, K., Noshirvani, H., Livanou, M., and Thrasher, S. (1998). Treatment of posttraumatic stress disorder by exposure and by cognitive restructuring: A controlled study. *Archives of General Psychiatry, 55,* 317-325.

McFarlane, A.C. and Papay, P. (1992). Multiple diagnoses in posttraumatic stress disorder in victims of a natural disaster. *Journal of Nervous and Mental Disease, 180*(8), 498-504.

Pitman, R.K., Orr, S.P., Altman, B., Longpre, R.E, Poire, R.E., and Macklin, M.L. (1996). Emotional processing during eye-movement desensitization and reprocessing therapy of Vietnam veterans with chronic post-traumatic stress disorder. *Comprehensive Psychiatry, 37*(6), 419-427.

Resick, P.A., Jordan, C.G., Girelli, S.A., Hutter, C.K., and Marhoefer-Dvorak, D. (1988). A comparative victim study of behavioral group therapy for sexual assault victims. *Behaviour Therapy, 19,* 385-401.

Resick, P.A., Kilpatrick, D.G., Dnasky, B.S., Saunder, B.E., and Best, C.L. (1993). Prevalence of civilian trauma and posttraumatic stress disorder in a representative national sample of women. *Journal of Consulting and Clinical Psychology, 61,* 984-991.

Resick, P.A. and Schnicke, M.K. (1992a). Cognitive processing therapy for sexual assault victims. *Journal of Consulting and Clinical Psychology, 60*(50), 748-756.

Resick, P.A. and Schnicke, M.K. (1992b). Cognitive processing therapy for sexual assault victims. In E.B. Foa (Chair), *Treatment for PTSD: An update.* Presented at the eighth annual meeting for the Society for Traumatic Stress Studies, Los Angeles, CA.

Richards, D.A., Lovell, K., and Marks, I.M. (1994). Post traumatic stress disorder: Evaluation of a behavioral treatment program. *Journal of Traumatic Stress, 7,* 669-680.

Rothbaum, B.O. (1995). "A controlled study of EMDR for PTSD." Presented at the Association for the Advancement of Behavior Therapy, Washington, DC, November.

Rothbaum, B.O., Foa, F.B., Riggs, D.S., Murdock. T., and Walsh, W. (1992). A prospective examination of post-traumatic stress disorder in rape victims. *Journal of Traumatic Stress, 5*(3), 455-475.

Shapiro, F. (1995). *Eye movement desensitization and reprocessing: Basic principles, protocols, and procedures.* New York: Guilford Press.

Shore, J.H., Vollmer, W.M., and Tatum, E.I. (1989). Community patterns of posttraumatic stress disorders. *Journal of Nervous and Mental Disease, 177,* 681-685.

Taylor, S. and Koch, W.J. (1995). Anxiety disorder due to motor vehicle accidents: Nature and treatment. *Clinical Psychology Review, 15,* 721-738.

Thompson, J.A., Charlton, P.F.C., Kerry, R., Lee, D., and Turner, S.W. (1995). An open trial of exposure based therapy on deconditioning for post-traumatic stress disorder. *British Journal of Clinical Psychiatry, 34,* 407-416.

Tolin, D.F., Montgomery, R.W., Kleinknect, R.A., and Lohr, J.M. (1996). An evaluation of eye movement desensitization and reprocessing (EMDR). In L. VandaCreek, S. Knapp, and T.L. Jackson (Eds.), *Innovations in Clinical Practice, 14,* (pp. 423-437). Sarasota, FL: Professional Resources Press.

Veronen, L.J. and Kilpatrick, D.G. (1982). "Stress inoculation training for victims of rape: Efficacy and differential findings." Presented at the Association for the Advancement of Behavior Therapy, Los Angeles, CA.

Wolpe, J. (1958). *Psychotherapy by reciprocal inhibition.* Stanford, CA: Stanford University Press.

Chapter 6

Short-Term Treatment of Simple and Complex PTSD

Louis Tinnin
Lyndra Bills
Linda Gantt

INTRODUCTION

This chapter presents a brief treatment method that uses video technology as a therapeutic tool in in-session treatment procedures and as homework. This approach permits controlled, nonabreactive processing of traumatic memories. It protects the patient from retraumatization and allows the trauma work to commence without undue delay.

Video-assisted therapy uses recursive reviews of the treatment sessions. Every session is videotaped—including those sessions reviewing previous tapes—and the patient owns the tapes. The patient conducts much of the therapy independently by studying the tapes at home. This treatment also uses video recording and replay in *video dialogue,* a specific procedure to diminish dissociation, and permits externalization of an individual's inner dialogue. The principles of video-assisted trauma therapy can be applied without video recording, but using the video camera, if the treatment is to be brief, is recommended.

THE HISTORY OF VIDEO-ASSISTED TRAUMA THERAPY

The method is based on two assumptions: (1) dissociated traumatic memories must be resolved before healing can occur; (2) abreaction is not necessary to resolve traumatic memories. These conclusions were reached in 1989 after conducting seventy-seven amytal interviews over two years. The amytal interview relies on an intravenous infusion of the sedative drug, sodium amytal, to produce a state of conscious sedation which allows the patient to talk with less inhibition (Naples and Hackett, 1978). These interviews help the patient construct a verbal narrative of a past traumatic experience. They are videotaped and later reviewed by the patient and therapist.

Many of the patients improved after reviewing the tapes and, contrary to initial expectations, the improvement did not correlate with emotional catharsis, but rather with completion of a verbal narrative about the trauma experienced. Many patients who improved developed a perspective of the trauma as historical past. They attributed the improvement to a sense of closure gained by reviewing the videotape.

Other forms of videotaped conscious sedation, in the search for a safe and practical method for trauma processing, also were tried. Nitrous oxide, the dentist's "laughing gas," was equally effective. However, the use of conscious sedation is expensive and requires cardiorespiratory monitoring, usually in a hospital. In comparing clinical outcomes, hypnosis was shown to be just as effective as amytal or nitrous oxide and had the advantage of safe use on an outpatient basis. This finding made it possible to develop and test an outpatient procedure that the authors called "recursive anamnesis," a term which refers to the process of a videotaped verbal reconstruction of traumatic memory fragments into a narrative. "Recursive" means making a tape of the patient watching the previous tape while improving the narrative to achieve full closure and avowal.

The Trauma Profile

Many hospitalized patients who had past trauma suffered psychotic symptoms and were admitted with the diagnoses of atypical schizophrenia or bipolar disorder. They were often unaware of their traumas and could not be tested directly about their symptoms of intrusion, avoidance, and arousal. A group of self-administered questionnaires that has been designated the "trauma profile" was used to screen for posttraumatic conditions indirectly and to measure change over time. Included were: (1) the Dissociative Experiences Scale (DES), a twenty-eight–item scale that is widely used to screen for posttraumatic disorders (Bernstein and Putnam, 1986); (2) the Symptom Checklist-45 (SCL-45) (Alvir et al., 1988) to measure global distress; (3) the Toronto Alexithymia Scale (TAS) (Taylor et al., 1988) to look at the reversal of alexithymia (Appel and Sifneos, 1979) as a good measure of recovery after treatment; and (5) a six-item test for ego regression, the Dissociative Regression Scale (DRS) (Tinnin, 1994).

Development of the Treatment Procedures

The initial recursive anamnesis using hypnosis was tested in a Veterans Affairs medical center on 115 combat veterans who had been evaluated for treatment in the PTSD programs of the medical center. Thirteen of the veterans did not follow through after their initial evaluation. Thirty veterans were admitted to the inpatient program. Twenty-five volunteered for the recursive anamnesis. The remaining forty-seven veterans were assigned to the PTSD day treatment program consisting of daily group therapy and activities, Monday through Friday, for four weeks. Measures of the outcome of treatment showed no improvement in the day treatment program group while the recursive anamnesis group experienced a twenty-one percent reduction (from a mean of 73 to 58) of PTSD symptoms as measured by the Clinician Administered PTSD Scale (CAPS) (Blake et al., 1990). The trauma profiles revealed no change in the dissociation or alexithymia scores. Furthermore, there was a tendency to relapse in three to six months. One-third of those who had improved lost their gains by six months.

Focal Psychotherapy Added

A group of twenty civilian outpatients treated at West Virginia University showed a similar partial response to treatment, although their reduction in PTSD symptoms was more robust, averaging 44 percent (from a mean of 81 to 59). The outcome of treatment changed dramatically, however, after six sessions of video-assisted focal psychotherapy were added to the recursive anamnesis for a group of sixteen subjects. There was a reduction of the DES scores from an average of 26 to 11, and TAS scores from 71 to 60 at six months. Twelve of the sixteen met criteria for recovery (absence of intrusive symptoms, DES < 20, TAS < 74).

The Problem of Dissociative PTSD

The addition of focal psychotherapy to the recursive anamnesis did not improve the outcome with the veterans. Upon reexamination of the original data, in a search for the explanation of their relatively poor response to the procedures that were so effective with the civilians, almost two-thirds of the veterans had noted that they heard voices. They endorsed the statement, "I hear voices that others do not hear" on the SCL-45 and a similar statement on the DES (item no. 27). The veterans had kept their auditory hallucinations secret before they completed these questionnaires; none of them had been diagnosed with schizophrenia (Holmes and Tinnin, 1996).

The trauma-profile questionnaires revealed that 65 percent of the 115 combat veterans admitted hearing voices. Their mean DES was 42, compared to 18 for those without hallucinations. Ninety percent of the veterans scoring 30 or above on the DES heard voices while 82 percent of those scoring less than 30 denied voices. They were uniformly alexithymic with a mean of 85 on the TAS, while 91 percent scored over 73, placing them in the clinical alexithymia range (Taylor et al., 1988). These veterans were highly distressed as evidenced by a mean score of 128 on the SCL-45.

Examination of the questionnaire results of a group of civilian patients (N = 62) who had suffered a wide variety of traumas, including child abuse, assault, accident, and medical traumas, found that 37 percent (N = 23) reported hearing voices. Sixty-four percent scoring 30 or above on the DES heard voices, while 80 percent of those scoring less than 30 did not. The mean scores of the hallucinating group were: DES = 36 (compared to 20 for those without voices), SCL-45 = 100, TAS = 79 with 70 percent scoring in the alexithymia range. Although there seemed to be a dissociative PTSD syndrome in the veterans, characterized by auditory hallucinations, high dissociative experience (DES > 30), and alexithymia, this pattern was not as pronounced or as consistent in the civilians.

The phenomenology of PTSD patients hearing voices (Holmes and Tinnin, 1996) indicated that these voices talked to the patients and expressed a point of view with intentions and opinions different from the patients' avowed intentions. The voices responded to an examiner's questions and the patients could hear the response and report the words. These voices invariably dated back to a past traumatic experience and usually began as a helping influence, changing over time to a more or less adversarial role. They may have been experienced as command hallucinations that urged suicide. The patients would usually feel an automatic obedience to the voices and would strive willfully to defy the commands. Much of the time, the voices would object to clinical treatment and try to prevent the patients' participation.

Video Dialogue Added

These hallucinations represent a posttraumatic dissociation that might interfere with a person's response to treatment for PTSD. The treatment of dissociative PTSD may require reduction of dissociation before the person can recover. This conclusion led to the development of the video dialogue procedure. Outcome data is not yet available to present, but the use of video dialogue seems to diminish dissociation and to manage command hallucinations. The veterans responded to video dialogue with an immediate reduction of their automatic obedience to the voices, and the procedure quickly eroded the dissociative boundaries between their executive consciousness and the voice (Holmes and Tinnin, 1996).

When using the video dialogue procedure to resolve the dissociative splitting that occurs in complex PTSD, the same benefit observed in the veterans with dissociative PTSD occurred. The complex PTSD patients found that their victim mythology (to be described) also responded, almost in lockstep with the reduction of splitting.

PRINCIPLES OF TIME-LIMITED TRAUMA THERAPY

The model of treatment that finally emerged consists of three components: *trauma work* which involves narrative processing of traumatic memories; *video dialogue* which repairs dissociative splits that usually remain after trauma; and *videotherapy* which treats the posttraumatic victim mythology.

Management of Trauma Phobia

One reason that conventional trauma therapies are prolonged is that therapists regard the patients' anxiety about describing the trauma as a gauge of their inability to deal with the traumatic emotion that might be elicited. Many psychodynamic therapists were trained in the belief that the patient must eventually abreact the trauma and achieve catharsis of the noxious affect. The usual strategy is to strengthen the patient's coping skills and then approach the traumatic memory bit by bit. This strategy has been hard on patients and therapists, sometimes retraumatizing both of them.

However, trauma phobia is not related to strangulated traumatic emotion. It is an anxiety that increases in proportion to the reversals of approach and avoidance of the traumatic memory over time. It dissipates entirely when narrative closure to the trauma is achieved. It can be minimized by competent explanation of the procedure for memory processing and the assurance that the trauma is not to be relived in the process. If the patient has already undergone abreactive therapy and reacts excessively, then trial runs of hypnosis or art therapy without trauma work may help diminish the fear.

Treat Ego Regression First

Ego regression occurs as a complication of trauma and is frequently seen in complex PTSD. With this form of regression, a person loses the normal capacity for self-regulation because of the failure of one or more fundamental psychological functions (Tinnin, 1989). The person may experience a weakening of *identity* with a loss of mental unity or self-sameness over time. The person may lose a reliable sense of *time* (including duration and sequence) or lack the capacity for *volition* or will. The person might experience a diffusion of *self-boundary* and have difficulty distinguishing self from other. When ego regression is present, the individual often has difficulty with *verbal symbolization* and may become literal-minded. These difficulties make it impossible to benefit from verbal psychotherapy that relies on psychological insight. The processing of traumatic memories also must be deferred until the regression is reversed.

Although the severity of ego regression can be evaluated by clinical signs alone, it is helpful to use a testing instrument. The trauma profile provides this by using two measures, the DRS (Tinnin, 1994) and the DES. The DRS scores the six autonomous ego functions of identity, time, volition, self-boundary, body image, and verbal symbolization. The presence of regression is indicated by the score on the DRS exceeding the score on the DES. If the DRS score is 50 or above and if it is higher than the DES score then the patient is significantly regressed and trauma work should be deferred until the regression is reversed. However, even if elevated above 50, the DRS score will not indicate regression as long as it does not exceed the DES score. Once a baseline DES score is established, the DRS (which is a brief, six-item questionnaire) can be repeated as often as needed to monitor regression.

Complex PTSD and Victim Mythology

Most traumatized people develop a pattern of attitudes that colors their beliefs and behavior. Living with dissociated traumatic memories that are repeatedly reenacted in a context of present experience, they come to regard themselves as damaged and vulnerable and the world as threatening. If the person's trauma was a single episode and resulted in simple PTSD, the recovery from the complication of victim mythology may follow naturally from successful trauma work alone. Once the person's traumatic memories are processed, the person may be able to see the present world differently and experience himself or herself more realistically.

If the person suffers from complex PTSD, however, the victim mythology may constitute an entire way of life. Assumptions about the world are determined not only from reenacted traumas but from the developmental distortions of a traumatizing life. The individual has come to experience the world as alien and has learned to hide behind a defensive wall, using it as a safe retreat from the dangers that seem inherent in any interaction with the world. But, the stronger the defenses, the more alienated the world becomes.

A patient with complex PTSD is usually a victim of childhood trauma who feels small, weak, and inadequate in a world that seems increasingly unmanageable and overwhelming. In time, the victim feels not only vulnerable, but unacceptable, secretly concluding that he or she is unworthy of love. This conclusion undermines even the hope of being loved and results in an image of a weak, inadequate, unlovable victim facing an indifferent, cold, and essentially hostile world which will easily crush him or her.

Dire Expectancy

This victim mythology means that it is really impossible to live humanly, that one must resign oneself to a merely vegetative existence and renounce strivings for basic human satisfactions. The full acceptance of this belief results in despair and depression. Most often, the victim does a seemingly paradoxical thing. The person decides, as it were, to live and exercise basic functions in some roundabout way in a world in which it is impossible to exercise them directly. In the victim's mind, there is always a vague, ominous sense of approaching doom, but this dire expectation is not held with absolute certainty. A flicker of hope sustains the person.

General Characteristics of the Victim Mythology

"Safety first" is the motto and the main issue of life in victim mythology. The victim's entire life is devoted to the pursuit of safety, of protection against danger. Decisions are made on the basis of dangers to be avoided rather than the objectives to be achieved. The methods of defense can vary from the extreme of putting on a fierce mask to frighten the enemy, to the other extreme of advertising oneself as a weak, harmless creature who could not hurt a fly to avert the anger of the presumed enemy. Behind these defenses, fear always lurks.

The victim's sense of danger results in a desperate quality to the person's intentions, to "do or die," so that any interference is a threat. The victim cannot experience closure or fulfillment. The victim lives with a secret sense of entitlement to some future reward for past and present suffering. Life is not lived in the present, but in a continuous inner flight from the dangers and displeasures of today to the hoped-for satisfactions of tomorrow.

The "enemy" in the mythology is a dark and irrational force, a perpetrator who is utterly alien, with whom no communication or understanding is possible. This mythical conception usually attaches to certain selected people (such as those in authority, or all men) and becomes the basis for irrational attitudes toward them. The victim's responses to different people are stereotyped, repetitive, uniform, and indiscriminate.

All-or-None Thinking

The victim mythology of individuals with complex PTSD is not simply a pattern of attitudes. It is a global way of life. The person's entire worldview is determined by the basic assumptions of being a damaged victim in a dangerous world. This conception is all-or-none. There is no allowance for partial change. If the person is to change, then the entire worldview must change. Full recovery depends on a therapeutic demolition of this worldview.

The major step of healing is the acknowledgement of the hopelessness and futility of a way of life based on victim mythology. Often, this follows the unmasking of that mythology by repeated discoveries that all converge to the point that this way of life is doomed to failure. Only then can a new way of life develop.

Much of the unmasking of the victim mythology takes place at home when the patient studies the videotaped treatment sessions. In this independent work, the patient's viewing of the tapes promotes an observing ego and an opportunity for objective self-confrontation. Without the benefit of the videotapes, that unmasking usually requires long-term psychotherapy.

APPLICATIONS OF VIDEO-ASSISTED TRAUMA THERAPY

The following section introduces the programs of treatment for simple PTSD, dissociative PTSD, and complex PTSD. The procedures and techniques are described in greater detail in the next section.

Simple PTSD

The person who experiences uncomplicated PTSD with the triad of intrusive, avoidant, and arousal symptoms, has usually suffered a Type I trauma. As defined by Terr (1991), this form of trauma consists of one or more isolated episodes as opposed to the Type II form that is typical of prolonged child abuse or captivity. The consequence of Type II trauma is more likely to be complex PTSD or dissociative disorder. Simple PTSD is differentiated by the absence of hallucinations, only mild dissociative experiences (DES scores in the range of 20 to 30), and a relatively mild victim mythology. Only rarely will dissociative regression be a problem. The treatment of simple PTSD consists of the *core module* of trauma therapy.

The Core Treatment Module

There are three phases of treatment in the core module: trauma work by recursive anamnesis and art therapy, video dialogue, and focal videotherapy.

The first step of the trauma work is to gain access to the traumatic memory, including both verbal memory and wordless images, and to describe it in the form of a verbal narrative. When hypnosis is used, this is called a "dissociative imagery anamnesis." The entire narrative is processed in a single, ninety-minute session. The session is videotaped and the tape is reviewed within a few days in the presence of the therapist. That session is also videotaped to record the sound track of the first tape and any discussion or elaboration of the narrative. This tape is used for homework by the patient, unless the review was interrupted by excessive emotion or dissociation. In this case, the session is repeated and a second recursive tape is made for the homework review. The patient's task is to review and study the tape with the goal of owning the narrative as personal history.

Although a single cycle of the dissociative imagery anamnesis, recursive reviews, and homework reviews provides sufficient trauma work for many cases of simple PTSD, the routine is to follow with two repetitions. The first is a repeat of the same thing to make sure that there are no gaps in the narrative. The second iteration is to screen for any unacknowledged earlier traumas and to process the earlier trauma if it is present.

An art therapy anamnesis routinely completes the trauma work. The objective of this is to construct a graphic narrative of the trauma that includes all of the important images and to transform the nonverbal narrative to a verbal narrative.

After the trauma work is completed, the video-dialogue phase commences and usually continues for two to four sessions. The objective is to make sure that any traumatically dissociated self-state is liberated from the traumatic experience that had seemed frozen in time.

The final phase, focal videotherapy, is designed to resolve the victim mythology. In the case of simple PTSD, this is usually not a difficult problem once the trauma work is completed. The task is to achieve a videotaped description of the trauma-driven assumptions about the self as damaged and the world as dangerous. The patient's study of the tapes should be enough to resolve the mythology.

The total duration of trauma therapy for simple PTSD requires approximately fourteen office sessions and eighteen hours. The first recursive session following the dissociative imagery anamnesis is best done within five days, because of a tendency for anxiety to build up after that time if the review is delayed. Otherwise, the duration between all other sessions is not important. A concentrated schedule is just as effective as one spread out over time. The core module is completed in one week in the intensive outpatient program, with sessions scheduled four to six hours daily.

Complex PTSD

Patients with complex PTSD were usually abused as children. Their Type II trauma resulted in a pervasive victim mythology. They are differentiated from dissociative PTSD by the absence of hallucinations. However, it may well be that dissociative PTSD is a subgroup of complex PTSD. Both groups have dissociative experiences. The DES scores associated with complex PTSD range from 20 to 50 while they run 30 or above in dissociative PTSD.

The total treatment duration for complex PTSD ranges between 30 and 40 sessions and, although the core treatment module is used, it is modified in the sequence of phases. Treatment usually begins with video dialogue to avert resistance and sabotaging of therapy. The video dialogue engages two aspects of the patient's personality with opposite sentiments about treatment. The objective is for the pessimist and the optimist positions to negotiate about cooperation in treatment. It usually takes two to four sessions to achieve this, and when this is accomplished, the trauma work can begin.

Trauma work for multiple traumas does not require repetition for individual ones (as with single traumas). The trauma processing begins with the earliest traumas first and commonly begins with preverbal traumas that are remembered only as images. After several traumas are processed, the procedure can be condensed so that more of the reviews can be processed as homework, skipping the recursive session in the office. It also works quite well for the art therapy anamnesis to replace the dissociative imagery anamnesis as the patient becomes more experienced in trauma work.

When the trauma work is completed, it is followed by video dialogue to resolve dissociation and splitting. This usually takes about six sessions for complex PTSD. Another six sessions are usually required to address the victim mythology with focal videotherapy.

Dissociative PTSD

Dissociative PTSD seems to be a clear-cut syndrome in the veteran population. In the civilian population, it is defined by the presence of hallucinations and a DES score in the dissociative range of 30 or more (Carlson et al., 1993). This form of PTSD seems to be common following the most severe Type I traumas such as combat, disasters, and rape. It is common, also, after Type II traumas involving a sadistic perpetrator. Following combat trauma, these patients are almost always alexithymic. Seventy percent of our non-combat PTSD patients who heard voices were alexithymic.

The trauma therapy for dissociative PTSD is very similar to that for complex PTSD, but it is usually somewhat briefer, with a total duration of twenty to thirty sessions. It also begins with two to four sessions of video dialogue to achieve agreement to cooperate in treatment. The video dialogue involves negotiation with the hallucinated voice.

The core treatment module follows, and is applied to, multiple traumas, if they are present, in the same manner as for complex PTSD. The video dialogue to resolve dissociation will be about the same duration as for complex PTSD (about six sessions), while the focal videotherapy is usually only about four sessions. A concentrated, intensive outpatient program schedule completes this treatment for dissociative PTSD in two weeks, while about three weeks is needed for complex PTSD.

DESCRIPTION OF TREATMENT PROCEDURES

The Regression Regimen

The standard regimen for ego regression was originally developed by Tinnin and Gantt. It has four objectives. The first task is to provide a *stimulus barrier* via tranquilizing medications, if necessary, and by prescribing optimal stimulation with prohibitions against being alone, taking naps, or drinking alcohol. The second objective is to *reduce ambiguity* in the interactions with other people. To accomplish this, the therapist assumes an authoritative, directive role and prescribes the behavior of family members or others who will help care for the patient. These significant others are recruited as therapeutic assistants to achieve the third objective, which is to provide any necessary *auxiliary ego function,* temporarily doing for the person what the person cannot do for him or herself. This usually involves a "tough love" approach, which uses firmness to keep the patient active and on task. The final task is to *support the autonomous ego functions.* This can be accomplished with a rigid daily schedule for sleep, meals, and activities and the keeping of a daily log with the listing of time and activity. An autobiographical history of school and work helps to restore the sense of identity. In addition to restoring identity, these chores help to repair the autonomous ego functions of time and volition. Once the ego regression is reversed, this regimen is terminated and the trauma therapy begins. Whenever regression recurs during the course of trauma therapy, the regression regimen can be reinstated.

Trauma Work Procedures

Dissociative Imagery Anamnesis

The goal of this procedure is to gain access to the traumatic memory and integrate the implicit, nonverbal images with the consciously remembered elements into a verbal narrative that brings closure to the experience. A major objective is to provide emotional protection while the narrative is being constructed. A controlled altered state of consciousness produced by drugs or hypnosis can provide both access and protection. An alternative approach is to use nonverbal communication to bypass the verbal brain controls. Drawing pictures in art therapy can do this, since the art product offers protection from reliving the experience by its property of being an external object. Other forms of visualization or thinking in images can also provide access to nonverbal mental images while maintaining an emotional distance from the trauma.

Hypnosis provides an effective altered state for the dissociative imagery anamnesis. Clinical experience shows that almost every person who has suffered significant trauma is capable of experiencing a hypnotic trance. The more dissociative the person's trauma, the easier it is to achieve a hypnotic trance (Spiegel, Hunt, and Dondershine, 1988). The trance does not have to be deep. A light trance will promote the form of visualization needed for narrative processing of the trauma.

Either a hypnotic induction by progressive relaxation or an open-eyed vigilant induction by encouraging a "thousand-yard stare" followed by a second phase of visualization of an imaginary place are used. The induction promotes an "observer mode" (picturing the event from the perspective of an outside observer) by an imaginary exercise of stepping out of the body and looking back at the self (Tinnin, 1994). The subject then maintains that perspective while reviewing the traumatic event and narrating it, as if watching it occur.

The patient is encouraged to identify the traumatic altered state of consciousness and any changes of consciousness that might fragment the memory. The narrative should contain any thwarted intentions, bodily experiences during altered states, and an account of the end point and aftermath of the trauma. The hypnotic anamnesis is usually excluded from the video recording, but the entire trauma narrative is recorded for the later recursive reviews.

Recursive Anamnesis

The first recursive review of the trauma narrative should be done within a few days because the patient tends to become more anxious if the review is delayed beyond that point. It is usual to schedule that session within five days. The goal of the review is to assimilate the trauma narrative into verbal memory and to avow it as a historical memory. Until that happens, the traumatic memory is experienced as unfinished and as if in present time. Once closure is achieved, the memory is experienced as in the past.

The first review is done in the presence of a therapist and this session is itself videotaped. The therapist monitors the patient's attention, stopping and rewinding the tape as needed for full assimilation. The patient adds to and elaborates upon the narrative, seeking to own it as a memory of the past. The review session is also videotaped and then independently reviewed by the patient as homework. The patient completes at least three reviews at home to desensitize to the trauma and to gain a sense of full ownership of the narrative.

Art Anamnesis

The art anamnesis routinely follows the recursive anamnesis. When multiple traumas are being processed, the art therapy procedure becomes the primary means of narrative processing. It can also be used instead of hypnosis when the patient objects to hypnosis or when the therapist is not trained to use it.

The patient uses large sheets of paper (12 × 18 inches), markers, pastels, and crayons. No particular artistic skills are required. The artist is encouraged to use the paper liberally, one sheet for each picture, so that missing images can be added later. The objective is to integrate all of the dissociated images into a graphic narrative that depicts the entire traumatic experience as a historical event. The patient reviews the pictured event, puts it into words and avows it as personal history. Once narrative closure and verbal coding is achieved, the images are no longer dissociated.

The major difficulty in achieving this is that the conscious mind has its own verbal memory of the trauma that usually does not admit the existence of other images. Thus, it seals over any gaps of recall. The repressed memory might yield to a verbal probe but not the dissociated memory. It is not verbally coded and so remains unconscious, in parallel with the repressed memory. The problem is how to bypass the verbal mind with all of its conscious and repressed content, to gain access to dissociated nonverbal memory.

The graphic narrative gains access by drawing. Although the verbal mind claims total ownership of the body and its actions, it fools itself about drawing. When a person draws, the hand obeys nonverbal commands on a par with the verbal. Both hemispheres of the brain have input into the motor commands for each hand. The nonverbal motor control can equal, and sometimes exceed, the verbal motor control. Therefore, a person's drawing may be influenced as much or more by unconscious, nonverbal intention as by conscious, verbal will.

Emotional distance. The patient runs the risk of emotional reenactment when drawing the dissociated images. This risk finally diminishes when the point of narrative closure is reached. Excessive abreaction of emotion would interrupt the trauma work and risk regression or a dissociative state before closure is achieved. The fastest and most effective trauma work is accomplished without emotional reliving of the traumatic events. Fortunately, the nature of the drawing task itself creates some emotional distance from the event since the pictures can be viewed at a physical distance, "out there."

There are other ways to help the patient avoid being drawn into the trauma scenes. It helps to maintain emotional distance if the entire graphic narrative is drawn in the observer mode. That is, the patient draws his or her self in every picture and avoids drawing a scene "as seen" at the time of the trauma. It also helps to draw both "before" and "after" pictures that depict initial safety and final survival. Sometimes an additional "safe place" picture to turn to while working on other pictures will help the patient feel grounded. A patient may draw the same safe place scene (for example, a peaceful forest scene) at each sitting and use it for a soothing effect while working on traumatic images.

Memory fragments. As the patient draws, the therapist helps to identify points of potential breaks in the narrative. The most important points to consider are the onset and offset of the freeze state, the beginning and end of the altered state or of any change in consciousness, and, finally, the aftermath of the trauma. There is often a specific "thwarted intention" (usually to take some protective action) or "fixed idea" (such as "I'm going to die") just before the onset of the freeze state when the victim feels trapped. This suspended urge or notion may later haunt the survivor as an intrusive symptom. The patient can resolve the unfinished intention or idea by simply assimilating it into the narrative, so that he or she can easily see what comes next.

Usually, a dual story line occurs when the victim experiences the traumatic altered state of consciousness. An altered state takes many forms. It might be a benumbed bodily state, a fantasy experience of being somewhere else, or an out-of-body experience in which the victim watches the event as if it were happening to someone else. The patient should include both experiences—that of the body and that of the altered state—in the pictures. The bodily sensations experienced during the altered state will tend to recur as intrusive body memories and may lead to misdiagnosis as physical ailments.

The hand remembers. The patient might begin a graphic narrative of an unremembered trauma by drawing a dream image or a flashback image or even a scribble and then expanding it with what "must have come next." The artist allows images to emerge with the faith that "the hand remembers though the head forgets." One may overcome a block to progressing by doing a map picture, depicting a bird's eye view, or drawing a zoom picture enlarging an element of a picture.

The patient can similarly gain access to preverbal images that were laid down in memory during infancy, before language developed and before verbal coding of memory. The intrusive symptoms arising from preverbal traumatic memories usually reenact bodily experience in symptoms such as smothering sensations (originating, for example, in infantile apnea or smothering or surgical anesthesia); diffuse pain with focal points in pelvis, genitals, or rectum (from infantile sexual abuse by probing or penetration, enemas, painful medical procedures, etc.); or other bodily distress. This reenactment of bodily sensation is often referred to as "body memories." The patient might construct the nonverbal narrative by first depicting the sensation and then allowing spontaneous drawing to elaborate the body memory into a picture narrative. These body memories cease as soon as the trauma is narratized and verbally avowed.

Re-presenting. When the patient comes to own the narrative as personal history, the traumatic dissociation has been resolved and the experience has been verbally coded and assimilated. Completing the drawing of the narrative does not automatically accomplish this avowal. The patient may still see the event as happening to someone else, or may still be unable to believe that the trauma happened.

The patient can most easily affirm and own the narrative if it is "re-presented." Simply displaying the pictures in narrative sequence at a distance beyond arm's reach begins the re-presentation. The patient beholds the picture story "out there" as an external depiction of a past event and begins to own the event, usually in gradual increments. The therapist assists the patient's verbal assimilation by "reading" the pictures and dramatizing the story in words. The therapist's rendition might begin: "One day in the life of . . ."

Because the avowal usually occurs in increments, it is helpful for the patient to have repeated representations. This is easily accomplished if the re-presentation by the therapist is videotaped for the patient's homework reviews using the home recorder and television. If the video equipment is not available, it is wise to repeat the re-presentation by the therapist at least once in a later session.

Video Dialogue

This videotherapy procedure was originally used to externalize communication between alter personalities of patients with dissociative identity disorder. In this procedure, the alter personality speaks to the host personality, looking into the eye of the videocamera. The recorded segment is then replayed with the host watching. Then, the host videotapes a response, looking into the eye of the camera. After that segment is replayed for the alter to watch, the exchanges continue, with each taking turns speaking and watching. This simple procedure has been found to be a breakthrough treatment. It allows the therapist to avoid multiple individual relationships with alter personalities without sacrificing communication between the alters and the host personality. The therapist relates to the host and the host relates to the alters through the externalization procedure that promotes logical verbal communication and negotiation. The video monitor shows the patients their true image, even when their mirrors reflect only their deluded image of alter personalities as physically different people. This makes it much more difficult for the personalities to deny the fact that there is only one body for all of them. The experience of talking out loud and listening to the other, in turn, profoundly changes the nature of the patient's subsequent internal communication between alters.

Command Hallucinations

Because video dialogue was found to be so useful with dissociative identity patients, it was natural to try it with a serious problem that is often nearly impervious to treatment—command hallucinations. Most of the time, patients with this problem feel compelled to obey what are known as command hallucinations. Some patients with voices commanding suicide go on to kill themselves after thwarted treatment interventions using behavioral measures and medications. The inspiration for using video dialogue with these patients came as a result of learning that most combat veterans with PTSD hear voices and those voices often engage in an inner dialogue (Holmes and Tinnin, 1996). Once they were persuaded that hearing voices did not mean that they were crazy, these veterans readily entered into externalized dialogues and their voices readily participated.

It only takes one experience of an externalized dialogue with a voice to eliminate the automatic obedience that the patient feels. It demystifies the voice and introduces a negotiation mode for resolving conflict. The external negotiation of internal conflict has the effect of diffusing dissociative boundaries as the person and voice reach agreements and inevitably become more alike to each other.

Impulsive Problems

Video dialogue is now being used for a variety of other problems. In patients with episodic aggression, impulsive suicide attempts, and self-mutilation, there is often an inner part (a voice or an ego state) that generates the impulse. That part is capable of participating in a video dialogue. The patient talks "for" that part until the part talks for itself. The impulsive act then becomes a matter of will and subject to negotiation.

Dissociation

When the negotiation of an externalized video dialogue leads to some agreement, no matter how minor, this institutes an irresistible change in the relationship between the person and the part. The change diminishes differences and therefore diminishes the dissociation. This seems to hold equally for alter personalities, ego states, introjected objects, and even bodily pains.

How to Conduct a Video Dialogue

A video camera, a videotape, a video recorder for rewinding and replaying the tape, and a television monitor are needed for conducting a video dialogue. A lapel microphone helps to achieve good sound quality. The therapist can operate the remote control to begin with, but may relinquish the control to the patient later.

The first task is to determine who will participate in the dialogue and to address that "part" directly before beginning the videotherapy procedure. The therapist asks questions of that participant and the patient reports what the participant answers. For example, the therapist asks:

"Are you listening?"
"Can you learn?"
"Will you cooperate?"

Any response, positive or negative, assures the success of the venture. If the patient detects no inner response, a dialogue may not be possible at the time. If the need is urgent, the therapist should not be deterred and should press on for a dialogue, if not with the chosen participant, then with the hidden observer or some other part that is willing to participate. If the therapist demonstrates the procedure, playing the part of the patient and then playing the part of the participant, the patient's resistance may melt away.

The actual video dialogue usually begins with the patient inviting the participant to dialogue. The patient looks into the camera and invites the other to respond. The tape is rewound and replayed for the participant to watch and prepare to speak in turn. The therapist facilitates the transition from one speaker to the other by some regular ritual such as counting. The therapist might say, "Close your eyes while I count to seven and then 'Voice' will open your eyes and look into the eye of the camera and respond." Instead of counting, the therapist might suggest changing chairs, or, simply say, "Now you talk for Voice." The therapist relates to the host personality and encourages negotiation and agreement while avoiding relating to the participant if possible. The patient reviews the tapes of the dialogue sessions at home, and may continue the video dialogue at home as a self-help measure.

Video Dialogue for Simple and Complex PTSD

Even in cases of simple PTSD there is often a self-state or ego state that experiences being frozen in time and locked into the timeless traumatic experience. Although successful trauma work makes it possible for this experiential state to become unfrozen, the dissociation may persist until directly addressed. For example, if the patient nearly died, there may be a dissociated state of mind that feels dead. Similarly, the experience of being overwhelmed and utterly helpless may be dissociated as a paralyzed self or a demoralized self. A dialogue with one or the other traumatized self diminishes dissociation and promotes relinquishing of the victim mythology.

A person with complex PTSD usually experiences pervasive, dissociative splits between personality aspects such as dependency/independency, pessimist/optimist, or victim/perpetrator. Video dialogue is effective in reducing this kind of polarity, particularly if the therapist does not take sides.

Focal Videotherapy for Victim Mythology

Focal videotherapy is a videotaped, brief, focused psychotherapy. It is focused on the patient's victim mythology and it is designed to provide the opportunity for the patient to gain an objective and independent grasp of the self-defeating effect of that mythology.

The sessions are face-to-face and are devoted to exposing the patient's fearful, assumptive world. Between sessions, the patient reviews and studies the tapes and chooses a segment to review at the next session. The therapist's task is to facilitate a clear formulation of the victim mythology and its effect on the patient's way of life.

Relinquishing the Illusion of Invulnerability

Trauma demolishes the illusion of invulnerability that many of us hold, even into adulthood. The traumatized person often feels super-vulnerable and totally unprotected and may believe that nothing short of magical invulnerability could provide for a sense of safety. The wish for magic can block the person's rejection of the victim mythology and attainment of a reasonable sense of safety. The survivor of trauma is often faced with the need to relinquish and grieve the illusion of invulnerability. Once the patient has talked about the issue and has it on tape to study at home, it becomes possible to face it and decide on a realistic course of action.

Shame and Guilt

Inappropriate guilt often complicates the recovery from trauma and is often a defense against shame. In every trauma there is a moment of utter helplessness when the impulse to fight or flee is thwarted. The memory of that helplessness is infused with shame in many survivors and the individual may assume an unjustified sense of responsibility just to maintain an illusion of choice. Guilt, then, is the price for relief from shame. When the survivor accepts the fact of being frozen in helplessness and that it occurred in the past, shame usually ceases to be a problem.

Entitlement

It would seem appropriate justice for one who has suffered the cruel blow of trauma to receive reparation. There should be some reward or some blessing for great suffering. The helpless victim may come to hold that expectation as life-affirming and as giving meaning to suffering. The promise of future relief may become incorporated into the victim mythology as entitlement. This can interfere with the survivor's self-help by emerging as a feeling of entitlement to rescue or recompense by the therapist. The major emphasis on self-help in this therapy and the opportunities for discovery of self-defeating assumptions during videotape reviews facilitate the patient's relinquishing of the illusion of entitlement.

Relinquishing Victim Mythology

In the case of simple PTSD, the patient is able to identify and to quickly correct the excessive reliance on the motto "safety first," once it has been formulated and captured on tape in the therapy session. In the case of complex PTSD, it is not so easy to unmask the victim mythology, but the principle is the same. The patient reviews the tapes and learns through repeated discoveries that it is futile to wish for happiness while endeavoring merely to survive. However, many times, the opposing trends of hopeful aspiration and pessimism are firmly organized as dissociated self-states with blind loyalty to their codes. They do not easily accede to the discoveries of the viewer. Video dialogue is a solution to this problem. The dissociated separation of those opposing trends is readily undermined by externalized vocal communication. Their dialogue, negotiation, and agreement make it possible to substitute a new way of life for the bankrupt victim mythology.

CONCLUSION

Video-assisted trauma therapy makes it possible for a patient to transform dissociated traumatic memory to historical memory without having to relive the trauma. The process allows the patient to get through the necessary memory processing rapidly and to resolve dissociation using specific procedures. It makes it possible to treat complex PTSD with the same basic procedures used for simple PTSD. A major part of the treatment is done by the patient independently, away from the therapist's office, using the home equipment.

The videotapes belong to the patient. If there is a need to repeat the treatment at a later time, it can be done by the patient without having to return to the therapist. The patient can review and study the tapes all over again and learn to use an externalized dialogue (by videotape, audiotape, or writing, for example) as a self-help measure for a variety of problems.

REFERENCES

Alvir, J., Schooler, N., Borenstein, M., Woerner, M., and Kane, J. (1988). The reliability of a shortened version of the SCL-90. *Psychopharmacology Bulletin, 24,* 242-246.

Appel, R. and Sifneos, P. (1979). Alexithymia: Concept and measurement. *Psychotherapy and Psychosomatics, 32,* 180-190.

Bernstein, E. and Putnam, F. (1986). Development, reliability, and validity of a dissociation scale. *Journal of Nervous and Mental Disease, 174,* 727-735.

Blake, D., Weathers, F., Nagy, L., Kaloupek, D., Klauminzer, G., Charney, D., and Keane, T. (1990). A clinician rating scale for assessing current and lifetime PTSD: The CAPS-1. *Behavioral Therapy, 13,* 187-188.

Carlson, E., Putnam, F., Ross, C., Torem, M., Coons, P., Dill, D., Loewenstein, R., and Braun, B. (1993). Validity of the Dissociative Experiences Scale in screening for multiple personality disorder: A multiple center study. *American Journal of Psychiatry, 150,* 1030-1036.

Holmes, D. and Tinnin, L. (1996). The problem of auditory hallucinations in combat PTSD. *Traumatology E-Journal.* Available online: <http:llwww.rdz.stjohns.edu/trauma>.

Naples, M. and Hackett, T. (1978). The amytal interview: History and current uses. *Psychosomatics, 19,* 98-105.

Spiegel, D., Hunt, T., and Dondershine, H. (1988). Dissociation and hypnotizability in post-traumatic stress disorder. *American Journal of Psychiatry, 145,* 301-305.

Taylor, G., Bagby, R., Ryan, D., Parker, J., Doody, K., and Keefe, P. (1988). Criterion validity of the Toronto Alexithymia Scale. *Psychosomatic Medicine, 58,* 500-509.

Terr, L. (1991). Childhood traumas: An outline and overview. *American Journal of Psychiatry, 148,* 10-20.

Tinnin, L. (1989). The anatomy of the ego. *Psychiatry, 52,* 404-409.

Tinnin, L. (1994). *Time-limited trauma therapy for dissociative disorders.* Bruceton Mills, WV: Gargoyle Press.

Chapter 7

Life After Trauma:
Finding Hope by Challenging Your Beliefs
and Meeting Your Needs

Dena Rosenbloom
Mary Beth Williams

INTRODUCTION

A survivor's experiences of trauma shake the very foundation of his or her being, including that survivor's sense of safety, trust, control, self-worth, and connection with oneself and others. Traumatic events shatter illusions about how safe the world really is and how much control any individual has over his or her life. To help survivors heal from the impact of those traumatic events, the authors developed a workbook, *Life After Trauma: A Workbook for Healing* (Rosenbloom and Williams, 1999), designed to help challenge the beliefs that traumatic experiences modify or change. In other words, this workbook is a guide to facilitate the rediscovery of order in the posttrauma world. It also is designed to help survivors make sense of posttrauma reactions through definitions, explanations, and opportunities for self-examination; to understand personal responses to traumatic experiences through answering questions and completing exercises; and to experience positive life changes in areas of trauma-related difficulties through text and exercises which examine and test assumptions and core beliefs.

The workbook is based on the ideas of McCann and Pearlman (1990), presented in their book *Trauma and the Adult Survivor.* McCann and Pearlman identify five basic emotional needs for the self and for the individual as that individual interacts with others: to be safe, to trust, to feel some control over life, to feel self-worth, and to feel close. These five basic needs,

---

Portions of this chapter are based on D. Rosenbloom and M. B. Williams, 1999, *Life After Trauma: A Workbook for Healing,* New York: Guilford Press.

when met, function as a cushion to protect the self against or help provide some buffer in the face of traumatic events. A traumatic event usually involves actual death or fear of death, or serious emotional or physical injury. However, what is most important about the trauma is not necessarily the aspects of the event itself (length, duration, location, agency) but how the survivor experiences them. A goal of the workbook, therefore, is to help survivors better understand the lens through which they see and experience traumatic events and the relationship between those events and their subsequent lives.

There are no right or wrong ways to respond to traumatic life events. Some survivors withdraw into silence; others seek out support. Some feel drained of all energy, never feeling as if they have gotten enough rest; others have seemingly unlimited nervous energy. Each individual reacts uniquely to a traumatic event, depending on the particulars of the trauma and the individual's unique self and history. Exposure to violence, brutality, death, and atrocity, however, are all factors which also shape a reaction and may lead to its intensity of impact.

IMPACTS OF TRAUMA

As a physical stressor, trauma affects how the body reacts and how the central nervous system functions. Traumatic events may cause physical signs of rapid heart beat, nervousness, sleep difficulties, and changes in brain chemistry. Trauma also leads to many mental reactions, including

1. changes in thoughts about the self and self-attributes, including the inability to control fate and feelings of fearfulness and vulnerability;
2. changes in thoughts about the world, as explanations for tragic events become difficult or impossible to find;
3. disruptions in thoughts, as traumatic images "pop" into the survivor's mind unwanted and, seemingly, out of that individual's control;
4. feelings of being overly alert and aware of the surroundings (hypervigilance);
5. feelings of being "spaced out" or disconnected from the self; and
6. confusion about a sense of history, including uncertainty concerning what happened or who was involved in particular events.

Trauma also leads to many emotional disruptions, including

1. the inability to feel safe;
2. difficulty trusting one's own feelings, views, or impressions;
3. difficulty trusting other people;

4. diminished self-esteem, often accompanied by shame and self-hate;
5. feeling helplessness rather than feeling in control;
6. feeling chronically empty;
7. the inability to feel (alexithymia); and/or
8. the inability to modulate (blunt or amplify) feelings.

In addition, behavioral reactions to traumatic events include being unable to be close to or intimate with others; avoidance of places or situations that are reminiscent of the traumatic event; and the use of activities or actions such as addictions, workaholism, self-harm or harm to others to avoid feeling the impact of a traumatic event.

The Process of Accommodation

Traumatic events disrupt or change beliefs through a process called accommodation. Through accommodation, beliefs change to "fit" the circumstances of a particular trauma. In normal, everyday life, beliefs frequently are held onto firmly when they seem essential to safety, well-being, and existence, in spite of challenges to them. Still, what a person learns from experience does influence beliefs. Accommodation is an automatic and often unconscious process of checking out whether the experience of the trauma fits with existing beliefs about the self, others, or how the world works. The occurrence of unexpected traumatic events or the repetitive occurrence of events that could be seen as traumatic often disrupt or challenge existing beliefs. Resulting beliefs may change to accommodate or "fit" the circumstances of the traumas. These new, trauma-based beliefs are not easy to change and often remain strong, in spite of contradicting evidence. If these beliefs are formed during childhood, they may be even more difficult to challenge or test, Beliefs also may be entrenched if they have been reinforced by people or experiences.

An important task for a trauma survivor is to examine what might hold that individual back from testing and changing assumptions and beliefs. Developing that understanding may free the survivor from being "stuck" and help institute change. Understanding can lead to self-forgiveness and lessening of self-blame.

One goal of the workbook is to help survivors better understand the lens through which they view their traumatic experiences, events, and relationships. Once that understanding is developed, the individual may choose to examine alternative viewpoints and try new experiences that might support or challenge those beliefs and assumptions.

THE MEANINGS OF TRAUMATIC EVENTS AND COPING

Traumatic events may seem to carry their own inherent and objective meanings. However, this is not the case. Events and the facts that describe them need to be interpreted and given meaning. Each individual has a way of finding meaning and making sense of his or her experiences, including the traumatic events that have occurred. The first step in dealing with a traumatic event is to begin to make sense from the residue of jumbled feelings, thoughts, and beliefs about one or more of the basic human needs to be safe, to trust, to feel some sense of control over life, to feel self-worth, and to feel close, with the self, others, and the world. The goal is to be able to know, generally, what happened, what emotions occurred in response to what happened, how those feelings could be managed, how to cope with the experience in a more positive manner, and how to take care of oneself following a trauma. Together, these form the foundation for working through a traumatic experience. Historically, strategies for coping during a traumatic experience often fit, or were designed to adapt to, the specific event. They include specific strategies to manage the particular circumstances and aspects of that event. However, those coping strategies may not be appropriate to maintain once the event has ended. Other styles of coping may be more appropriate.

What can facilitate coping more easily with the occurrence of and fallout from a traumatic event? Thinking things through by using a variety of skills, abilities, and techniques makes it easier. A survivor's intelligence allows him or her to analyze the impacts or effects of the trauma on current situations or characteristics. Willpower and initiative will help him or her stick with the goal of transforming trauma and to even "get going" with the work. Other strategies that help with coping include holding onto a future perspective, maintaining insight or awareness of personal needs while looking inward or introspecting, and empathizing with self and others while, at times, viewing life with a sense of humor, even when in a great deal of pain. Maintaining some flexibility also helps by increasing creativity and enlarging the range of options for action.

Another important aspect of coping is striving toward personal growth. Striving helps provide a sense of hope and meaning and pushes the individual toward healing. In the workbook, respondents are asked to look at how they think things through by answering questions such as the following:

- Are you able to delay immediate desires for the sake of a longer-term goal? (willpower)
- Do you stick with projects or new things or do you give up easily?
- What future do you envision for yourself?

- Are you aware of your own personal needs? If so, what are some of them?
- Do you have a sense of humor? How flexible are you?
- What is your understanding of the words "personal growth"?

Another way of coping is making choices that are self-protective. Trauma survivors frequently feel helpless, confused, and out of control after traumatic events. The needs of the survivor frequently change during a traumatic event. Some needs recede, while others can become more prominent. Needs for safety or connection with other people, for example, may grow more pressing if feelings of vulnerability or isolation follow the traumatic event. Protective coping skills include anticipating consequences by planning or thinking ahead about what might possibly result from particular behaviors and entering into mutual give-and-take relationships. Many trauma survivors have experienced relationships marked by significant power differentials and abuse; these survivors may not know or be aware of their rights or how to develop equal, mutually respectful future relationships. Part of this awareness includes maintaining appropriate interpersonal boundaries, another self-protective coping skill. Traumatic experiences frequently involve boundary violations. Natural responses to violations may include withdrawal, fear, or feeling shame, self-blame, a loss of power and/or control. The ability to create and maintain good physical and emotional boundaries can provide protection from feeling vulnerable to further victimization. The workbook contains exercises to help trauma survivors understand personal boundaries as a means to develop some sense of control in their relationships. Issues of personal space, touch, and emotional distance are addressed.

An additional coping ability is making self-protective judgments. Traumatic experiences frequently undermine one's sense of effectiveness, competence, or faith in personal judgment. Repeated, failed attempts to protect oneself can lead to feelings of self-defeat and can hinder a willingness to try to protect oneself in new situations. The workbook helps survivors to make choices and determine options as part of "gray thinking" rather than black-white thinking.

Relationships with the Self

The workbook also guides trauma survivors in looking at their relationships with themselves, including how they think and feel about their emotions, how they respond to personal feelings, if they accept personal feelings, and how they treat themselves when experiencing feelings. There are six aspects of a survivor's relationship with the self. The first is being able to hold onto a sense of connection with others, even when those others are not physically present. Trauma survivors often feel isolated, desolate, hopeless, and abandoned; these feelings lead to further feelings of loneliness and internal emptiness. Trauma survivors often feel alone with their pain and separate or different from others. The second aspect is the ability to be alone without being lonely, including viewing time alone as a gift to enjoy. The third aspect is being able to comfort, care for, and do nice things for oneself.

The final three aspects of the relationship with the self are tolerating or lessening the intensity of extremely difficult or painful feelings, the ability to handle feedback from others without being devastated, and having positive self-esteem. Traumatic experiences often leave residual feelings of shame and self-hatred or self-loathing that can be particularly overwhelming. A major goal of the workbook is to help lessen these feelings; exercises are provided to facilitate that process. Trauma survivors frequently have "thin skins" and are very sensitive to the comments of others. Learning to handle positive feedback or constructive feedback from others without taking offense or viewing comments as an attack is another protective coping skill. Finally, experiencing and/or witnessing traumatic events, particularly if an individual was unable to take protective or defensive action, often erodes or damages that person's sense of self-esteem. An entire chapter of the workbook discusses self-esteem and helps the survivor work on building a positive view of self.

Spirituality

Spirituality, or a sense of life's meaning, hope for the future, and purpose or mission in life may be disrupted by trauma. Spirituality also includes a sense of altruism (doing for others), idealism, and the belief that something or some dimension of experience exists that is greater than or beyond the self. Spirituality is the awareness of the nonmaterial, existential aspects of experience. Traumatic experiences may lead to changes in spiritual beliefs. Some survivors see their spiritual beliefs challenged, if not dissipated, by what happened; others find new meaning and strength in spirituality, and look for the coincidences that occurred or the lessons that can be learned. Exercises in the workbook help survivors examine their spiritual beliefs as a way to cope with what happened and reengage a sense of hope and connection.

Assumptions That Underlie Beliefs

Assumptions are underlying beliefs that influence and often guide decisions, reactions, and relationships. Often people are not aware of their assumptions. Traumatic events seem to challenge what was once taken for granted and bring many beliefs into more conscious awareness. These assumptions may not be totally accurate or correct. However, it is possible to question the origin of the assumption and check if the assumption is accurate.

WORKING THROUGH TRAUMATIC EVENTS

After a traumatic event occurs, the goal for both the victim and therapist is to be able to know, generally, what happened, how the individual felt in response to what happened, how the individual managed ensuing feelings and coped with the experience, and how the individual cared for himself or herself. These aspects of the goal of self-knowledge form the basic foundation of "working through" a traumatic experience. The person who works through a traumatic event successfully is able to do the following in many situations:

- Tolerate or lessen the intensity of painful feelings
- Counter self-blame
- Hold onto a sense of connection with present and absent others
- Be alone without being lonely
- Self soothe when distressed
- Anticipate consequences of events
- Set and maintain appropriate interpersonal boundaries
- Enter into mutually supportive, give-and-take relationships

In general, feelings get attached to beliefs (in particular) when beliefs have been learned or acquired through traumatic experiences. If an individual wants to test a belief and experiment with alternatives, the attached feelings may make the difference between a willingness to try out alternatives or an unwillingness to take a risk to see things differently. These beliefs, impressions, and feelings may become so compelling that they get interpreted as facts and absolute truth. However, one person's "facts" may be uniquely different from another person's factual understanding because the filter of unique experiences differs for each person. Traumatic events can change (or at least modify) that filter and can leave a victim feeling unsafe, out of control, guilty, mistrustful, and isolated, among other personal experiences. As mentioned earlier, willpower and initiative, insight, empathy with others, a sense of humor, flexible thinking, striving toward personal growth, and a willingness to see shades of gray help individuals cope with trauma.

TESTING BELIEFS

Testing beliefs about the five basic needs for safety, trust, power/control, esteem, and intimacy requires taking chances. These needs, according to Contextualistic Self-development Theory as originally developed by McCann and Pearlman (1990), and further developed by the staff of the Traumatic Stress Institute (TSI) in South Windsor, Connecticut, are defined as follows:

1. *Safety:* the need to feel reasonably invulnerable to harm inflicted by self and others; the need to feel that valued others are reasonably invulnerable to harm inflicted by self or others.
2. *Trust:* the need to rely on personal judgment; the need to rely on others to meet one's needs.
3. *Power/Control:* the need to feel some influence over what happens to oneself; the need to feel some influence over what happens to others.
4. *Esteem:* the need to feel a good sense of connection about oneself; the need to value others.
5. *Intimacy:* the need to feel close to oneself; the need to have a close relationship with others.

Testing beliefs in these five areas will offer the individual the opportunity to make choices. If an individual does not assume or decide what is factual before checking out each situation, then that person can be more creative in interpretation and/or response. What appears to be factual is actually colored by individual interpretation.

Process for Testing a Belief

But how does one test beliefs? The following format presents a series of questions that, used in part or whole, guides one through the process of testing a belief. First, state the belief you wish to examine more closely or better understand.

1. Describe a situation that has led you to question why and when you have . . . (the belief).
2. How did you interpret this situation and what do you think it meant to you? What do you think it meant to others? What do you think it meant about your world?
3. What does the situation tell you about yourself and your beliefs about . . . ?
4. When did you start to believe this? When and how did you learn it? When did you start to believe this about others? When did you start to believe this about your world?

5. How does this belief make you feel? What feelings about yourself arise?
6. How does believing this protect or help you?
7. How does this belief hold you back or get in your way?
8. How could you check to see whether or not what you think is true?
9. What is the worst thing that could happen if you test what you believe? Could testing the belief hurt you? Could it hurt someone else? Could it kill you? Could it kill someone else?
10. What good things might happen if you test what you believe?
11. Are there other ways to interpret what happened? What else could the situation mean? Is there an alternative to what you think about yourself? Is there an alternative to what you think about others? Is there an alternative to what you think about the world?
12. What positive feelings do you have when you think about this alternative meaning?
13. What negative feelings do you have when you think about this alternative meaning?
14. Has this process helped you change the way you see and understand yourself? Others? The world and how to make sense of it?
15. Will testing the belief really matter ten years from now? How would testing the belief and possibly changing it help with your future?

Examining and Testing Beliefs About Safety

Traumatic events may rob an individual of a sense of safety and security in the world. Some individuals who have been traumatized experience this belief about their lack of safety only fleetingly or during situations that are reminiscent of the traumatic experience. Other individuals may believe that they are completely unsafe the majority of the time. This is particularly true when the individual has grown up in an unsafe world. Experiencing a traumatic event later in life, postchildhood, may disrupt a previously strong sense of safety. Witnessing a traumatic event, even when an individual is not in direct, immediate danger, often erodes a sense of personal safety. Indirect exposure to traumas experienced by others can evoke images of events and their accompanying feelings.

A lack of perceived safety may leave an individual more vulnerable to future emotional injury and at greater risk for harm. Exercises provided in the workbook give respondents the opportunity to examine beliefs about safety, as well as the origins of those beliefs.

Traumatized individuals may have black and white thinking about safety. They may see things as all or nothing, for example, feeling completely vulnerable or completely protected. In reality, safety is *not* an either/or proposition and involves choices and variations. Safety may become an accessible goal if not thought of in the either/or manner and include differing degrees of vulnerability.

In the workbook, the respondent answers a series of questions about safety. These questions may challenge the respondent to reflect upon and, at times, tolerate strong feelings, intense thoughts, and (possibly) destructive impulses. The containment process offered within the workbook helps the individual separate past traumatic experiences from present events and circumstances. Containment strategies help the respondent self-soothe while healing beliefs about safety and self-protection. As the individual examines in depth at least one belief about safety of self, safety of others, and safety in the world, through a variety of strategies, opportunities for making changes arise repeatedly.

DISCERNING THE MEANING OF TRUST

Trust and safety are related. It is impossible to trust others if an individual does not feel safe. Also, if an individual cannot trust others, it is difficult to feel safe. Trusting others helps an individual to feel more secure and less alone in the world. Traumatic events can shatter a sense of trust. Even one traumatic event can disrupt trust in self (e.g., the way one behaved in the face of trauma) and trust in others.

A definition for "trustworthy" is provided as a guide to help readers to allow themselves permission to look or ask for certain things in others in their relationships. For example, a trustworthy person is consistent, reliable, available, and able to follow through. A trustworthy person is honest and does not violate physical or emotional boundaries. Many traumatized people blame themselves for some aspect of the trauma that happened to them. They may mistrust themselves, questioning their own decisions. They may stop listening to themselves and their own intuition. They may not pay attention to internal alarms or feelings, and they may cut off access to important information that might help in decision making, in gathering information, or with asking questions. When one ignores internal alarms or feelings, one loses access to important information that might help at the time or later. Ignoring internal messages makes it difficult to protect and care for oneself.

Many trauma survivors have learned that others do not keep their word and cannot be trusted with information about them, the survivors. In this workbook, survivors are asked to complete a series of questions about trust in self, others, and the world. Some of those questions examine the topic of independence. Once the respondents answer these questions, they are asked to identify themes and patterns about trust as well as the feelings and thoughts that accompany those patterns. Then, they are asked to choose one or more beliefs about trust to examine and test. They are also asked to develop affirmations about trust—positive statements about themselves and others.

GETTING CONTROL

Trauma survivors often have had their environments or bodies invaded by either events or other people. In many instances, a passive response enabled the individual to survive; in others, fighting back and struggling was to no avail, or even seemed to intensify the trauma. In other instances, belief in personal power was destroyed or, at least, challenged. Control, then, seemed as if it belonged to others and any aim to regain a measure of control was an impossible, if not illusive, goal.

One way to conceptualize the words "power" and "control" involves thinking about the ability to have control over some aspect of the self (words, actions, reactions) and/or to have an impact on others. Possession of a skill or ability empowers an individual to position the self to be heard or seen. A true sense of control and power begins with self-acceptance and self-knowledge, personal limits, and access to what does or does not "feel" right. Having control without needing absolute control is important.

The fear of talking about a traumatic experience and becoming or being seen as out of control is silencing and leads to feelings of powerlessness. Silence can also amplify one's emotional experience, since there is no direct route for expression and release or feedback and support from others. Learning how to be assertive, in contrast to being passive or aggressive, meets the needs of everyone involved and aims to create equal relationships. Assertiveness takes courage to implement. When a traumatic event leads to a loss of control over forces or other people, the traumatized individual may respond with feeling helpless or with attempts to try to control everything in the environment, no matter the cost. Ironically, trying to control things that cannot be controlled typically results in feeling completely out of control. Being able to clarify and focus on what is possible to control actually leads to some measure of personal power.

It is impossible to control the actions of others; attempting to do so may result in feelings of frustration and helplessness. It is possible, however, to give voice to or state a feeling of preference that might influence another person.

Constructing a Personal Shield

Certain words, licenses, credentials, items, or other objects may stand for or symbolize an individual's personal power. These symbols represent aspects of an individual's strength as well as available resources. When feelings of helplessness and powerlessness arise, drawing these symbols into awareness or looking at or touching actual physical symbols may reconnect a trauma survivor with a sense of personal power. In the workbook, survivors are given the opportunity to construct a Personal Shield that contains these symbols of personal power. The shield a survivor creates is designed to protect the survivor in times of crisis, challenge, or fear by reminding or recommending him or her to strengths or resources. The following topics, statements, goals, and aspects of self might be included in a shield. This list is not exclusive, but provides suggestions by asking the survivor completing the workbook to complete the following statements:

- My life's motto is . . .
- The symbol(s) of the sources from which I draw energy to survive is/are . . .
- The people to whom I owe allegiance or feel closest are . . .
- The symbol(s) of my personal resources is/are . . .
- My safe or protected place(s) is/are . . .

BELIEVING IN YOURSELF AND OTHERS

Traumatic experiences can devastate the way a survivor views, interprets, judges, and feels about himself or herself. Feeling good about oneself and others is a basic need and is necessary for valuing or having faith in oneself, for thinking about oneself positively, or feeling valued by others. In the absence of self-esteem, one might believe that he or she was responsible for the traumatic events that occurred, or that he or she was fated or destined to suffer for past acts or sins. These beliefs may lead to feelings of guilt, shame, and depression, as well as self-destructive acts. In reality, the terror of the traumatic event most likely led to shock, confusion, paralysis, total focus on basic survival, and fight, flight, or freeze reactions. Feelings of blame lead to feeling stuck; a belief in control when no control was possible interferes with healing and moving beyond the trauma.

Low self-esteem leaves an individual vulnerable to criticism; it may also influence that person to react in a critical, blaming manner toward others. Negative feelings about oneself make it difficult to develop friendships, let alone a feeling of intimacy. If others get too close, they may learn of the survivor's perceived sense of "badness" and not want a relationship. This can lead to withdrawal from others, further exacerbating the negative impact of the trauma.

Traumatic events that include degradation, demoralization, torture, and disregard for the victim's humanity are particularly damaging to self-esteem. Internalization of the perpetrator's negative messages of worthlessness, particularly if conveyed to a child, can remain over the life span unless actively explored, examined, or challenged.

People with high self-esteem are less judgmental of both themselves and others. This section of the workbook helps survivors identify present assumptions about their value and esteem for self and others. Survivors are invited to complete an exercise in which they identify words or phrases that equate to positive self-esteem in general, and then indicate which of those phrases or words apply to them personally. Once this is done, the survivor is asked to combine the words or phrases with an "I am" to create affirmations about self-worth. Words or phrases that are not circled or identified in the list may be identified as goals for later attainment.

FEELING CLOSE TO YOURSELF; GETTING CLOSE TO OTHERS

Intimacy with oneself is a sense of closeness to and acceptance with that self as well as acceptance of personal feelings, impulses, thoughts, preferences, and limitations. The chapters in the workbook prior to this chapter are designed to help a survivor approach the goal of self-knowledge and self-acceptance.

Trauma can take an individual away from himself or herself, making it difficult to understand emotional and behavioral reactions, and to identify feelings or make sense of what happened. Following a trauma, some people experience an inability to recognize their inner experiences as familiar. Survivors of trauma may cut themselves off from feelings to protect themselves from feeling overwhelmed. Alienation from feelings may lead to vulnerability since they often seep out in a disguised or indirect manner. Others seek quick fixes through addictive behaviors to keep feelings buried. Suggestions for developing an intimate relationship with oneself include the following:

- Slow the pace of your life to have time to notice feelings and reactions.
- Take time to check in with yourself and ask, "How do I feel about that?" or "What is my opinion or stance on this?"
- Make plans to allow time to relax and reflect.
- Remain drug- and alcohol-free.
- Spend time with friends; turn to them for support if a "listening ear" is needed.
- Use touch in appropriate, healthy ways without violating others' or your own boundaries.

- Use personal belongings for self-soothing.
- Keep in mind the twelve-step slogan "You can control by letting go."

Intimacy with others is also important. Wanting to fit in with and feel connected to others is natural. However, the very nature of trauma and exposure to pain, cruelty, betrayal, or destruction can damage a sense of connection with or attachment to others. As noted, trauma makes it difficult to trust; however, in order for a truly intimate relationship to develop it is necessary to trust another. A traumatic loss of a significant individual also can undermine a sense of connection to others. Experiencing the death of another person can lead to a loss of innocence, fear of loving again, or the sabotage of potentially close relationships, all in an effort to protect oneself from future loss. It might also be difficult to imagine that anyone else could understand the depth of one's pain or other aspects of experience in the wake of trauma, thereby furthering withdrawal or the sense of alienation from others.

Intimacy with another person requires revealing thoughts, feelings, strengths, flaws, dreams, and vulnerabilities. Sharing involves taking risks. Learning to know another person intimately takes time. The following statements describe some experiences that are part of loving, intimate relationships. Those completing the workbook are asked to think about each statement and then develop steps to achieve those statements that are not present in their intimate relationships. Among the statements found in the workbook are the following:

- We take time to be together without distractions; we do not let other things get in the way.
- We each pay attention to and talk about our feelings.
- We respect each other's need to spend some time alone.
- We enjoy spending time as a couple with friends.
- We are able to enjoy physical intimacy in a manner that feels safe and respectful to both of us.
- We generally try not to control one another's feelings or actions.
- We have fun together.
- We respect growth and change in each other.
- We feel supported by each other.

The workbook also includes exercises designed to help the survivor examine his or her worldview or fundamental beliefs about the world, why things happen in the world, beliefs about one's identity, and a general sense of self and what the self represents.

CONCLUSION

Traumatic life events can be devastating. Surviving them and going on in a day-to-day manner reflects strength on the part of survivors. It is extremely important for the trauma survivor to remember that he or she is not alone. Others have similar problems, fears, and frailties. Sharing experiences with supportive others helps to build connections and is worth the risks involved.

Traumatic events also may cause the survivor to develop a sense of connection to a power greater than the self, whether nature, community, or some form of religion. A spiritual sense of connection may help combat alienation, disconnection, and disappointment while providing a sense of protection in a world that no longer seems safe. It also provides a sense of somewhere to place faith and trust, in a world that seems unpredictable; a sense of being loved, in a world that feels harsh and uncaring and out of control; a sense of connection when all else feels fragmented.

An important task of trauma resolution is making meaning out of what happened and what has changed as a result. As stated earlier, things are not always as individuals want them to be. Life can be unjust and unfair. Bad things do happen to good people. There are no absolutes in the world. Making sense of trauma may be a life-long task. However, how a person makes sense of the events in the present is more within control when a new perspective and a different level of self-knowledge is possible. Completing the workbook *Life After Trauma: A Workbook for Healing* (1999) may help the survivor gain unexpected gifts, including

- a new awareness of inner strength;
- a different set of priorities;
- a heightened appreciation for daily life;
- respect for others who have also survived;
- a sense of awe at nature and the cycles of life;
- a deepened emotional life;
- a philosophy of life that explains tragedy and makes sense of the unexpected;
- comfort with what was once too frightening to contemplate;
- understanding or enhanced acceptance of life's complexities; and
- confidence in the ability to survive anything.

REFERENCES

McCann, I. L. and Pearlman, L. A. (1990). *Trauma and the adult survivor.* New York: Brunner/Mazel.

Rosenbloom, D. and Williams, M. B. (1999). *Life after trauma: A workbook for healing.* New York: Guilford Press.

SECTION III:
GROUP TREATMENTS

Chapter 8

The Development of a Group Treatment
Model for Post-Traumatic Stress Disorder

Gordon Turnbull
Tosin Clairmonte
Stuart Johnson
Colina Hanbury-Aggs
Bo Mills
Walter Busuttil
Adrian West

INTRODUCTION

It would not be possible to describe the Group Treatment Programme for post-traumatic stress disorder (PTSD) at Ticehurst House Hospital without first briefly tracing its initial development at RAF Wroughton. The Programme, which was originally developed within the Royal Air Force, is fully described by Busuttil et al. (1995).

The RAF Wroughton Programme was conceived and designed during the early stages of the Gulf War (Operation Desert Storm) in 1991. At that time, RAF psychiatric services were mobilized. Massive numbers of battle-stress casualties were anticipated, including those who had developed PTSD (Brandon, 1991a). The Royal Air Force Medical Service had been interested in the effects of stress on its personnel since its inception, because of the nature and the task of the organization. However, there had been consid-

The authors wish to express their thanks and gratitude to the following people for their tireless energy, enthusiasm, support, and inspiration in the further development of the PTSD Group Treatment Model at Ticehurst—Dr. Anthony Goorney, Margaret Cudmore, Louise Orpin, Jan Fright, Margaret Egner, Ian Dennis, Christine Miller, Patricia Young, and Anne Davies—and to the following people for the pioneering work at RAF Wroughton—Group Captain (RAF, retd.) John Rollins, Sergeant Nick Blanch, Sergeant Ronald Herepath, and Wing Commander Leigh Neal.

erable changes in ideas concerning the causation and management of stress reactions during the life span of the Service over almost eighty years of its history. At each stage, changes in states of knowledge and prevailing attitudes, as well as the needs of the Service, were reflected in the evolution of practical management of the problems created by stress reactions. Likewise, the RAF Wroughton Programme was based on established theoretical concepts of PTSD and was influenced by the requirements of the situation during the Gulf War. Perhaps, most importantly, the program reflected the varying degrees of successful outcomes of many years of attempts to manage traumatic stress reactions.

POST-TRAUMATIC STRESS DISORDER

Post-traumatic stress disorder (PTSD) is currently defined in the fourth edition of the *Diagnostic and Statistical Manual of Mental Disorders* of the American Psychiatric Association (APA, 1994) and in the tenth edition of the *The ICD-10 Classification of Mental and Behavioral Disorders* of the World Health Organization (WHO, 1992). PTSD has been recognized since 1980 in the DSM-III (APA, 1980). It has undergone two slight revisions in the DSM-III-R (APA, 1987) and the DSM-IV (APA, 1994), but the initial concept proved itself to be robust and has been upheld.

PTSD occurs in individuals who have been exposed to a catastrophically stressful event which is said to be "traumatic." This event presents such a major blow to the psyche that it overwhelms psychological defense mechanisms to the extent that it cannot be responded to in an effective way. It is not enough, in itself, for an individual to have been exposed to war-zone stress or other traumatic experiences such as rape, motor vehicle accidents, child abuse, or natural disasters to be diagnosed with PTSD in the latest revision of the concept (DSM-IV). It is also necessary for the exposed individual to experience strong emotional reactions such as intense fear, terror, horror, helplessness or a belief that they might have died. This additional aspect represents an important change in the diagnostic criteria and in the meaning of the term "trauma."

The full description of a traumatic event is encapsulated within Criterion A of the DSM-IV definition of PTSD. Appropriately, this has been called the "Gatekeeper" Criterion. Criterion A states:

1. the person experienced, witnessed, or happened upon an event or events that involved actual or threatened death or serious injury, or the event was a threat to the physical integrity of the self or others
2. the person's response involved extreme fear, helplessness, or horror.

When it has been established that a person has been traumatized, three major symptom clusters develop (Criteria B, C, and D).

The first (B) is called the *reexperiencing* cluster of symptoms. Traumatic memories essentially continue to recur either in spontaneous daytime thoughts, nightmares, and in dissociative states known as "flashbacks." These recollections may also be triggered by stimuli that are reminiscent of the trauma.

The second cluster (Criterion C) is characterized by *avoidance and numbing.* PTSD sufferers find the reexperiencing symptoms so disturbing and intolerable that they develop a number of cognitive and behavioral strategies to reduce the number and the intensity of the intrusive recollections. *Avoidance* symptoms include avoidance of situations that remind the individual of the trauma, and the *numbing* symptoms include shutting down emotional expression, dissociation, psychogenic amnesia, and social withdrawal.

The third and last cluster of symptoms are those representing hyperarousal (Criterion D). Although they closely resemble the symptoms of most anxiety disorders, including insomnia and irritability, their characteristic feature is hypervigilance. Those who have been traumatized never want to be traumatized again.

Underlying driving forces of intrusive recollection versus avoidance of traumatic memories mean that PTSD may develop de novo many years after the sensitizing traumatic experience. This is called "delayed-onset PTSD." PTSD appears to be a unique anxiety disorder which involves many of the cognitive, psychological, and psychobiological mechanisms that are important in coping and adaptation and may have an intense survival emphasis.

ETIOLOGICAL THEORIES

Peterson, Prout, and Schwartz (1991) wrote a comprehensive review of the main etiological theories for PTSD. Both the psychological aftermath of the Vietnam War and the DSM-III provided the background for an intense focus for research into the effects of combat-related traumatic stress reactions. The result was a rapid expansion of the PTSD literature and parallel development of several etiological models from different theoretical perspectives, none of which appears to be able to fully explain the etiology of PTSD. Any attempt to construct a comprehensive understanding of etiology needs to include an analysis of the relative contributions of the following factors:

1. The nature and dimensions of the trauma
2. The biological experience of the trauma, i.e., its neurochemical and neurophysiological substrates

3. The subjective experience of the trauma, including variables such as personality traits, cognitive style, past experience, and immediate sensory perception, which influence the way in which stressful events are perceived, appraised, and processed (Turnbull, 1994a)
4. The nature of the recovery environment, including its cultural adaptation to trauma (Harel, Boaz, and Wilson, 1993)

Friedman (1988) suggested that PTSD is the quintessential psychological disorder in which exposure to a stimulus (catastrophic stress) is followed by a conditioned emotional response maintained by avoidance behavior. This is in accord with Mowrer's Two Factor Learning Theory (Mowrer, 1960) in which the traumatized individual is distressed by memories of the threatening aspects of the traumatic event. A wide range of neutral cues that are present at the time of the trauma become classically conditioned by the process of higher order conditioning and stimulus generalization. In this way, a victim may become conditioned to a wide spectrum of stimuli present at the time of the trauma, but not directly related to it, including sounds or the time of day (Foa, Steketee, and Rothbaum, 1989). At the same time, the individual learns that avoidance of trauma-associated cues minimizes anxiety so that extinction becomes impossible.

In behavioral terms, the nondisclosure of traumatic experiences may be regarded as an avoidance reaction which prevents resolution and adaptation. Ramsay (1977) reviewed behavioral treatments for bereavement and noted the general agreement in the literature that grief had to be worked through. If it is not worked through, the individual continued to suffer emotional distress of some type. Ramsay conceptualized unresolved grief as avoidance behavior similar to that seen in phobics. He stated that "stimuli and situations which could get the grief work going, which would elicit the undesired responses so that extinction could take place are avoided," so that the person becomes "stuck" in the grief reactions (Ramsay, 1977, p. 131). Ramsay also advocated repeated confrontation with prolonged exposure and response prevention to accelerate grief work and reported positive results. This work was supported by the findings of Mawson et al. (1981).

Rachman (1980) introduced a theory of emotional processing which was consistent with a behavioral explanation, a theory often cited as a rationale for treatment of grief and PTSD. Rachman used emotional processing to describe processes "whereby emotional disturbances are absorbed, and decline to the extent that other experiences and behaviour can proceed without disruption" (p. 51). When an emotional disturbance is not absorbed satisfactorily, then, according to Rachman, "the central, indispensible index of unsatisfactory emotional processing is the persistence or return of intrusive signs of emotional activity" (p. 51). Rachman provided a list of "signs" of inadequate processing including obsessions (Rachman, 1978), disturbing dreams (Bandura, Adams, and Beyer, 1977), and unpleasant intrusive thoughts (Horowitz, 1975). Indirect signs were thought to include an inability to concentrate, excessive restlessness, and irritability. The similarity between this group of symptoms and some of those within the definitional rubric of PTSD is apparent. Rachman (1980) also suggested that there were certain personality, stimulus, and associated environmental factors which might be connected with difficulties in emotional processing. Among Rachman's list of factors which were likely to impede processing, the refusal or inability to talk about the disturbing stimuli ranks high. Pennebaker and Susman (1988) hypothesized that inhibition results in increased autonomic nervous system (ANS) activity which, over time, increases the probability of psychosomatic illness. They presented the results from several studies "that indicate that talking about—or in some way confronting—traumatic experiences is psychologically and physically beneficial" (p. 327).

Psychodynamic formulations have historically emphasized that prevulnerability to traumatic reactions depends upon the accentuation of certain vulnerable personality traits following exposure to high magnitude stresses. These concepts have *not* proved to be of value in the explanation or understanding of traumatic stress reactions and are not supported by the statistical evidence provided by studies of the victims of combat stress. In these studies, training and selection aspects did not coincide with the concept of prevulnerability in personalities (Chemtob, Baker, and Neller, 1990).

Freud (1919) and Kardiner (1941) used psychoanalytical theories to explain the combat neuroses of soldiers. However, more recent psychodynamic contributions focusing on the concept of information overload have proved to have more practical value and have been developed into information processing/cognitive-appraisal models of PTSD (Janoff-Bulman, 1985). Horowitz (1979) contended that, because traumatic events are outside the realm of usual human experience, the individual does not already possess built-in schemata for the assimilation and integration of the new information. The inability to process the information in the cognitive sense creates anxiety which is further compounded by the subjective interpretation of threat. Information models generally propose a phasic response as an adaptive attempt to assimilate the traumatic experience; the individual alternates between denial and numbing as a defensive maneuver to hold the traumatic information in the unconscious and avoid intrusive reexperiencing of vivid imagery of the trauma. The phasic response facilitates a gradual processing of that information. Janoff-Bulman (1985) focused on the disruption of established assumptions that permit the world to be viewed as predictable, stable, controllable, and safe.

The aim of treatment, therefore, is to complete the processing of information rather than induce a catharsis by abreaction (Peterson, Prout, and Schwartz, 1991; Horowitz, 1979).

Positive evidence for the beneficial effects of disclosure of traumatic experiences comes from Fowlie and Aveline's (1985) questionnaire study of 175 RAF aircrew officers who had survived emergency ejection from fast-jet aircraft. Fowlie and Aveline found that 40 percent of the respondents described prolonged emotional disturbance. However, 31 percent of the survivors indicated that sympathetic guidance and counseling during rehabilitation had been crucial to their emotional recovery. In contrast, a predictor of poor outcome was an expressed inability to talk about the ejection and its consequences. Fowlie and Aveline recommended that confidential counseling of ejection survivors should be routine since "this can reduce prolonged emotional morbidity" and "adverse consequences may be limited" (p. 609).

Biopsycho-physiological evidence to date is consistent with the hypothesis that chronic PTSD is a hyperarousal state associated with autonomic nervous system (ANS) hyperactivity and hyperreactivity (Friedman, 1988). Van der Kolk et al. (1985) focused on the importance of the locus ceruleus as the primary source of norepinphrinergic innervation to the limbic system, cerebral cortex, cerebellum, and to a lesser extent, the hypothalamus as a controlling mechanism in the development of coping responses for stressful stimuli. They observed that the central nervous system exerted hierarchical control over the ANS, based on studies of inescapable shock in animals. Van der Kolk et al. (1985) concluded that clinical symptoms of hyperarousal (with exaggerated startle response, explosive outbursts, nightmares, and intrusive recollections) suggested the development of chronic catecholamine hypersensitivity. It seemed likely that massive trauma precipitated a vulnerability to respond with excessive autonomic reactivity by the alteration of the activity level of the locus ceruleus. Similarly, Friedman (1988) proposed that acute stress affects neuroendocrine systems in a manner that maintains the vigilant posture at an abnormally high level and lowers the threshold of arousal. Yehuda et al. (1995) further extended this theory in her work on the elucidation of acute biochemical and humoral responses to overwhelming stress.

An important psychophysiological area of research is the animal model of learned helplessness postulated by Maier and Seligman (1976). This model is based upon the experimental observation that animals exposed to inescapable aversive conditions such as pain, loud noise, or cold water go on to show difficulty with new learning and show chronic evidence of distress. Friedman (1988) noted remarkable similarity between hyperalertness and avoidant behavior following the exposure of animals to experimental stress and clinical PTSD. Learned helplessness studies have demonstrated when an organism learns that response and escape are not interdependent. ANS responses become excessive and nonspecific. This condition leads to interference with cognitive responses to stressful stimuli (Strian and Klicpera, 1978). In human terms, this translates as anxiety becoming the initial response to stress. If there is no way to control the situation or decrease the stress, that anxiety is replaced by depression (Seligman, 1975).

Cognitive-behavioral theory proposes that emotional disorders, in general, stem from dysfunctional interpretation of environmental events. Cognitive-behavioral therapy (CBT) aims to challenge the maladaptive interpretations, leading to a change in the prevailing emotional state. Foa and Kozak (1986) proposed that the concept of meaning (not incorporated into traditional learning theories) is both essential and central to the understanding of the human experience of trauma. They argued that to change a dysfunctional fear structure, two steps are required. First, the fear structure has to be activated as completely as possible; second, new information of an adaptive quality needs to be incorporated into the structure which is incompatible with some of the elements already present. The concept is based on the perception that the common denominator for the feared situation in PTSD is the "perceived threat." In CBT, perceived level of threat is seen to be a better predictor in the development of PTSD than are objective measures of trauma, and a theoretical position which incorporates the element of meaning is required to explain the PTSD phenomenon.

Research on sleep and dreaming suggests that there may be a unique biological pattern associated with PTSD. For example, Vietnam veterans with combat-related PTSD exhibit sleep abnormalities such as increased REM latency, less REM sleep, diminished stage 4 sleep, and reduced sleep efficiency (Kramer, Kinney, and Scharf, 1982). In addition to an abnormal sleep pattern, disturbed dreaming is a prominent abnormality in chronic PTSD (Ross et al., 1989). These investigators speculated that dream disturbances associated with PTSD may be relatively specific to the disorder, hence, PTSD may be fundamentally a disorder of REM sleep mechanisms.

From the evidence examined, it therefore appears that catastrophic exposure to trauma may be followed by stable biological alterations in the ANS, neuroendocrine system, and the sleep/dream cycle. Such alterations seem to be unique to PTSD, distinguishing it from other psychiatric disorders (Friedman, 1988; Yehuda et al., 1995).

THE PTSD GROUP TREATMENT PROGRAMME

The Ticehurst PTSD Group Treatment Programme closely adheres to the core principles of the model originally developed at the Royal Air Force Hospital Wroughton. However, continuous reappraisal of the model, in light of evolving clinical experience in a mainly civilian population of patients, has led to modifications in the techniques used. A biopsychosocial approach to treatment has been maintained. The program utilizes a highly structured initial two-week residential phase of group work as the cornerstone of treatment, supplemented by one year of follow-up, which includes three formal group day reviews at six weeks, six months, and twelve months. Psychological debriefing (PD) techniques are adapted to the needs of PTSD sufferers traumatized by a wide variety of different experiences. The population at Ticehurst ranges from civilians to retired military personnel to active-duty service personnel.

THE DEVELOPMENT OF THE TRADITION
OF GROUP APPROACHES

There has long been a tradition of utilizing group treatments to alleviate the effects of exposure to traumatic stress in the military world. A full description of the evolution is beyond the scope of this chapter. Tom Main introduced the "therapeutic community" concept in Birmingham, England. His group work encouraged spontaneous emotional interaction between patients and staff (Katz, 1985; Clark, 1977; Harrison and Clarke, 1992). Maxwell-Jones rehabilitated British ex-prisoners of war in London (Katz, 1985).

In the United States, during the aftermath of the Vietnam War, there was a slow realization that veterans were suffering from significant traumatic stress reactions. The history of this period has been traced by Tiffany (1967), Bourne (1970), Collbach and Parrish (1972), Van Putten, Warden, and Emory (1973), Shatan (1973), and Lifton (1978). The introduction of the self-help organization, the Vietnam Veterans Against the War (VVAW), and "rap" groups promoted affinity, mutual availability, and the need to take responsibility for one's own life (Shatan, 1973; Lifton, 1978; Egendorf, 1975). "Rap" groups continued to flourish (Walker, 1983; Henden and Pollinger-Haas, 1984) and the awareness of mental health professionals, especially those working within the Veterans' Administration (VA) medical system grew steadily (Scaturo and Hardoby, 1988; Parson, 1984; Scurfield, Kenderdine, and Pollard, 1990; Peterson, Prout, and Schwartz, 1991). Formal treatments for combat veterans in VA hospitals were based upon highly structured models (Scurfield, 1993).

Gordon Turnbull, hosted by the VA Hospital in Palo Alto, was given permission to study the group treatments available to veterans at the National Center for PTSD in late 1990. This permission was given in anticipation of the need to develop similar programs of treatment for traumatized British combatants in the imminent Gulf War. Lessons learned at Palo Alto were quickly put to good use in the early development of the RAF Wroughton Programme. The three main strategies for the delivery of treatment for PTSD adopted by the Wroughton psychiatric team were:

1. development of a comprehensive assessment process;
2. creation of rapid, cost-effective, efficient, and simply delivered treatment; and
3. essential use of a multidimensional (biopsychosocial) approach.

The full description of the Wroughton Programme is contained in Busuttil et al. (1995). Modifications of this technique, faithful to core philosophies, were used in debriefings of the released British prisoners of war in the 1991 Gulf War and also the released British hostages from Lebanon (later that same year) (Psychiatric Division of the Royal Air Force Medical Service, 1993; Turnbull, 1997). Between 1994 and 1998 further development of the group treatment model for PTSD took place at Ticehurst House Hospital.

ASSESSMENT

In 1991, program developers gave careful consideration to available PTSD rating instruments to distinguish PTSD from other battle stress-related disorders. Core psychological tests found to be of value in both British and international research included the General Health Questionnaire-28 item version (GHQ-28) (Goldberg and Hillier, 1979), the Impact of Event Scale (Horowitz, 1979), and the Symptom Checklist-90 (Derogatis, Lipman, and Covi, 1973). The SCL-90 was later dropped from this list because group candidates felt that it took too long to complete, compared with the other relatively brief, self-report questionnaires. The Clinician-Administered PTSD Scale (CAPS), which assesses both current and lifetime PTSD, and also intensity and frequency of core symptoms of PTSD, was also used throughout the development of the group model (Blake et al., 1990). The Minnesota Multiphasic Personality Inventory (MMPI) PTSD Subscale (Keane, Malloy, and Fairbank, 1984), was originally selected because it was specifically designed to identify PTSD in war veterans, but its usefulness waned when the development moved to Ticehurst because of the increased heterogeneity of the groups. The Beck Depression Inventory (Beck et al., 1979) was used to screen for comorbid depression. In addition, caffeine, alcohol, and other substance usage was quantified using a simple questionnaire.

Further clinical evaluation included mental state examination, which was undertaken by a psychiatrist. Full assessment is usually completed in three hours or less.

A wide range of psychological tests were chosen initially because most of the published research in the late 1980s and early 1990s focused on studies of American and Israeli combat veterans. Little was known about cut-off levels for making the diagnosis of PTSD in the various instruments in a U.K.

population. A concurrent project assessed these levels. Findings of this research strongly supported convergent validity for the tests which the Wroughton team decided to use (Neal et al., 1996).

EFFICIENCY

Highly structured group psychotherapy was the cornerstone of the program, and has remained the primary method of treatment. A twelve-day residential program includes provision of a midprogram weekend break for the completion of "homework" tasks. The weekend also provides an opportunity for "time-out" for rest and relaxation after the intense, focused work of the preceding week. Formal work sessions span a total of sixty-three hours. The program is designed for a minimum of four and a maximum of eight patients; the optimum number has been found to be six patients. The course is run by two dedicated primary therapists/debriefers and one support therapist/debriefer. Primary debriefers become attached to the group and guide them throughout the entire program, and while the debriefers do not become fully integrated into the group, they do facilitate and foster the dynamic group work which starts up very rapidly. Primary and secondary debriefers are experienced in group work and can identify points in the development of the group process played out in their presence. The support (or "secondary") debriefer is always available to debrief the primary debriefers, although this tends to occur once a day after the formal group work has been completed.

When the group program was first conceived during the Gulf War (1991), large numbers of combat-stress casualties were anticipated and treatment was designed to meet this possibility. The preference for group rather than individual management was based on this expectation and also upon previous experiences of relatively poor outcomes for PTSD patients treated in a one-to-one design (insight-orientated, cognitively based therapy) at RAF Wroughton. The opinion was that group work offered distinct advantages by mobilizing therapeutic group dynamics in a homogeneous population (Yalom, 1975).

For reasons of efficiency, and also to test potential advantages of managing heterogeneous groups, it was decided to treat survivors of different traumatic events together in the same group. According to Scaturo and Hardoby (1988), treating sufferers in heterogeneous groups reduces

1. feelings of uniqueness,
2. feelings of isolation, and
3. avoidance and social withdrawal characteristics of PTSD.

The groups now run exclusively at Ticehurst are heterogeneous in terms of trauma, age, gender, religion, ethnicity, etc., but are homogeneous for PTSD. However, more than one survivor from any one specific event should not become involved in a mixed group of survivors. Individual perceptions of what happened may lead to conflict and avoidance issues.

Patients consistently reported that sharing traumatic experiences with survivors of different traumas was specifically helpful to reinforce the growing awareness that reactions to traumatic experiences were stereotyped and universal. The impact of the traumatic event was seen to be more important as a determinant of outcome than were individual variations in personality or coping style.

In selecting group candidates, care was taken to exclude "singletons," i.e., those who would "stick out like a sore thumb." Yalom (1975) described the following advantages of closed, homogeneous groups:

1. Rapidly "get" together
2. Are more cohesive
3. Get more immediate support from group members
4. Have less conflict
5. Offer more rapid relief of symptoms

The strictly adhered-to assessment procedure strongly reinforced group cohesion. The group appeared to represent a "rite of passage" for participants.

BIOPSYCHOSOCIAL STRATEGY

The biopsychosocial approach has been found to facilitate flexible management of PTSD. Burgess-Watson, Hoffman, and Wilson (1988) noted the multifaceted nature of PTSD and observed that it might only be understood properly by a "biopsychosocial approach." Tricyclic medications were initially used to reduce the severity of more intense reexperiencing symptoms (McFarlane, 1989), but, gradually, their use gave way to SSRIs (selective serotonin reuptake inhibitors), drugs consistently found to be superior to tricyclics in this respect. Peripherally acting beta-adrenergic receptor blocking agents (beta-blockers, e.g., propranolol) and centrally acting alpha-adrenergic blocking agents (e.g., clonidine) have proven to be of value incontrolling autonomic nervous system hyperarousal. Benzodiazepines (BZPs) have seldom been used during the daytime but have occasionally been found to be of value as hypnotics. In cases where self-harm, profound guilt, and profound depression have been expressed, major tranquilizers have been used sparingly and almost exclusively when disinhibition has been a potential problem. Mood-regulating drugs such as lithium and carbamazepine (CBZ) have hardly ever been employed. Overall, the use of drugs has been uncommon, both during the initial group management and subsequent follow-up phases.

Psychosocial elements in the treatment strategy are evaluated at the time of the initial assessment. For example, an intrinsic part of each assessment has been an explanation of the theory of PTSD. Those entering the group commonly have misconceptions about the disorder. Explanation of PTSD theory has proven to be of considerable value to patients and family members. Relatives responded positively to explanations of the behavioral changes that they had witnessed in patients. This illumination usually leads to a more enlightened approach to interactions, especially after the initial residential phase when patients return home.

At Wroughton, information leaflets were of two types: one specifically focused on the patient, and the other focused on the relatives. Leaflets included a "crisis" line telephone number. A new leaflet has since been designed and recommends the increasing number of popular books on the subject of PTSD (Kinchin, 1997; Skynner and Cleese, 1983).

Follow-up evaluation after the initial residential phase of treatment has been found to be invaluable and necessary, from both clinical and research perspectives. Originally, this satisfied the occupational requirements of the tight-knit military community where operational capacity was of paramount importance. Follow-up now is especially important in the treatment of individuals who are involved in personal injury litigation (for purposes of prognosis) and for emergency service personnel.

It was decided at the outset that formal group reassessment reviews would be organized at predetermined, postresidential intervals of six weeks, six months, and twelve months. Extra outpatient reviews for individuals, couples, or families were also made available upon request by the patient, a close family member, or the general practitioner to deal with the successive extensions of the victimization process, the so-called "ripple effect" (Symonds, 1980; Figley, 1985).

The Gulf War provided few acute battle-stress casualties. Once hostilities ceased, a steady trickle of Gulf War veterans were referred for assessment to Wroughton. All those who proved positive for PTSD were included in the program. The program also admitted patients who had been traumatized in other critical incidents and wars. These patients included war veterans and civilians from the Falkland Islands conflict of 1982, the Rhodesian monitoring operation of 1980, the Cyprus emergency of the 1970s, the Aden and Malayan emergencies of the 1950s, and the endemic, terrorist operations in Northern Ireland. PTSD victims who were traumatized by the Lockerbie, Scotland, air disaster (1988), the Hillsborough Football Stadium disaster (1989), the Hungerford shooting (1987), road traffic accidents, assaults, and other traumatogenic incidences were also included. Released hostages were also involved (notably victims of the Iraqi "human shield"). The work with released hostages has continued to develop at Ticehurst (and with prisoners who have subsequently been discovered to have been unjustly imprisoned and are conditioned to behave like hostages).

The initial research on the efficacy of the Wroughton version of the group treatment program was based on an evaluation of progress made by a total of sixty-four patients. The program proved to be popular with referring agencies because of the excellent clinical results, and led to a noticeable increase in the referral rate of PTSD patients traumatized in incidents that had occurred before the Gulf War. This also represented an increased awareness of PTSD as a diagnostic entity among general practitioners working both in and out of the military community. Also, these practitioners had begun to believe that effective treatment of PTSD had become a realistic and practical option. Furthermore, increased publicity and medical education (Brandon, 1991a,b) indirectly benefited these forgotten victims. Especially relevant to combat veterans, was the explanation that their covert PTSD had been exacerbated by media coverage of the Gulf War, which may have caused reappearance of symptoms as a result of reminders of their own traumatic experiences. In some, the PTSD symptoms appeared de novo and verified the concept of delayed-onset PTSD.

TECHNIQUE

The Residential Course

The Setting

Group work is carried out in a self-contained, deinstitutionalized living and therapy area ideal for promoting group cohesion. Geographical separation from the general psychiatric treatment unit reinforces the process of "normalization." Group members and therapists are of mixed gender. The variations and mixture of gender-determined attitudes, insights, and perspectives are intrinsically beneficial in promoting normal social relations and behavior.

Therapists and Monitoring of Progress

Group work is facilitated by two primary therapists (primary debriefers). Throughout the development of the model, all primary therapists are trained mental health professionals and include psychiatric nurses, psychiatrists, and clinical psychologists. All therapists have previous experience in group psychotherapy and a firm grounding in the group dynamic process; most also have experience with Psychological Debriefing (PD), also known as Critical Incident Stress Debriefing (CISD).

A supporting therapist (secondary debriefer) carries out a systematic review of the group work with the primary debriefers on a daily, or more frequent basis. This provides an opportunity for ventilation of intense feelings experienced within the group by the primary debriefers. At Ticehurst, the introduction of an experienced and trained group analyst has been shown to significantly enhance the quality of secondary debriefing. Supervision and monitoring of group processes and group dynamics can be facilitated by a secondary debriefer. The primary debriefers are given an opportunity to understand the dynamics and processes of the group as it evolves over the twelve-day period. The secondary debriefer also ensures that objectivity is maintained.

Close contact is maintained with group participants to track their progress. First, each patient is requested to keep a daily journal noting his or her feelings, emotions, and a self-report on progress. These journals are read and discussed by all three therapists each morning before sessional work commences. Second, each patient is interviewed individually by all three therapists on three occasions as part of the course program. These individual meetings reassure the patient that, although he or she is being treated in a group, the integrity of the individual is also valued. This helps to allay fears of being submerged by the group. Meetings are intended to give patients the opportunity to bring to light any self-perceived problems, including those which might not otherwise be brought up during the group sessions. If problems come to the surface that might have significance for the group as a whole and which might stimulate further recovery of the group member who has vented them, therapists attempt to encourage that individual to bring the material up in the group sessions. However, the content of individual journals could also steer group discussions so that the divulged material might be included. It should be pointed out that the content of individual journals is kept strictly confidential and is never discussed during group work. Journals also allow participants to record personal impressions and insights. Reference to the journals after the initial residential phase, during the year of review, has often been very useful. Journals reassure patients about progress they have made, remind them of insights gained, of plans they have made for the future, and whether they are on course with these plans.

The residential course incorporates five main phases which are listed and briefly explained as follows. The same format has been retained in the Ticehurst program.

Phase 1: Introduction and Group Integration

On arrival, patients meet each other informally. This first meeting is important because it represents an unprecedented opportunity, in most cases, for group members to meet other PTSD sufferers. The gradual realization that each one shares the same symptom pattern, despite a wide diversity of traumatic experience, appears to have a remarkable impact, in itself, on reducing anxiety levels. The informality helps to reduce tension and dispel the inevitable apprehension that is bound to develop in those who have committed themselves to the group process.

Introductions to all three therapists occur in the first work session. This session is a very important part of the process; it acts as a "container" for the group by setting boundaries, instills hope (a therapeutic factor described by Yalom, 1975), and normalizes PTSD. It also leads to feelings of trust and safety. The therapists explain the goals of the program, help to draw up a list of the expectations of the group members, request that the journals are used to record them, and circulate a work timetable and a list of boundaries. The first work session also emphasizes the voluntary nature of participation, confidentiality, the absolute necessity of attending all sessions, the prohibition of all nonprescribed drugs including alcohol, and the closed nature of the group.

Therapists also explain monitoring techniques and the role of the support debriefer. The support debriefer departs at this point. A simple "trust exercise" follows to promote further integration, feelings of mutuality, and the formation of alliances within the group. Primary therapists also take part in the trust exercise and begin their relationship with the group.

Each group participant then has an opportunity to meet with all three therapists in a private-room session. The goals of this meeting are to reenforce motivation and offer encouragement. The therapists undertake a relaxed but full mental state examination to screen for and establish the presence or absence of current symptoms, including suicidal risk.

This introduction to the program emphasizes education about trauma and the importance of learning about the processes involved. The "old" medical question, "What is *wrong* with you?" is replaced by what is considered to be the more enlightened "What *happened* to you?"

Phase 2: Personal Accounts

The psychological debriefing (PD) phase is then introduced. Group members listen to a twenty-minute audiotape in which authentic disaster victims describe their experiences and emotions. This tape acts as a template for each group member who, in turn, describes in detail, the facts, emotions, and sensory perceptions surrounding their own traumatic experience, which are the three fundamental components of PD. PD techniques (similar to CISD techniques described by Mitchell, 1983) were originally designed to be utilized in homogeneous groups of disaster victims or emergency workers in the aftermath of a single, unifying disastrous event (Dyregov, 1989). The intention of PD is to facilitate reconstruction assimilation and integration of actual evidence, sensory perceptions, and emotions to promote information processing and, possibly, to prevent PTSD in the long-term. The study of the Piper Alpha disaster body handlers (Alexander and Wells, 1991) has strongly supported the observation that PD techniques represent an effective preventative measure. PD is now entering a period of critical reappraisal (Bisson and Deahl, 1994).

The incorporation of PD as part of the treatment program is essential in light of information-processing theory. The PD technique used does not represent a simple "disclosure" of impressions of the traumatic experience. The use of PD in a heterogeneous group of chronic PTSD sufferers does not appear to cause problems. Diverse traumatic events share common themes and "cross identification" is not difficult. The life threat, the loss of control and dignity, the destruction of the "myth of invulnerability," the "shattered assumptions" (described by Janoff-Bulman, 1985), the misinterpretations regarding personal performance and the handling of the disaster by those in authority, are identified with relative ease in the group. The same applies to the stereotyped PTSD symptom clusters. This helps group members to release previously repressed memories by listening to other group participants. The group should always insist on highly detailed personal accounts which prompt a clearer recollection of each individual trauma and restore a sense of "being in control." The use of PD, therefore, promotes strongly cohesive, supportive alliances. After completion of formal group work, group members often continue to discuss the information revealed during their "own time." Fellow sufferers possess more credibility as empathetic listeners than do therapists. After completion of this phase, reexperiencing symptoms appear to diminish in intensity and there is a noticeable reduction of anxiety levels and avoidance/numbing symptoms.

Before the original development of the group treatment program, similar PD techniques were used within the framework of individual treatment. However, using the PD techniques in a group format (as was originally reported by Mitchell, 1983) optimizes information processing because of the shared learning experience.

Throughout the continued evolution of the program at Ticehurst, a realization of the importance of nonverbal communications in relating the impact of the trauma within the group has occurred. Although obvious "body language" expressions have been recognized for a long time, it is only relatively recently that powerful, unconsciously motivated reenactments of the trauma are frequently used to express what has occurred. Reenactments are perceived to be of most significance when the trauma has an interpersonal basis.

"Survivor guilt" was categorized as an associated feature of PTSD in the DSM-III-R definition. The phenomenon of "survivor guilt" is more common in combat veterans than in any other category of PTSD patient (Crocq et al., 1993). Survivor guilt has a particularly corrosive quality on self-esteem and is often closely associated with profound depression (Williams, 1987). The group process appears to be especially effective in dispelling "survivor guilt." This appears to be the result of the dispelling of perceptual distortions on which survivor guilt is commonly based. Distortions are challenged by other group members. Permitting the venting of overcontrolled anger, which has become introjected, also helps to lessen this guilt. In fact, some patients who have gone through this group program eventually begin to regard their traumatic experiences as having provided an unfortunate, yet imperative opportunity for personal growth.

Phase 3: Didactic Teaching and Discussion

Three topics are included in this teaching:

1. Stress and its management
2. Post-traumatic stress disorder
3. Drugs commonly used and abused by PTSD sufferers

The aim of this phase is to supply information, dispel misconceptions, and promote the identification and discussion of common problems. Group members make notes of insights gained and lessons learned in their journals.

Stress and its management. Group members identify both the psychological and the physical symptoms of anxiety. Therapists emphasize the cognitive theories of anxiety and develop the theme that external stressors are fundamentally important as triggering factors in the evolution of PTSD. The "Gatekeeper" (Criterion "A" in the DSM-IV, APA, 1994) is used to make the point that not only does the stressful event need to be perceived as threatening, it also needs to produce a powerful emotional reaction of fear, terror, or helplessness for the event to become truly traumagenic. Therapists use the Yerkes-Dodson law (Yerkes and Dodson, 1908) to illustrate the relationship between arousal and performance, including the impact on concentration, and emphasize the need to be able to recognize stress/arousal levels in all facets of day-to-day life including occupational, social, and family stresses. By acknowledging that stress exists in everyone's life and needs to be self-managed, therapists can introduce practical concepts of how to prevent and reduce stress. This may include planning a schedule, achieving a balance between work and leisure, appropriate allocation of work, the importance of physical exercise, constructive personal debriefing and emotional ventilation, "worry work," and anxiety management. To provide a contrast to this constructive attitude to living and minimizing stress levels, therapists describe negative, stress-laden lifestyles that are characterized by a lack of awareness of stress and maladaptive stress-reduction behaviors.

A session of formal Anxiety Management Training (AMT) by means of deep muscular relaxation (Jacobson, 1962) demonstrates that stress relief is possible. Thereafter, muscular relaxation training sessions become a daily event. Upon discharge, each patient is given an audiotape of the exercise that is best suited to himself or herself and is guided to use it as frequently as possible. A physical exercise session each day of the program helps to reduce stress, build group cohesion, and encourage distraction as secondary goals. At Ticehurst, aromatherapy and reflexology sessions have been found to be helpful also.

Post-traumatic stress disorder. Therapists discuss the current definition of PTSD in the DSM-IV and put this into proper historical perspective. The full history of PTSD helps group members to appreciate the crucial importance of the DSM-III to the crystallization of modern concepts, but also makes them aware that traumatic stress reactions have been recognized since ancient times and have been regarded as part of general experience known as the "human condition." Therapists make the distinction between acute stress disorder (ASD in DSM-IV) and post-traumatic stress disorder (PTSD in DSM-IV). ASD is explained as a transient reaction presenting within one month of exposure to a traumatic experience, while PTSD represents a chronic disorder, often heralded in by ASD, which shares the same or very similar symptom clusters. PTSD becomes the "cocoon" that encapsulates the unprocessed memories of a traumatic experience which may continue to exist interminably. Therapists emphasize that a proactive approach to the processing of the traumatic memories becomes necessary once PTSD has developed, and that a passive fading away of symptoms over time does not appear to happen in most cases. The group is encouraged to "normalize" reactions by discussing the inevitability of the ASD/PTSD response (if the "Gatekeeper" criterion is satisfied), and to be aware of high prevalence rates for PTSD both in the United Kingdom (Jackson, 1991) and in the United States (Helzer, Robins, and McEvoy, 1987).

Drugs commonly used and abused by PTSD sufferers. Therapists discuss drug abuse and dependency and an explanation of withdrawal syndromes with group participants. Alcohol, caffeine, nicotine, minor tranquilizers (e.g., benzodiazepines), and minor analgesics (often containing opiates in proprietary, "over-the-counter" preparations which do not require medical prescription) have a specific relationship to biological "underpinnings" of

PTSD (van der Kolk et al., 1985; Ochberg, 1993) and therapists make special mention of these factors.

Phase 4: Personal Audit

The primary aims of a personal audit are to promote self-awareness and personal responsibility and to encourage group participants to improve the degree of self-control in their lives. Two simple exercises have been developed for use in the course. These are the "Lines" and "Ladders" exercises.

Lines exercise. Group members are asked to plot a time graph of their lives as a "homework" task during the weekend break in the middle of the residential period. Members note all significant high and low points and plot positive and negative events on the vertical axis (including a neutral midway point representing zero). Age in years is represented on the horizontal axis. Members chart the whole of their lifetime experience as well as the critical period of exposure to the traumatic stressor and use their journals to help them to present their own significant life events to other group members in an easily grasped, graphical, step-wise, and coherent way. Therapists at Ticehurst have noted that it is not helpful for group members to involve others in the construction of their Lines initially because perspectives become confused and the process can become contaminated. Initially, the Lines exercise is intended to be a private, personal, self-audit which is then shared with other group members. Group members are encouraged to discuss their traumatic experiences and the meaning of their PTSD symptoms with their families and partners during the weekend break. The weekend also serves to further reduce the risk of dependency on the therapists and fosters a sense of personal responsibility for the resolution of symptoms.

After the weekend break, group members are shown a video depicting authentic PTSD sufferers talking about their traumatic experiences and coping strategies. The goal of this video at this stage in the group process is to enhance self-awareness of different coping styles when confronted by distressing material. Characteristically, most group participants have tended to avoid any media coverage of distressing events because it has reminded them of their own trauma. Some high-profile cases have actually been reported by the media. The showing of the video follows the principles of classical behavioral exposure. At the outset, everyone agrees to switch off the video on request, although group participants contract to watch the entire film, no matter how distressing and how long it takes. The film brings into sharp perspective the contrast between positive and negative coping styles that have been used by those who have been filmed. Group participants identify the "adaptive" and "maladaptive" coping styles that they have utilized in their own attempts to process traumatic experiences, share these insights, and compare and contrast them with what they have seen on the film.

Each group member presents the Lines exercise on a white board to other members and invites their comments and criticism. The Lines exercise has two major therapeutic benefits for group participants. For the first time, the traumatic event is fitted into the context of whole-life experience and is compared with other high and low points. A new perspective is gained. Second, the graphical representation allows therapists to help the individual identify positive and negative behavioral coping patterns brought about by significant life events other than the trauma. These patterns of behavior often prove to have considerable resonance for other group members and become highly significant entries in the journals. The group becomes increasingly aware of inherent coping styles, and maladaptive patterns can be identified as maintaining factors for the PTSD. Group discussion highlights the effects of these maladaptive patterns of behavior on other aspects of their lives, their families, and social contacts.

Ladder exercise. The Ladder exercise permits the individual to plan his or her future by identifying short- and long-term goals which the participants then present to the entire group for discussion and reality testing. Plans need to be as realistic as possible, and in keeping with the individual's coping styles identified in the Lines exercise. The individual's own coping styles are adopted into future planning, with the emphasis on using positive coping strategies and abandoning maladaptive strategies.

In this exercise, group participants draw a ladder with several rungs on a large sheet of paper. On the top rung they place their long-term goal, and on the bottom rung the lowest point in their lives. The intervening rungs are filled in by the individual as "steps" to be taken to achieve the ultimate goal. The Ladder exercise needs to be multidimensional. Dimensions include marital, family, social, occupational, and financial aspects of living, and vary according to individual need. Each individual presents the plan to the group to facilitate reality testing. The Ladder may be modified through positive feedback from other group members and is then incorporated into the individual's journal for future reference and updating during the year of review. The Ladder exercise enhances powers of self-criticism, self-awareness, and self-esteem and makes maximum use of local support networks. At Ticehurst, solution-focused brief therapy (as cited in de Shazer, 1985) is of especially practical value in translating the Ladders exercise from theory into practice. It helps to define firm and detailed goals and identify the "preferred future." The Lines exercise, hopefully, has previously identified positive coping strategies and strengths which can be used as tools to achieve goals at this stage, as the individual attempts to build a picture of life without PTSD.

Phase 5: Family Reintegration

Family reintegration is the final phase of the course. Family members, including spouses, children, and partners attend this session by invitations made by group participants. This phase starts with a review of the basic concepts of PTSD and the impact that it has on individual survivors. The discussion then expands to include a description of the impact of PTSD on partners and families (not forgetting children) and on other important social and occupational relationship patterns.

The discussion covers a variety of psychological models including primary survival emotions (Mills,1998), human relating models, Transactional Analysis, and Family Systems. Group members and their partners and families then both take part in an active discussion facilitated by a primary debriefer and a member of the trauma team with experience in relationship work. Therapists see spouses, partners, family members, etc., privately, if they wish, or, perhaps, together with the relevant group member. A key concern of the group members at this stage is the difficulties that they experience in sharing details of their trauma reactions with family members, something they have already accomplished with fellow group members. Research conducted at Ticehurst has revealed that 90 percent of group members have been unable to share their traumatic experiences with their families and partners before entering the group (Mills, 1998). Reasons for this include

- protection of partners,
- desire to keep the family system uncontaminated,
- avoidance, and
- fear of receiving an inappropriate response.

Family members gain insight into the psychological mechanisms that underpin the failure of communication and this helps them to look at their relationships in a new light. Further specialist help with relationship and intimacy issues for couples and individuals is available if deemed necessary.

Before this phase is concluded, "safety nets" are discussed which will help group members and their families to deal with any future crises. Ideally, local facilities should be utilized to minimize dependency on the trauma unit, and empowerment of group members and their family systems should also be emphasized. The group disperses after setting a suitable date for the first review (which occurs at six weeks) and after circulating the crisis telephone number.

Reviews

The group reassembles to review progress at six weeks, six months, and one year postresidential phase. Assessments identical to those carried out at the initial point of contact are repeated. Each review includes group discussion with emphasis on residual symptoms of PTSD, what problems have been solved and how, and on progress up the rungs of the Ladder exercise. The primary debriefers concentrate on the maintenance of nonjudgmental attitudes and offer positive and constructive criticism throughout reviews.

DISCUSSION

The Group Treatment Programme at Ticehurst for PTSD has been cost effective. The wide geographical dispersion of patients is compatible with an inpatient approach, at least in the initial phase of the program. The efficacy of the program is fully described in a published article (Busuttil et al., 1995). Results have shown that 83.5 percent of patients no longer fulfill the DSM-III-R criteria for PTSD at the one-year review. The high success rate indicates that further controlled studies designed to evaluate the value of psychological debriefing (PD) techniques in the treatment of established PTSD are required. Preliminary results of a study of the evolved technique used at Ticehurst show recovery figures that are not dissimilar to the Wroughton study, demonstrating the "portability" of the program from a predominantly (though not exclusively) military population of patients to a predominantly civilian population.

Therapists involved in the evolving design of this group program continue to remain convinced that the initial residential phase is a very important contributing factor to highly successful outcomes. The residential setting rapidly and consistently generates a safe and trusting environment which facilitates Psychological Debriefing and the processing of traumatic memories. Group participants appreciate that they make rapid progress, even though they may have been suffering from PTSD for a considerable time. This is very encouraging, and provides a new optimism for recovery. Results indicate that this optimism is borne out in approximately 75 percent of cases. It is very unusual for patients not to make at least a partial recovery, and of those who do not recover within the year of review, some make slower progress over a longer period of time. Often, they have a specific obstacle to overcome before they make a full recovery. Hurdles have included involvement in personal injury litigation, marital problems, unresolved legal proceedings over custody and visitation disputes regarding access to children following divorce, and decisions about premature retirement on the grounds of ill health. In other cases, the presenting traumatic stress reaction has unveiled previous traumas, including both "simple" and "complex" traumatic experiences. The latter includes childhood abuse, an event not previously recognized as a source of symptoms or, in some cases, an event completely repressed by patients themselves.

GROUP PROGRAM FOR COMPLEX PTSD

A new group treatment program was established at Ticehurst in 1997 to treat individuals exposed to multiple severe psychological trauma. Patients included those subjected to torture, repeated battery in marriage, repeated abuse in childhood, several adverse experiences in an emergency work environment, and others who had developed complex PTSD. Complex PTSD is a concept that was developed after extensive field trials in the United States by the American Psychiatric Association. Field trial studies demonstrated that victims of multiple trauma not only suffer classical symptoms of PTSD (persistent reexperiencing, persistent avoidance and emotional blunting, and hyperarousal, especially hypervigilance), but also changes in character, repetitive self-harm, and putting others at risk. Assessment includes full clinical evaluation and a series of validated self-report and clinician-administered questionnaires. The goal of assessment is to identify presence and severity of core PTSD symptom clusters. Social and occupational impact, comorbid depression, illicit drug use, excessive use of commonly used substances such as alcohol, caffeine, and nicotine are also evaluated.

A structured, ninety-day rehabilitation program has been developed which includes a combination of group and individual work, embraced by a milieu therapy environment. The program is comprised of three "blocks," each lasting one month. These are psycho-education, disclosure, and cognitive restructuring. Follow-up consists of three group reviews at six weeks, six months, and twelve months. Preliminary evaluation has demonstrated very favorable outcomes for reduced hospital readmission, improved function, and symptom reduction.

CONCLUSION

Elimination of emotionally crippling symptoms is the primary goal of treatment approaches in PTSD. The group treatment model described in this chapter tackles biological, psychological, and social dimensions of the disorder. Its high rate of success may reflect this biopsychosocial approach which leaves "no stone unturned."

REFERENCES

Alexander, D.A. and Wells, A. (1991). Reactions of police officers to body handling after a major disaster. A before and after comparison. *British Journal of Psychiatry, 159,* 547-555.

American Psychiatric Association (1980). *Diagnostic and Statistical Manual of Mental Disorders,* Third Edition (DSM-III). Washington, DC: APA.

American Psychiatric Association (1987). *Diagnostic and Statistical Manual of Mental Disorders,* Third Edition, Revised (DSM-III-R). Washington, DC: APA.

American Psychiatric Association (1994). *Diagnostic and Statistical Manual of Mental Disorders,* Fourth Edition (DSM-IV). Washington, DC: APA.

Bandura, A., Adams, N., and Beyer, J. (1977). Cognitive processes mediating behavioral change. *Journal of Personality and Social Psychology, 35,* 125-139.

Beck, A.T., Rush, A., Shaw, B.F., et al. (1979). *Cognitive Therapy of Depression.* New York: Guilford Press.

Bisson, J.L. and Deahl, M.P. (1994). Psychological debriefing and the prevention of post-traumatic stress. *British Journal of Psychiatry, 165,* 717-720.

Blake, D.D., Weathers, F.W., Nagy, L.M., et al. (1990). A clinician rating scale for assessing current and lifetime PTSD: The CAPS-1. *The Behavior Therapist, 13,* 187-188.

Bourne, P.G. (1970) Military psychiatry and the Vietnam experience. *American Journal of Psychiatry, 127,* 481-488.

Brandon, S. (1991a). Advice to psychiatrists concerning casualties repatriated to NHS hospitals from the Gulf. *British Journal of Psychiatry, 158,* Advice enclosure.

Brandon, S. (1991b). The psychological aftermath of war. *British Medical Journal, 302,* 305-306.

Burgess-Watson, I.P., Hoffman, L., and Wilson, G.V. (1988). The neuropsychiatry of post traumatic stress disorder. *British Journal of Psychiatry, 152,* 164-173.

Busuttil, W., Turnbull, G.J., Neal, L.A., West, A.G., Blanch, N., and Herepath, R. (1995). Incorporating psychological debriefing techniques within a brief group psychotherapy programme for the treatment of post-traumatic stress disorder. *British Journal of Psychiatry, 167,* 495-502.

Chemtob, C.M., Baker, G.B., and Neller, G. (1990). Post-traumatic stress disorder among special forces Vietnam veterans. *Military Medicine, 155,* 16-20.

Clark, D.H. (1977). The therapeutic community. *British Journal of Psychiatry, 131,* 553-564.

Collbach, E.M. and Parrish, M.D. (1972). Army mental health activities in Vietnam: 1965-1970, In *The Vietnam Veteran in Contemporary Society,* Washington, DC: Veterans Administration.

Crocq, M.A., Macher, J.P., Barros-Beck, J., et al. (1993). Post-traumatic stress disorder in World War II prisoners of war from Alsace-Lorraine who survived captivity in the USSR. In *International Handbook of Traumatic Stress Syndromes,* eds. J P. Wilson and B. Raphael (pp. 253-261). New York: Plenum Press.

de Shazer, S. (1985). *Keys to Solutions in Brief Therapy.* New York: Norton.

Derogatis, L.R., Lipman, R.S., and Covi, L. (1973). SCL-90: An outpatient psychiatric rating scale—Preliminary report. *Psychopharmacology Bulletin, 9,* 13-28.

Dyregov, A. (1989). Caring for helpers in disaster situations; psychological debriefing. *Disaster Management, 2,* 25-30.

Egendorf, A. (1975). Vietnam veteran rap groups and themes of post war life. *Journal of Social Issues, 31,* 111-124.

Figley, C.R. (1985). From victim to survivor: Social responsibility in the wake of catastrophe. In *Trauma and Its Wake: The Study and Treatment of Post-Traumatic Stress Disorder,* Volume 1, ed. C.R. Figley (pp. 398-415). New York: Brunner/Mazel.

Foa, E.B. and Kozak, M.J. (1986). Emotional processing of fear: Exposure to corrective information. *Pyschological Bulletin 99,* 20-35.

Foa, E.B., Steketee, G., and Rothbaum, B. O. (1989). Behavioural/cognitive conceptualisations of post-traumatic stress disorder. *Behaviour Therapy, 20,* 155-176.

Fowlie, D.G. and Aveline, M.O. (1985). The emotional consequences of ejection, rescue and rehabilitation in Royal Air Force aircrew. *British Journal of Psychiatry, 146,* 609-613.

Freud, S. (1919) Psychoanalysis and war neuroses. In *Sigmund Freud, Collected Papers,* Volume 5, ed. and trans. J. Strachey (pp. 83-87). London: Hogarth Press.

Friedman, M.J. (1988). Toward rational pharmacotherapy for post-traumatic stress disorder: An interim report. *American Journal of Psychiatry, 143,* 281-285.

Goldberg, D.P. and Hillier, V.F. (1979). A scaled version of the general health questionnaire. *Psychological Medicine, 9,* 139-145.

Harel, Z., Boaz, K., and Wilson, J.P. (1993). War and remembrance: The legacy of Pearl Harbor. In *International Handbook of Traumatic Stress Syndromes,* eds. J. P. Wilson and B. Raphael (pp. 263-274). New York: Plenum Press.

Harrison, T. and Clarke, D. (1992). The Northfield experiments. *British Journal of Psychiatry, 160,* 698-708.

Helzer, J.E., Robins, L.N., and McEvoy, L. (1987). PTSD in the general population: findings of the epidemiological catchment area study. *New England Journal of Medicine, 317,* 1630-1634.

Hendin, H. and Pollinger-Haas, A. (1984). *Wounds of War: The Psychological Aftermath of Combat in Vietnam.* New York: Basic Books.

Horowitz, M.J. (1975). Intrusive and repetitive thoughts after stress. *Archives of General Psychiatry, 32,* 1457-1463.

Horowitz, M.J. (1979). Psychological response to serious life events. In *Human Stress and Cognition,* eds. V. Hamilton and D.M. Warburton (pp. 235-263). New York: Wiley.

Jackson, G. (1991). The rise of post-traumatic stress disorders. *British Medical Journal, 303,* 533-534.

Jacobson, E. (1962). *You Must Relax.* New York: McGraw-Hill.

Janoff-Bulman, R. (1985). The aftermath of victimisation: Rebuilding shattered assumptions. In *Trauma and Its Wake: The Study and Treatment of Post Traumatic Stress Disorder,* Volume 1, ed. C. R. Figley (pp. 15-35). New York: Brunner/Mazel.

Kardiner, A. (1941). *The Traumatic Neuroses of War.* New York: Hoeber.

Katz, S.E. (1985). Psychiatric hospitalisation. In *Comprehensive Textbook of Psychiatry,* Volume 1, eds. H.I. Kaplan and B.J. Sadock (pp. 1576-1582). Philadelphia: Lippincott Williams &Wilkins.

Keane, T.M., Malloy, P.F., and Fairbank, J.A. (1994). Empirical development of an MMPI subscale for the assessment of combat-related post-traumatic stress disorder. *Journal of Consulting and Clinical Psychology, 52,* 881-891.

Kinchin, D. (1997). *Post-Traumatic Stress Disorder: The Invisible Injury.* London: Successunlimited.

Kramer, M., Kinney, L., and Scharf, M. (1982). Sleep in delayed stress victims. *Sleep Research, 11,* 113.

Lifton, R.J. (1978). Advocacy and corruption in the healing profession. In *Stress Disorders Among Vietnam Veterans: Theory, Research and Treatment,* ed. C.R. Figtey (pp. 209-230). New York: Brunner/Mazel.

Maier, S.F. and Seligman, M.E. (1976). Learned helplessness: Theory and evidence. *Journal of Experimental Psychology; General, 105,* 3-46.

Mawson, D., Marks, I.M., Ramm, E., et al. (1981). Guided mourning for morbid grief: A controlled study. *British Journal of Psychiatry, 38,* 185-193.

McFarlane, A.C. (1989). The treatment of post-traumatic stress disorder. *British Journal of Psychiatry, 62,* 81-90.

Mills, C.S. (1998). *Heads I Win, Tails You Lose: The Impact of Traumatic Life-Events on Relationships.*

Mitchell, J.T. (1983). When disaster strikes: The critical incident stress debriefing process. *Journal of Emergency Medical Services, 8,* 36-39.

Mowrer, O.H. (1960). *Learning Theory and Behaviour.* New York: Wiley.

Neal, L.A., Busuttil, W., Rollins, J.R., Herepath, R., Strike, P., and Turnbull, G.J. (1996). Convergent validity of measures of post-traumatic stress disorder in a mixed military and civilian population. *Journal of Traumatic Stress, 7,* 447-455.

Ochberg, F.M. (1993). Post traumatic therapy. In *The International Handbook of Traumatic Stress Syndromes,* eds. J.P. Wilson and B. Raphael (pp. 773-783). New York: Plenum Press.

Parson, E.R. (1984). The role of psychodynamic group therapy in the treatment of the combat veteran. In *Psychotherapy of the Combat Veteran,* ed. H.J. Schwartz, (pp. 153-220). New York: S. P. Medical and Scientific Books.

Pennebaker, J.W. and Susman, J.R. (1988). Disclosure of traumas and psychosomatic processes. *Social Science and Medicine, 26,* 327-332.

Peterson, K.C., Prout, M.F., and Schwartz, R.A. (1991). *Post-Traumatic Stress Disorder: A Clinician's Guide.* New York: Plenum Press.

Psychiatric Division of the Royal Air Force Medical Service (1993). The management of hostages after release. *Psychiatric Bulletin, 17,* 35-37.

Rachman, S. (1978). An anatomy of obsessions. *Behavioural Analysis and Modification, 2,* 253-278.

Rachman, S. (1980). Emotional processing. *Behaviour Research and Therapy, 18,* 51-60.

Ramsay, R.W. (1977). Behavioural approaches to bereavement. *Behaviour Research and Therapy, 15,* 131-135.

Ross, R.J., Ball, W.A., Sullivan, K.A., et al. (1989). Sleep disturbance as a hallmark of post-traumatic stress disorder. *American Journal of Psychiatry, 146,* 697-707.

Scaturo, D.J. and Hardoby, W.J. (1988). Psychotherapy with traumatised Vietnam combatants: An overview of individual, group and family treatment modalities. *Military Medicine, 153,* 262-269.

Scurfield, R.M. (1993). Treatment of post-traumatic stress disorder among Vietnam veterans. In *International Handbook of Traumatic Stress Syndromes,* eds. J. P. Wilson and B. Raphael (pp. 879-888). New York: Plenum Press.

Scurfield, R.M., Kenderdine, S.K., and Pollard, R.J. (1990). Inpatient treatment for war-related post-traumatic stress disorder: Initial findings on a longer-term outcome study. *Journal of Traumatic Stress, 3,* 185-201.

Seligman, M.E.P. (1975). *Helplessness: On Depression, Development and Death.* San Francisco: C. A. Freeman.

Shatan, C.F. (1973). How do we turn off the guilt? *Human Behaviour, 2,* 56-61.

Skynner, R. and Cleese, J. (1983). *Families and How to Survive Them.* London: Methuen.

Strian, F. and Klicpera, C. (1978). Significance of autonomic arousal for the development and persistence of anxiety state. *Nervenarzt, 49,* 576-583.

Symonds, M. (1980). Victim responses to terror. *Annals of New York Academy of Sciences, 347,* 129-136.

Tiffany, W.J. (1967). Mental health of army troops in Vietnam. *American Journal of Psychiatry, 123,* 1585-1586.

Turnbull, G.J. (1994a). Debriefing of released British hostages from the Lebanon. *National Center for PTSD Clinical Quarterly, 4,* 21-22.

Turnbull, G.J. (1994b). Sensory deprivation in hostages. In *The Neurological Boundaries of Reality,* ed. E.M.R. Critchley. Ferrand Press: London.

Turnbull, G.J. (1997). Hostage retrieval. *Journal of the Royal Society of Medicine, 90,* 478-483.

van der Kolk, B.A., Greenberg, M.S., Boyd, H., et al. (1985). Inescapable shock, neurotransmitter and addiction to trauma: Towards a psychobiology of post traumatic stress. *Biological Psychiatry, 20,* 314-325.

Van Putten, T., Warden, H., and Emory, M.D. (1973). Traumatic neuroses in Vietnam returnees. *Archives of General Psychiatry, 29,* 695-698.

Walker, J. (1983). Comparison of "rap" groups with traditional group therapy in the treatment of Vietnam combat veterans. *Group, 2,* 48-57.

Williams, T. (1987). Diagnosis and treatment of survivor guilt. In *Post-Traumatic Stress Disorders: A Handbook for Clinicians,* ed. T. Williams (pp. 75-92). Cincinnati: Disabled American Veterans.

World Health Organization (1992). *The ICD-10 Classification of Mental and Behavioural Disorders: Clinical Descriptions and Diagnostic Guidelines.* Geneva: WHO.

Yalom, I.D. (1975). *The Theory and Practice of Group Psychotherapy.* New York: Basic Books.

Yehuda, R., Kahana, B., Binder-Byrnes, S., Southwick, S., Mason, J., and Giller, E.L. (1995). Low urinary cortisol excretion in Holocaust survivors with posttraumatic stress disorder. *American Journal of Psychiatry, 152,* 982-986.

Yerkes, R.M. and Dodson, J.D. (1908). The relation of strength of stimulus to rapidity of habit formation. *Journal of Comparative Neurological Psychology, 18,* 459-482.

Chapter 9

Developing and Maintaining a Psychoeducational Group for Persons Diagnosed As DID/MPD/DDNOS

Mary Beth Williams
Sandra Gindlesperger Nuss

INTRODUCTION

Little has been written or presented concerning group treatment of Multiple Personality Disorder/Dissociative Identity Disorder (MPD/DID) clients (Caul, 1984; Coons and Bradley, 1985; Putnam, 1989; Caul, Sachs, and Braun, 1986; Kluft, 1989; Hogan, 1992; Turkus and Courtois, 1994). Ross and Gahan (1988) believe that group therapy is nonessential, and that the group is an adjunct to individual psychotherapy. Buchele (1995) has written that group therapy is "quite helpful to most patients . . . at some point during the recovery process . . . usually most effective when combined with individual psychotherapy" (p. 86). The ISSD (International Society for the Study of Dissociation) *Guidelines for Treating Dissociative Identity Disorder (Multiple Personality Disorder) in Adults* (Barach, 1994) notes that group therapy is not the primary means of treatment but can be useful as an adjunct treatment method.

One form of group therapy is the educational support group. According to the International Society for Traumatic Stress Studies (ISTSS) treatment guidelines in *Group Psychotherapy for Posttraumatic Stress Disorder* (ISTSS, 1999), supportive group therapy is a type of "covering" therapy designed to maintain interpersonal comfort within a context of present-focused coping. This type of group brings persons with like or similar diagnoses together in a bond of commonality of experience and need. Studies of group treatment, the guidelines suggest, provide potentially effective assistance to trauma survivors (based on fourteen studies). Because individuals diagnosed with DID frequently have a high level of anxiety arousal, suicidality, and fear of self-disclosure, a more "uncovering" type of group treatment would not be appropriate.

Group membership reduces feelings of isolation, emphasizes commonality, lessens the sense of stigmatization and deviance, and helps build an identification with others (Briere, 1989). For example, many persons diagnosed with DID state that their condition is exhausting. Hearing this belief from others is normalizing. Yalom (1985) has concluded that group participation can instill hope, impart information, provide a sense of universality, teach socialization techniques and imitative behavior, build interpersonal learning, and correctly recapitulate the primary family group, among other factors. From the humanistic viewpoint, groups are supportive environments for the sharing of experiences and provide opportunities to give mutual self-help and develop interpersonal coping skills.

According to Overbeck and Overbeck (1995), support groups have many functions. Among them are to provide a safe, nonjudgmental setting for sharing with peers and to provide ideas and avenues for members to begin to regain control over their lives. Support groups also provide opportunities for formation of new support relationships outside the group and opportunities for members to share knowledge and experience. The New Jersey Support Group Clearinghouse (1990) identified four characteristics of support groups:

1. Mutual help through pooling knowledge and sharing experiences as members try to help one another
2. Peer support gained through sharing of common problems or stressful life situations, resulting in an "you're not alone" sense
3. Affordability through either no-fee or minimal-fee structures
4. Exclusivity when groups are run by members without professionals

The ISTSS treatment guidelines (ISTSS, 1999) add that supportive approaches

a. acknowledge and validate the traumatic exposure;
b. normalize traumatic responses;
c. utilize the presence of other individuals with a similar history to dispel the idea that a therapist without a similar history cannot be helpful because that therapist has not shared the experience; and
d. adopt a nonjudgmental stance toward survival behavior required at the time of the trauma. (p. 3)

Supportive groups do not focus on the details of "what happened," when validating the actual impact of the trauma. Group interventions can be helpful in exploring "middle range affects of frustration, sadness, happiness, hurt" (ISTSS, 1999, p. 5) to diffuse more extreme affects related to hyperarousal (rage, terror). Support groups generally help members maintain some level of personal comfort with a fairly low level of demand (p. 5). In addition, groups orient clients toward current coping, assist members to mobilize strengths and competence, and "reduce or control interference from symptoms and trauma-based attitudes, as they affect social, emotional, occupational, recreational, and health-related functioning" (p. 5). Groups also provide support for concurrent individual treatment. However, support groups do tend to be less flexible in accommodating to individual needs, although supportive group therapy may be better for less stable individuals than a more uncovering type of group therapy.

Turkus (1991) writes that group treatment for clients diagnosed with MPD must occur within a structure. Goals of a group include identification of distorted perceptions and dysfunctional thinking, and helping clients to learn self-management of and behavioral techniques for control of symptoms. Groups, therefore, function as a setting for responsible alters to practice control and express emotions in a constructive way while members creatively help one another. In addition, groups help members establish boundaries for themselves, set limits, and build social networks. Members experience the reality factor of sharing common experiences in a confidential environment that fosters group problem solving and practicing of communication skills. In addition, members who are further along in treatment (e.g., who have mapped their systems, have integrated or fused some alters, who have been able to maintain employment while healing) serve as resource persons and role models for those who are newly diagnosed or have less developed self-knowledge or coping skills.

HISTORY OF THE GROUP

The educationally oriented outpatient support group described in this chapter was established by a private psychiatric facility, Dominion Hospital (Falls Church, VA), as a community service in September 1993. The group was supported by Dominion Hospital until January 1997. At that time, at hospital direction, it was changed to a self-pay group. However, most of the members of the group were unable to maintain even a low fee and membership decreased dramatically. The group continued through the summer of 1997 with a general membership of five to seven persons. When it was formed, the hospital staff envisioned the group as a way to assist members to deal with emotional stresses by teaching new coping skills, educating members about the problem or illness, supporting one another in dealing with new problems, and encouraging one another in treatment outside the group.

The group was originally open-ended, with open membership and no screening of members. It was advertised in the local newspaper as a walk-in group for anyone with the MPD/DID diagnosis. Members were expected to be in individual therapy; however, there was no follow-up to see if this was the case or if attendees actually had an MPD/DID diagnosis. New members could enter each week, on a continuing basis. This policy was extremely stressful and led to extreme emotional reactivity in many members.

Initially, a totally open format and lack of screening, though undesirable to the leaders, was the preferred method of service delivery by the hospital. However, it was not until a group member who was not in treatment and did not have a confirmed diagnosis was arrested for stalking another group member, among other charges, that the policy was changed. Group leaders were then able to insist that members be screened through the hospital's First Step Program (an initial screening and diagnostic component), that signed authorizations for participation be given by each member's individual therapist, and that membership be limited to no more than sixteen members at any one time. A series of screening questions were developed by the group members and leaders as a formal screening interview (Yalom, 1985).

COMPOSITION AND STRUCTURE OF THE GROUP

Between the time of its creation until its termination in 1997, the no-fee group met for approximately seventy-five minutes weekly and was open to new members on the first session of the month. Members developed a group contract which encouraged them to attend regularly and be on time. If members were going to be absent for extended periods of time, they notified the leaders. There were no age or gender requirements. The youngest group member was twenty-one; the oldest, mid-fifties. Members of the group had a diverse phenomenology. The majority presented with high levels of guilt and shame concerning their diagnoses as well as with many interpersonal problems with family members, peers, spouses, co-workers, and fellow students. They frequently exhibited dissociative symptoms during group when painful material was introduced or when they were triggered. Their symptoms were similar to those reported in a variety of research studies of trauma survivors (Briere, 1992; Briere and Runtz, 1988; Brown and Anderson, 1991; Chu and Dill, 1990; Courtois, 1988; Jehu, 1988; Saunders et al., 1992; van der Kolk, Perry, and Herman, 1991; Williams, 1990). The majority were socially isolated; a few members who had been hospitalized together had occasional out-of-group social contacts with one another. The amount of additional outside contact was decided by the group (Watson, 1994). Members who chose to exchange phone numbers often used one another as a support system when crises occurred and provided each other with specific, situation-oriented information (e.g., what to do when, how to cope with . . .) in a very here-and-now-oriented manner. Members also helped one another problem solve, a technique used consistently in group sessions.

The group had coleaders; however, the second leader was not licensed and could not lead the group on her own. Because group members would not accept a substitute leader, when the first leader was out of town, for example, the group did not meet. Co-leaders offered each other mutual support and picked up on each other's blind spots, thereby decreasing vicarious traumatization. One leader was able to work with individuals who had dissociated to "bring them back," while the group continued under the leadership of the second leader (Benjamin and Benjamin, 1994a).

As noted, the members of the group had a diverse presenting phenomenology, diverse histories, and were at various stages of the healing process. Because the group was a support group, members did not share their abuse histories or trauma histories. The focus of the group was on present healing and coping, not on uncovering work. Some members were newly diagnosed; others had begun some type of integration. At least five members of the group were receiving disability and did not work; other vocations included a university professor, an attorney, a therapist, and several business women. Only five of the regularly attending group members were married; several were recently divorced. Many of the members were socially isolated except for limited contacts with fellow group members.

Throughout its existence as a no-fee group, the group had a core of at least six to eight members who attended weekly. Others stayed for a few sessions or had periodic attendance because of work commitments or the need to "take a break." Numerous group members had repeated hospitalizations, particularly as a safety measure when suicidality became intense. Group members consistently exhibited symptoms of hyperalertness (when new persons joined the group, when someone slammed a door at the foot of the stairs, when a child screamed on the inpatient ward above the conference room used by the group). The level of mistrust for new members decreased with the development of stricter screening procedures, group rules, and the group contract. Self-destructive behaviors were not permitted during the group, and anger control by group members was generally good. However, when certain members became exceedingly angry because they had been triggered, other members of the group reacted negatively by shutting down, staying away from sessions, or dissociating. When members began to discuss the behavior of one another when angry, the leaders suggested that particularly volatile members needed to take a sabbatical "time out" from the group while they worked on their trigger issues in individual therapy. Members included a statement in their group contract that encouraged them and gave them permission to intervene if a member was too disruptive or monopolizing of group time, thereby censuring that member while requesting her or him to cease the behavior.

GROUP PROCESS

Although the group is no longer in existence, in order to describe the group process, it will be discussed as if it were still in operation. In this way, others may find it easier to use this chapter as a model.

The first meeting of the month is the "check in" meeting. During this meeting, each member has the opportunity to share experiences and issues from the past month. The location of this meeting, due to hospital commitments, is in a different room. To ease the transition between locations and to help in the entry of new members, group members have a monthly birthday celebration (with cake) at this meeting. Having food seems to make the change and the entry easier. This meeting takes place in the locked section of the hospital. If members need to use a restroom during group, they must exit and enter through the locked doors. The group leaders place the key on the table around which group members sit so that they can have free access. This setting is in contrast to the setting for the other meetings throughout the month, which include restrooms, several "nooks and crannies" for privacy should a trigger reaction occur, and no locked door.

The check-in meeting also is used to acquaint new members with group rules, procedures, and other members. It also generates topics for later meetings. At meetings other than the check-in meeting, the group begins with the discussion of a topic, review of homework from the present meeting, or focus on previously decided discussion topics. Earlier in the group's history, members wanted to deal with personal issues or topics that needed immediate attention at the beginning of the group session. This open discussion sometimes became too involved to "cut off" in thirty minutes and the topic for the evening was not addressed as a consequence. As a result, the exercises, homework discussions, and topic discussions now last approximately forty-five minutes. Members then can bring up topics and problems, if so desired. Open discussion of a specific member's concern enables everyone to share similar situations and solutions. This supportive approach helps members think of alternative problem-solving methods and strategies and also challenges maladaptive belief systems and schemas. If no topics are presented, then the leaders introduce other, more educationally oriented topics. At the time this chapter was written, the group was working on two general areas using written materials: containment techniques, and identification and modification of belief systems (Rosenbloom and Williams, 1999). No member is forced to participate in any aspect of the discussions.

BASIC PRINCIPLES IN CONDUCTING
A PSYCHOEDUCATIONAL SUPPORT GROUP

Kluft (1993) identified a series of principles in his article "Basic Principles in Conducting the Psychotherapy of MPD" which also apply to some degree to a psychoeducational support group and the roles of group leaders. These principles are presented as suggestions for persons who are seeking to develop an educational support group for DID/DDNOS individuals.

1. Leaders need to set a secure frame and firm, consistent boundaries. Through trial and error, and over time, leaders and group members establish a more secure frame and the group becomes a "safer place" for its members. The group described in this chapter established group rules and a contract which are available upon request.

2. Leaders need to encourage members to focus on the achievement of mastery. Involving group members in planning topics to be discussed helps in this task. Members of the group described in this chapter were encouraged to give input into the content and process of the group in respectful, assertive ways. They worked together to develop the contract and group rules. Some of the topics they discussed and wrote about included management of anger, self-mutilation alternatives, and mapping. Materials developed by the group on these topics are also available upon request.

3. Leaders need to recognize and constantly stress to group members that safety and trust are the keys to building a group alliance. Making the group a safe place for members must be a major concern of leaders and members alike. Initiating screening procedures through procedures such as the First Step Program, requiring new members to furnish the name and phone number of their individual therapists, and establishing group rules have helped promote feelings of safety. Threats to the safety of the group are taken seriously and discussed openly. The group must change location the first meeting date of a month, the date on which new members join the group because the normally used room is occupied by staff doctors. Allowing group members to choose among possible locations for that meeting helped to lessen anxiety about the change.

4. Because it is a support group, it is not necessary for members to "tell their stories" to one another or discuss their traumas. If a member begins to present too graphic details of abuse, leaders intervene and explain that presentation of such material might lead to abreactions in others and that sharing of traumatic material is not to occur in the group. Leaders need to be aware that contagion of symptom presentation can occur; a flashback in one client can lead to dissociative symptoms in another. For example, in this group, a single word (e.g., "shackles") led to an unexpected abreaction in another group member. Should an abreaction occur, leaders need to ground alters as quickly as possible to minimize symptom contagion. When child

alters appear, leaders need to ask (in a calm, firm voice) for the child to return to a safe place. Leaders may also ask others in the system to assist in this process. The presence of overwhelmed or frightened child alters is disruptive to the group and triggers other members to dissociate.

Members need to provide leaders with safety mechanisms (pictures, cue words, directions) to help them return to an adult or older teen (more responsible) alter, should switching occur. When members have been hospitalized together, they often are knowledgeable about one another's process and may help one another "come back" to the group. In this group, members provided leaders with drawings, lists of cue words that trigger switching, hypnotic induction techniques, and other methods to assist in grounding. Members are encouraged to deal with issues and memories triggered by group members or events outside of group with their individual therapists, rather than in the group setting.

5. Leaders need to model good communication skills as they build communication networks with each person's individual system. Leaders can model communication through appropriate self-disclosure and the use of "I" statements as well. They also need to encourage communication between members of the group. Members are encouraged to discuss the topic among themselves, to express themselves assertively, and to discuss the impact that they have upon one another.

6. Leaders need to be consistent, open, understanding, and warm. However, they also need to set limits and inform hostile alters who are abusive that they are not welcome in the group because their presence is too disruptive. Leaders need to reiterate as often as is needed that working on abuse issues per se is not the function of the group. Members who push those limits need to be reminded of group rules and boundaries on a regular basis.

7. Leaders need to provide hope and give positive feedback. They are in a position to help members identify maladaptive beliefs, develop more adaptive beliefs, and thereby help members restore shattered basic assumptions, and to verbally identify, praise, and reinforce positive beliefs. Members in this group have begun a workbook that identifies and helps them change (if necessary or desired) belief systems about safety, trust, power/control, esteem, and intimacy (Rosenbloom and Williams, 1999). This structured format helps members identify and correct cognitive errors (e.g., the belief that self-harm to one alter does not hurt the system); it also provides an opportunity for members to recognize that others in the group do have positive beliefs about these five need areas (including the group leaders). Information about the workbook is available upon request.

8. Leaders need to pace the process of the group. If a topic becomes too overwhelming (e.g., self-mutilation), leaders encourage members to ground themselves or leaders may end the discussion, postponing further comments until a later time. The level of structure facilitated by the leaders varies ac-

cording to the needs of members and the topics being presented (Watson, 1994). Members do a "check out" at the close of group as a grounding strategy. This technique is used to ensure that each member is in a "safe place" before leaving group and is a means for a responsible alter to be present and in control to ensure safety on the trip home.

9. Leaders need to model and teach self-responsibility, cooperation, consistency, commitment, assertive communication, problem solving, and other social skills. They need to take an active, warm, therapeutic stance within the group (Dolan, 1985). Group leaders also need to be active in and feel comfortable with strong emotions as they arise in the group. They should be nondirective and nonreactive unless they must function to protect an individual member or the group as a whole.

Additional roles of group leaders in a psychoeducational support group mirror those stated by Donaldson and Cordes-Green (1994): messenger, monitor, mediator, and member. Although they are discussed separately in this chapter, these four roles generally occur simultaneously. As messengers, group leaders model helping skills, teach conceptual information and theory both directly and indirectly, analyze behavior and teach appropriate emotional expression, and teach assertiveness skills and maintenance of boundaries. Leaders are resource persons, not authorities, who answer questions and provide information according to their knowledge. Group members, as well, serve as messengers, and provide one another with information and resource materials about trauma, PTSD, DID, and other related topics. If knowledge is not close at hand, leaders and messengers obtain information and provide the group with handouts, articles, and resource materials. As Turkus (1991) noted, education has a normalizing function. Handouts can serve as the impetus to valuable discussions and activities (e.g., development of a Trigger Mapping Ladder, available upon request).

As monitors, leaders should attempt to be vigilant to all areas of process and content of the group. They observe triggers for group members to topics chosen, reactions of members to one another, silences, eye contact, nonverbal behaviors, and other process aspects of the group. They also analyze the "whys" of process and talk between themselves before or after the group concerning what they see, hear, and conclude. As mediators, the leaders give feedback and information, ask questions, make observations, facilitate group problem solving, and seek to offer help in difficult situations. As members, they are genuine, responsive participants who are emotionally available during the group and, at times, by phone outside the group. They also are learners who are constantly seeking professional knowledge and are examining the impact of the group on their own issues, processes, and selves, with an awareness in mind of vicarious traumatization and compassion fatigue.

BENEFITS OF SUPPORT GROUP
PARTICIPATION FOR MEMBERS

Criticism of the use of group interventions with persons with MPD/DID often centers around issues of group contagion. Some critics suggest that a group for persons with this diagnosis serves as a breeding ground of symptom suggestion and memory suggestion. However, structure and format as a psychoeducational group, not a therapy group, limits such contagion. Screening interviews for group membership were conducted by the hospital's First Step program. In the majority of cases, leaders are not aware of the specifics of members' trauma histories. Trauma history and abusive experiences are not topics for discussion during the group. Instead, group discussion and process is designed to deal more with educationally based issues, coping skills, and ways for members to take care of themselves both in group and in the world. Members encourage one another to take risks, to be assertive, to fight proactively for their rights (e.g., in a divorce, custody battle). The "victim mentality" is not encouraged or fostered within the group.

Therefore, one of the most helpful, and important, areas for discussion for group members concerns group and individual member safety. Safety includes the need to feel reasonably invulnerable to harm, and secure. Many members of the group do not feel safe under a wide range of conditions and situations. Some try to form rigid boundaries around themselves; others are constantly at risk for self-harm when they are threatened, when parts reveal information about the historical or perceived past, or when they encounter persons or events that remind them in any way of earlier abuse.

As Buchele (1995) has aptly noted, a group cannot function unless it is a "truly safe, predictable place" of sanctuary (p. 91). Williams' (1993a,b,c) and Williams and Sommer's (1994) techniques to provide safety in individual therapy can also be utilized in the group setting. Discussions of safety and ways to gain safety have assisted members in "outside group" life choices as well.

Many group sessions have also explored ways to develop coping mechanisms that would lead to a greater perception of safety and the creation of foolproof safety contracts. Several group members have made their own personal safety contracts available to the group as educational tools. (Examples of safety contracts are available upon request.)

Each member of the group is encouraged to develop or utilize a previously developed internal or external safe place to use should the material become overwhelming or should they begin to be triggered by another member. This place exists either in reality or fantasy, in nature or in a human-made location. If group members have become upset during a meeting and need time to "ground" before leaving the session and before the final "check out" occurs, group leaders may do a short relaxation exercise while asking each member to go to their safe place and regroup (Salston and Baker, 1993). Other external sources include written positive affirmations; safety objects such as geodes, stuffed animals or small toys; participation in activities which boost self-esteem (coursework, volunteer activities, peer activities); art activities; and reference to treasured items including photo albums, collages, and memorabilia.

Another positive benefit for group members has been their development of cognitive restructuring techniques to change maladaptive thought processes and maladaptive self statements about safety and self-harm. The group serves as a form to teach means to identify and attempt to utilize internal sources of self-soothing, including intuition, intelligence, inquisitiveness, willpower/determination, self-awareness, problem-solving abilities, religious values, and empathy for others (Feord, 1994). Group leaders model appropriate self statements, particularly those that involve assertive boundary-setting. Self-dialogue is taught to be simple and truthful and may include the statement "This is now, not then; I am safe" (Salston and Baker, 1993).

Another beneficial function of the group is discussion about and possible development of procedures, techniques, and strategies for containment of strong affects, compulsions to retraumatize the self, self-mutilatory urges and attempts, suicide gestures, or boundary violations (Miller, 1994). These techniques and strategies include the utilization of contracts, safety plans, self-soothing mechanisms, positive memories, visualizations, cue words, containers in which to place images and affects, and others. Containment (as well as appropriate expression) of anger is another major topic (Grame, 1995; Ross and Gahan, 1988). Different means to express rage in a non-harming manner include the use of "bop bags," weight lifting, controlled destruction of glass at a recycling center, batakas (bats), and other physical means to release the anger from its internalized storage places.

The group is not designed to be a member's lifeline; as has been noted, each member has an individual therapist. Generally, group leaders are available by phone to members only during a crisis, as a "last resort" if individual therapists are not available, or when other support systems fail. Leaders may also be available when members call concerning potential topics for group or to discuss members' reactions to a particular session when something that occurred left them feeling unsafe or wary. Members do not abuse phone contact with the group leaders and respect the boundaries concerning timing and length of phone contacts.

Many group discussions center around the topics of relationship building and boundary setting. Married members may have relationship difficulties that corroborate Putnam's (1989) suggestion that, in many cases, MPD clients often marry mates with significant psychological difficulties. Several of the group members have been involved in verbally or physically abusive relationships. Others have been abandoned by partners as they have progressed through the treatment process, or have partners who are unwilling to acknowledge the diagnosis, even after years of therapy for the partner.

Group members may also discuss the topic of boundaries. They may relate many instances in which they have been unaware of what constitutes appropriate boundaries and frequently have been unable to set limits (Horning, 1994). As a consequence, they begin to look for guidelines for intra- as well as interpersonal boundaries and separations and complete numerous exercises on this topic. Members have noted that discussions of boundaries and assertiveness have been some of the most helpful for them (Courtois and Leehan, 1992). They learn to confront one another about issues and behaviors in an assertive manner. However, new members may find this degree of interaction somewhat intimidating until they have acclimated to the group.

Many of the group members may believe that their diagnosis *must* be kept a secret and may be shared only with selected family members and/or close friends. The majority of group members do *not* believe that the diagnosis means that they have the "right" to be a victim. Those who are on disability learn ways to return to the workforce through successful use of containment strategies learned in the group. The group is not structured to encourage a nonactive response to symptomatology. In fact, the philosophy of the group is the development of coping skills that enable life "in the world." Several group members have returned to school to complete advanced degrees. Others have learned how to tap into special education and rehabilitation services under the Americans with Disabilities Act (ADA).

Members have related stories of how the revelation of their diagnosis was received by others. One participant related that her younger sister responded that she must be possessed by the devil and immediately contacted the family's minister and requested an exorcism. A second participant indicated that most people do not want to know about traumatic experiences in others because they fear contagion of the diagnosis. Several group members have consciously isolated themselves from family and friends because they believe that no one will understand. Group leaders have encouraged members to share their diagnosis only with persons who are supportive and compassionate. Members have also been encouraged to identify a support team of at least three persons and then use that team to develop a plan of action for crisis situations. However, members are also reminded that a spouse or other support person has the right to refuse to provide crisis intervention at a given time if he or she does not feel emotionally or physically able to do so (Williams, 1991; Williams, 1995). Soliciting support from others, however, does not give a member permission to forego the responsibility of self-care if at all possible. Group members are encouraged to educate their supportive individuals about triggers, specific wants and needs, unique patterns of presentation of alters, and necessary physical and emotional boundaries in a positive manner so as not to alienate them.

VALUES OF THE LEADERS

Leaders of a psychoeducational group need to believe in the values of support and consistency while constantly helping group members strive for personal safety. Their value orientation is to do no harm, to model assertiveness and flexibility, and to allow no destructive contacts between group members if at all possible (i.e., discourage contacts if negative). Leaders need also to value knowledge and seek continually to expand their own knowledge bases in the fields of trauma, dissociation, DID, and other related areas. They also need to have knowledge in the fields of systems theory and child development. Leaders in the group held at the hospital value an active style of leadership that involves education and sharing of knowledge. Leaders of any support group for persons diagnosed with DID need to realize that they are not automatically trusted by members and must earn trust over time. Therefore, they must utilize their intuitive, responsive, warm, genuine styles to work for the good of the group and be generally comfortable with material shared by clients and the emotions that they reveal. This does not mean that they are unaware of countertransference/vicarious traumatization issues, however.

AREAS OF CONCERN AND ETHICAL
ISSUES IN THE GROUP

Peer contact for persons with a similar diagnosis can provide validation and lead to a firmer acceptance of that diagnosis. Some individuals, however, believe that such contact can be contagiously iatrogenic and lead to false-positive presentations (Simpson, 1995). Thus, in the group setting, members may come to accept "without question the presence of distinct parts of themselves as well as the amnestic barriers among them . . . reinforcing a [sense of] fragmented identity . . . [and] emphasize the view of the diagnosis as a psychological showpiece . . . [from which] patients can receive considerable secondary gain" (Buchele, 1995, pp. 87-88). Group leaders as well as the members should structure a support group in such a manner that individuals remain, to the greatest extent possible, in responsible, adult alters or states. A strong group structure limits reinforcement and encourages a positive, proactive stance to life.

Leaders of any type of group for persons diagnosed with DID must be extremely good managers, particularly when members behave in bizarre or inappropriate ways. Over time, leaders learn to identify specific alters who may appear and become familiar with specific triggers for individual members or for the group as a whole. In this group, members recognize that certain phrases trigger others, and, therefore, make a conscious effort to avoid the use of those phrases or warn the individuals ahead of time prior to their use. This awareness decreases dissociation and switching. However, particularly when new members come to the group, it is possible for members to dissociate and leave in a tumultuous state without leaders even knowing (Linehan, 1993). This occurred in one instance when one member did not return home after group and was found hiding in the bushes outside the hospital several hours later. Initiating a one or two sentence check out by each member in an adult/responsible alter has countered this type of behavioral response.

Barach (1994) wrote that an open group may prompt acting out; new members whose histories are not known or whose styles of presentation of symptoms are not known can be very disruptive as they come and go in the group. This type of group, in other words, can lead to secondary traumatization in others as well as a contagion of symptoms. Although this is true, group structure can minimize disruptions. Group socialization occurs quickly. New members have rules and a contract to sign. The initial screening interview stresses that the group is not therapeutic and that abuse issues are not to be discussed or worked through; abreactions are not encouraged. Allowing new members to enter only once monthly also limits this type of disruption. Group membership was also limited to sixteen persons. Leaders believe it is unethical to have a larger group because the size would limit the participation of those present.

Members are encouraged to keep group confidentiality. A problem arose when one member called another and revealed information that could have been harmful to herself or others. In this instance, stalking was involved and the member who made the call did not share the information with the leaders as he had promised. To prevent this from happening again, group members are now encouraged (and expected) to reveal any potentially dangerous information to the group leader so that the leader(s) can deal with the person individually or get in touch with the person's therapist, hospital administration, or the authorities. This information also includes threats of suicidal actions revealed by one member to another. When such information is revealed, the group functions in a supportive role and encourages members to use their safety plans and to follow safety contracts. In more than one instance, the group has encouraged a member to seek hospitalization immediately following the meeting and the member has then gone to First Step and/or contacted the individual therapist. Group members encourage one another to share important information, particularly information about suicide threats and plans in the past and for the present, with their therapists.

This is particularly true when a member who has a new therapist has not disclosed self-mutilating or self-destructive behaviors to that new therapist.

Group members are not to give phone numbers, addresses, or information about other members to anyone without that member's permission. In one instance, a group member provided the police with names and numbers of other members. The police made calls to at least three members, unaware of their diagnoses, and the consequences were disastrous (two members were eventually hospitalized). The group leader eventually was able to contact the officer and explain the situation. Legal prosecution of the group member who was stalking the others had to take precedence. However, the officers did agree to allow group members to be interviewed in the presence/with the assistance of their therapists.

Because of these issues, a group for persons diagnosed as DID cannot be a walk-in group. It is essential for persons to have screening first and to provide the names/phone numbers of their therapists who have diagnosed them. This eliminates the arrival of persons who are known to be non-MPD or the attendance of persons who are too disturbed, too new to the diagnosis, or too fragmented to participate. Another issue centers around techniques used to deal with problem members or new members. As an ongoing group, the core members react to new members and to change of location and format. However, the adoption of group rules and set times when new members can join the group has helped modify this reaction. Leaders have dealt with members who are consistently tardy; who have wanted to "take over" as leader; who are excessively angry, thereby frightening other group members; who display inappropriate behavior; who begin to self-abuse with keys, plastic knives or other instruments; who demand too much time on a regular basis; who attempt to run out of the room or lock themselves in a bathroom and cause a disruption; who refuse to stop discussing too vivid or grotesque material; among others. Group leaders must establish their role as having authority to intervene in these instances. Group members also have intervened, e.g., members have asked persons who are tardy to be on time so they do not disrupt the process. Persons who are inappropriate in behavior or who abreact and cannot ground themselves quickly are taken to a hallway adjacent to the room by one leader while the other continues the group. Persons who are self-abusive are either addressed nonverbally or verbally by a leader. At times, other members may signal the leaders to what is happening if the leaders are not already aware. Members frequently believe that they are responsible when others react negatively to a statement they make and that statement acts as a trigger for acting out (anger, crying) or acting in (dissociation). They take on emotions of guilt and shame for their self-presumed responsibility in "causing" the behaviors. Leaders should discuss issues of responsibility of self and responsibility for others honestly and openly to help members confront these negative beliefs about presumed power.

Leaders should insist that implements which might be (or are beginning to be) used in a self-destructive manner are either put away or given to the leaders. Leaders can then use the grounding techniques that members have provided, if necessary. Members should also know that long visits to the bathroom (which is in one corner of the room) will eventuate in a knock on the door by a leader. Should no response be given, leaders have a key and will open the door. This is not seen as a violation of privacy and has prevented dissociative episodes from continuing, thereby enabling leaders to help members ground.

COUNTERTRANSFERENCE
AND VICARIOUS TRAUMATIZATION

Group leaders realize, as do many others (McCann and Pearlman, 1990a,b; Danieli, 1994; Pearlman and Saakvitne, 1995), that vicarious traumatization is inevitable and that exposure to traumatic material takes its toll on therapist as well as client. Leaders should limit the amount of grotesque, gruesome material that is shared by members to protect other group members from secondary traumatization and to protect themselves from those vicarious effects. By modeling appropriate behavior, leaders should also set personal boundaries. They should refuse to be abused verbally by alters, no matter their age. Verbal attacks by hostile alters can trigger many countertransference issues in both leaders and group members. Leaders, therefore, should take an assertive stance and react to hostility firmly, without becoming a transferential, negative parent. However, it is difficult to maintain a detached stance in the face of a disruptive tirade that then triggers other group members. Leaders may also experience frustration at the lack of movement of some group members or the resistance they have shown to do the work in group or as homework. Members who attempt to use dissociation as an excuse from doing group assignments are encouraged to examine the reasons behind the resistance. In addition, as Benjamin and Benjamin noted (1994a,b,c), helplessness, and the inability to cope exhibited by some group members may lead leaders to feel helpless and overwhelmed or may lead to rescue fantasies. Over time, members became less tolerant of members' retreats into helplessness or hopelessness. Instead, they became problem-focused and looked toward ways to problem solve and to find solutions.

An additional source of countertransference and vicarious traumatization occurs as a result of frustration when group members call a leader outside the group on a less-than-crisis basis and expect the group leader to provide therapeutic care. In these instances, the group leaders should redirect the client to his or her individual therapist and reinforce their roles as backups when "all-else" fails. However, leaders should also let members and therapists know that they do not serve as backup therapists when that individual therapist is out of town or unavailable. Several group members are in constant crisis and crisis intervention with them can be wearing, frustrating, and exhausting. This is particularly true in instances in which the individual therapist refuses to respond to a crisis phone call that is genuine. Leaders have then contacted therapists and worked out future response scenarios (Coons and Bradley, 1985).

A RETROSPECTIVE LOOK AT THE GROUP: WHAT DID IT ACCOMPLISH?

Since the group terminated, numerous group members have stayed in touch with either the therapist or the coleader on an intermittent basis. Most members, though, have not contacted either leader. A few members have continued in or entered into therapy with the primary group leader and have expressed their regret that the group is no longer available. They have affirmed the value they found in group participation. Group membership reduced their isolation, offered validation of the diagnosis, and provided an opportunity for them to be "real" without having to hide who they were (Riggan, 1998).

One advantage of the group was that it was ongoing in nature. Core members returned week after week and served as role models for new individuals. They actively welcomed these new members, explained the rules of the group, socialized new members into the group process, and formed their own outside-of-group social support system. Because of the ongoing nature of the group, members took an active part in planning topics and activities. In this way, they helped to meet their own needs (Overbeck and Overbeck, 1995).

The group was a community of peers in which members were committed to the formation of a social reference group that allowed them to form a sense of group identification (Roth and Batson, 1997). Group identification occurred quickly for most members. This bonding, as Roth and Batson (1997) wrote, "is based on an experiential knowledge of sharing a similar life tragedy, which evolves over time into a solid connection based as much on differentiation of experiences as on common ground" (p. 117). Advantages of the group mirrored those found by Webb and Leehan (1996). The group helped members to validate their diagnosis in an increasingly hostile therapeutic environment. As treatment for chronic conditions, including DID, becomes harder and harder to fund through insurance, and as The False Memory Association continues to attack the diagnosis, this validation has been extremely important. Validation built mutual acceptance of each other's symptomatology, difficulties, and solutions. Experiencing a common reality was legitimizing and encouraging. The safety of the setting and the supportiveness of leaders and fellow members were also positives of the group. The curative factors of this group were the same as those identified by Federle and Harrington (1990):

1. Validation through connection, "working through," and sharing of the pain of the past in a context of relationship
2. Empowerment through valuing and encouraging one another's abilities
3. Self-empathy and compassion for self and empathy for one another
4. Mutuality through listening and acting without being judgmental, through watching the survival of others, and through taking responsibility for personal risk

Finally, the group encouraged, supported, and fostered healthy interaction and communication between members and members and leader(s). This communication helped members to develop trust, discover the true caring that emanated from other members, to give support to one another to lessen isolation and denial, to receive and give attention, and to discover new ways of coping (Chew, 1998).

CONCLUSIONS

Providing information and facilitating discussion thorough the forum of a psychoeducational group helped members normalize their diagnoses, behaviors, symptoms, and life difficulties through contact with others. Providing members with opportunities to rehearse behaviors, problem solve, and build connections was a very worthwhile component of the group process, as was teaching them trauma and systems models. Structuring the group as a present-oriented, proactive forum limited the contagion effects of the "negatives" of DID: switching between alters, dissociative episodes, and acting-out behaviors.

Group leaders recognize that working with a group of persons with MPD/DID who are in a vulnerable state is risky; chaos can spread quickly, as can fear and grief. Leaders of any support group for persons diagnosed with DID must be constantly alert to the ways in which traumatic reenactments are frequently triggered through a choice of words, an action, or a reaction of other members, in spite of structure and group rules. Mutual triggering can occur in a fraction of a second. Leaders must also learn about the systems of each of the more regularly attending members. Leaders must recognize that dissociation is also very contagious and they must be constantly on the alert to "bring members back" to a more adult state.

Developing and maintaining a psychoeducational support group is an extremely rewarding adventure. As members build a sense of groupness and community, as leaders get to know them and their systems more intimately, a truly unique group structure and process evolves. Members teach one another and group leaders much about "what it means to be multiple." It is the writing of one group member (Feord, 1993) that reminds the reader of the impact of multiplicity on each and every participant.

> Although others may not understand multiplicity, they do understand human suffering. . . . Many family members or friends may avoid discussing the . . . illness because they don't know how to help. [Persons] diagnosed with MPD essentially want and need the same things all other people do. They need love, space, and the happiness that comes from knowing that they are making a worthwhile contribution to the world. However, because they are human, they cannot expect everyone to like them, support them, and express only positive sentiments toward them. Everyone is unique and has inherent attributes that appeal to some people while, at the same time, repel others. Multiples, like anyone else, need both positive and negative feedback from others in order to grow as human beings. Group members [have come to know that] each person is responsible for making his or her own happiness on earth. Multiplicity is not an excuse to deny oneself the right to be happy nor should it be used as a scapegoat for relationship problems. . . . Like anyone else [group members] can examine their lives and identify changes they can make now, and in the future, to fulfill their dreams.

It is one role of the group to help them in that process of growth.

The appendix at the end of this chapter includes the following. Each of these items is self-explanatory as to its purpose and function and is based on information found in the chapter.

- Support Group Welcome letter
- Group Rules
- Authorization for Support Group Participation
- Notification of Therapy Termination
- Getting the Most Out of Group
- Record of Alters
- Encouraging Alters to Remember
- Session 23: Grounding Techniques
- Session 7: Hospitalization
- Safety Plan: March 1994
- Steps to Immediately Follow When Suicidal
- Contract for Safety Issues
- Safety Contract

APPENDIX: GROUP HANDOUTS

SUPPORT GROUP WELCOME

Welcome to _____. We are happy that you have decided to attend our support group tonight.

Because there are so many types of groups available at _____, and in the _____ area, it can be difficult to choose the right group. We want to make sure that this group is right for you and fits your needs at this time. Allow us to share with you some thoughts that might help you determine if this group is the right one for you.

First, we would like to help you understand the difference between a support group and a therapy group. The distinction is important because the goals for each are somewhat different. In both cases, people come to these groups because they have some level of emotional distress. A support group assists members in dealing with emotional stresses by teaching new coping skills, educating members about the problem or illness, supporting one another in dealing with new problems, and encouraging one another in treatment outside of the group.

Group therapy, on the other hand, does many of the same things, but it encourages participants to go deeper into their problems, to resolve inner conflicts, and to confront issues that are long-standing. It may mean that anxiety, anger, conflict, and confrontation are pursued and explored in the group. Due to the emotional intensity, there are usually fewer people in a therapy group than in a support group. In fact, if you feel that a support group is not meeting your needs because of its size, it may mean that you would be better served in group or individual therapy.

We recommend that people use support groups to enhance their individual, group, or couples therapy, not to take the place of it. We think it is important to be in some kind of outside therapy while in a support group. If you need a recommendation, you should feel free to contact _____ at _____. A counselor can meet with you and, after talking with you, can make a recommendation for treatment that will complement the support group.

Once you have determined what group is the best for you, we encourage you to attend it regularly. This will make the experience more meaningful for you, and will be a greater support to others in the group. We also request that you consider only one support group, to allow others the chance to participate in a support group at _____.

The role of the group leader in a support group is to educate, to encourage members in their treatment, and to lend support when a group member is experiencing a difficult time. This might mean that the group leader would want the member to speak with a counselor for an evaluation and recommendation. This is why it is important for the group member to alert the group leader when he or she is feeling overwhelmed, confused, or distraught.

The group leader also reserves the right to:

1. ask the group participant to seek out an assessment immediately;
2. take a time out from the group if the participant's behavior becomes inappropriate;
3. recommend that the group member seek more time with his or her outpatient therapist; or
4. recommend another, more appropriate support group.

We congratulate you for reaching out for support. We hope that this group meets your expectations. If you have any questions about how the group can work for you, please don't hesitate to ask the group leader.

MPD PSYCHOEDUCATION/SUPPORT GROUP RULES
(AS OF AUGUST 24, 1994)

1. To participate, group members will provide _____ with a release from their treating therapists confirming their participation in regular outpatient therapy. In addition, if they may potentially dissociate during group time, effective grounding techniques used by their alters will also be provided.
2. Every topic discussed during group meetings is strictly confidential.
3. Participants must respect each other so that group meetings are a safe place for everyone to be in the here-and-now. Physical and emotional abuse of each other either during or outside of group time is not permitted.
4. In addition, self-destructive behavior is not allowed during group sessions.
5. Group members will protect each other by recognizing that the purpose of the group is psychoeducational and supportive, not therapeutic. Therefore, topics which include graphic details of abuse or other comments which may reasonably be expected to trigger other participants are not permitted. With the exception of these situations, however, participants will respect each others' right to speak and share without interruption.
6. On the first Wednesday of each month, new participants may briefly check in (usually not to exceed several minutes).
7. If an individual has a personal issue of importance to discuss on dates other than the first Wednesday, group time will be allotted to this topic if group members support this agenda. Otherwise, discussion topics will be decided in advance.
8. Participants must remain in the conference room until the meeting ends, and refrain from walking or running out without first checking out. If privacy is needed, however, participants may isolate in other areas of the conference room, but the foregoing rules continue to apply.
9. Each member also agrees to make every effort to be physically present in his or her body throughout the group meeting, and remain psychologically focused to the extent possible.
10. Touching other participants is permitted if permission is first requested and received.
11. When the group ends, each participant must be physically and psychologically capable of going home. To ensure that everyone is safe, and that an alter responsible for driving is present, members must check out briefly at the end of each meeting.
12. Contact with other group members outside of scheduled meeting times is permitted, but only with one another's permission.

AUTHORIZATION FOR SUPPORT GROUP PARTICIPATION

I hereby authorize my client/patient to attend the psychoeducational support group offered by _____ for individuals with dissociative disorders, and confirm that he or she is in continuing therapy with me at the present time. I agree to notify this group's facilitator, _____, using the attached form should therapy be discontinued for any reason. In the event that telephone contact is necessary, _____ can be reached at _____.

Client/Patient's Name: _____

Therapist's Printed Name: _____

Therapist's Address: _____

_____

_____

Therapist's Telephone Number: _____

Signature of Therapist: _____

Date of Authorization: _____

NOTIFICATION OF THERAPY TERMINATION

TO: _____

_____

_____

_____

_____

FROM: _____

(Therapist's Printed Name)

_____

_____

_____

(Therapist's Address)

RE: _____

(Client/Patient's Printed Name)

I hereby notify _____ that I am no longer treating the above-named client/patient, who was authorized by me to attend _____ psycho-educational support group for individuals with dissociative disorders.

DATE: _____

SIGNATURE: _____

GETTING THE MOST OUT OF A GROUP

1. You will get the most out of the group experience if you invest yourself. ACTIVELY PARTICIPATE!
2. Help build trust in the group early on by openly discussing how you feel, even about your nervousness and/or trouble you have trusting other members. Do not keep secrets from the group or "sit on" persistent feelings you have. It you feel bored, frustrated, withdrawn, or afraid, let others know about it.
3. For the group to be most helpful, you and the other members will need to feel safe. Learn how your group protects confidentiality, and respect it.
4. You will not be forced to reveal everything about yourself. Trust your own sense of balance and timing about how much, how, and when to disclose important things about yourself.
5. With early sessions, you may feel mostly confused or discouraged. That is a natural part of the process. Rather than giving up on the group at this point, try to stay with it, letting the group know how you feel.
6. At times you may feel frustrated, let down, or annoyed with the leaders. You may want help or answers that they do not give. Trust that the best help will soon come from other members.
7. Expect some discomfort within yourself. Also, don't be surprised if your life outside the group is disrupted. Making changes (whether in behavior or in self-discovery) may be disconcerting to you or others.
8. Expect to discover good things about yourself! Be open to receive support and encouragement from others.
9. Learn to listen carefully to other members. Do not automatically accept as truth or immediately reject outright; instead, consider and decide for yourself what does and what does not apply to you. Pay special attention to feedback that is consistent.
10. Let others know how specific things they do (behavior) affect you.
11. Avoid categorizing or labeling yourself or other members. Remember to differentiate between your reaction to what a person does and your judgment of them as a person.
12. Bring up topics or concerns that are important to you, even if painful or scary, early in the session; that way, you can receive the concern and attention you need. Do not wait until the last few minutes of group.
13. As much as possible, keep your discussion focused on the present: what is taking place "here and now" in the group session.

RECORD OF ALTERS

Name	Nickname	Age at Birth	Current Age	Has Awareness When Another Person Is Out	
				All the Time	Sometimes

Name	Event at Birth

Name	Descriptions

ENCOURAGING ALTERS TO REMEMBER

In your notebook, for each of the Alters identified, ask that Alter to discuss/draw/write about answers to the following:

I would like the others (both inside and without) to know about me/my experiences/my pain:

- I am . . .
- I like . . .
- I don't like . . .
- I want to keep as part of _____ (core) . . .
- I want to give to _____ (core) as part of her/him and his/her memories . . . (as a present)
- I do not need to keep as part of _____ (core) . . .
- I am now ready to . . .
- My purpose is (now) . . .
- My purpose was (when I was created) . . .
- My job (role) is . . .
- My job (role) was . . .

Draw a picture of what I see when I look inside me.

What is that symbol?

Draw a picture of me (This is me, I am).

Draw a picture of where I belong.

Draw a picture of what happened to me.

Draw a picture of me doing something with a family member (or members).

What is my symbol?

SESSION 23: GROUNDING TECHNIQUES
AND FORMATION OF ALTERS

After check-in, group time was devoted to discussing the events that occurred during last week's session and reestablishing a sense of safety for group members. The participant who reacted to the word "integration" apologized profusely for triggering other members, and expressed her concern about her continuing participation in the group. She was assured, however, that she is a respected, valued member of the group who would be sorely missed if she no longer participated.

Group members universally agreed that each participant reacts in varying ways to different triggers. It is not possible to prevent these reactions, particularly when triggers are unanticipated. Implementing the suggestions discussed in previous groups and learning one's system, identifying one's triggers to the extent possible, and developing effective coping mechanisms will maximize control, but will not ensure total control. Members were reminded that they should learn and practice grounding techniques so that these can be used to maintain control, to the extent possible, when faced with unexpected triggers.

The remainder of the group session was devoted to discussing how alters are formed. The leader again emphasized the need for each participant to map his or her alters. In addition to learning how and why each alter was formed, and what purpose he or she serves now, it is important to explore the memories and affect each alter holds. In many cases, feelings a group member is experiencing when confronting an anniversary and other triggers are caused by affect that is "bleeding through" from other alters in the system. Only by learning about one's system, and telling one's alter(s) that I'm ready to listen" or "I want to know" will a multiple be able to develop control over his or her response to these triggers.

During this discussion, members described the following types of alters they have identified:

1. Alters created to fill certain defined roles, or for specific purposes. These include to work, to have sex, or to hold specific memories or affect related to past trauma.
2. Alters which represent "introjects." One member described a persecutory alter who repeats statements made to her when she was a child by her father, and other members agreed that they also have alters who make similar statements at times.
3. Alters with the same name, or similar names as the host. The leader indicated that if a multiple has alters of varying ages who use the same name as the host, that treatment is less involved and integration is usu-

ally easier. One group member indicated that this is applicable to her situation.

4. Alters of the opposite sex. Many female participants have male alters, and the majority of these individuals indicated that these alters provide a protective function for the system as a whole.
5. Fragmentary alters. These come and go, and are integrated as memories are faced and associated feelings are abreacted and accepted. Several group members have identified fragmentary alters who formed from one abusive experience to hold limited memories or limited affect relating to the experience.
6. Three group members indicated that they are aware of alters who appear in the form of an animal.

Participants were vague when describing how alters were formed, and in most cases did not know. They also found it difficult to concretely describe where alters go or what they do when they are not "out." Several participants simply said that they go into an area which is similar to entering another room in one's house, or "hide behind the eyeballs." Members were encouraged to explore these questions when mapping their systems.

Until participants know their alters, and understand how and why each one reacts to triggers as he or she does, it is essential to practice and use grounding techniques. At times, group members must stop working with MPD issues to deal with circumstances occurring in the here-and-now. Increasing dissociation and chaos can result if unresolved problems in one's current life are not addressed in a timely manner. Participants generally agreed that, if triggered, a severe abreaction could result if they are unable to ground themselves. To establish safety, and start abreactive work, patients must be able to ground themselves so that a malignant abreaction can be promptly controlled. Group members discussed the following grounding techniques:

1. Use a journal to ask one's alters to allow the host to return during these times if this is possible.
2. Use Neuro-Linguistic Programming (NLP) techniques. One should focus on a part of one's body, to physically remind oneself that he or she is here. For example, the leader recommended that members feel and count their pulses to ground themselves. Focusing on external items in one's surroundings, such as the second hand used to count the pulse, aids in this grounding effort. Once one focuses on one item in the environment, and is comfortable doing so without dissociating, other items can be perused one at a time. Jewelry, such as a necklace, or other items worn by a patient can be very effective tools when used to ground oneself.

3. Concentrating on the senses by listing five things heard, seen, and felt, and then four, and then three, two, and one can be a very effective grounding technique. This exercise should be repeated until the participant feels controlled.
4. Smelling something pleasant will remind one that he or she is in the here-and-now. This technique should be used only if the member is reasonably certain that he or she will not encounter a negative trigger in the form of an odor.
5. Using audio tools to ground oneself can also be very effective. One group member repeatedly listens to a tape made by her therapist because simply listening to her voice on the tape helps the patient control herself. A second member has taped "stay grounded" statements and listens to them so that she will not dissociate when she encounters triggers. A third participant has taped stories which soothe her alters and she plays these when triggered. The leader suggested that group members ask each alter what he or she wants, and prepare tapes accordingly.
6. Several group members follow safety plans when feeling self-destructive or triggered. Because of the efficacy of this tool, participants were once again encouraged to work with their therapists to develop these plans.

A few participants once again stated that they cannot use a safety contract because their alters either won't sign it, or won't honor it. In conclusion, the leader suggested that they list each alter in the contract, and define his or her duty. For example, the alter who drives, works, etc., can be identified as such. This serves several purposes. First, it promotes understanding within the system. Second, alters are recognized and honored for the work that they each do. Also, it can facilitate control by clearly defining each alter's role and thus avert potential internal control struggles between them. If resistance is encountered while doing this, or executing the contract, the motivation behind the resistance must be identified. Members were encouraged to ask their alters who is resistant and why. Only then can this resistance be addressed. Effective contracting can be implemented if alters are clearly told that unless they step forward to address their concerns and object to the contract, they are bound by its terms. Members were encouraged to continue addressing unresolved contractual issues prior to the next session.

SESSION 7: HOSPITALIZATION

TOPIC: Effective Inpatient Treatment

Most patients with MPD need hospitalization at times during the course of their treatment. In many cases, repeated hospitalizations are required in crisis situations to control suicidal ideation and ensure the safety of the body. In some cases, hospitalization is planned to provide a safe setting for abreactive experiences, or to allow the emergence of persecutory alters.

Group members have varied experiences with inpatient treatment. Most participants have been hospitalized repeatedly to control self-abusive behavior. Group members who were ritually abused said that they sought the safety of an inpatient setting on key satanic holidays, while others sought the increased safety on anniversaries of their abuse. In one case, a patient sought hospitalization to control homicidal impulses.

The goal of inpatient treatment should be to resolve the presenting crisis as rapidly as possible, and strengthen the multiple's internal reserve so that safety can be maintained at home. Psychiatric patients often regress while inpatient and may become dependent on the vigilance of staff personnel to ensure their safety rather than focusing on their own need to develop effective coping strategies. MPD patients, in particular, may tax the resources of hospital staff who may perceive them to be manipulative and uncooperative. Staff may not understand that a patient's "mood swings" are actually due to emerging alters, rather than a desire to manipulate others. Group members described varying inpatient experiences, but universally agreed that effective hospitalizations typically occurred in facilities which specialized in treating dissociative disorders. The reasons given for this include the following:

1. Hospital staff accept the diagnosis of MPD. Those group members who were hospitalized in settings in which their diagnosis of MPD was not validated stated that their feelings of inadequacy, depression, and self-loathing increased, preventing them from developing the internal strength needed to commit to both life and continuing treatment.
2. Ward rules are established to allow a patient as much control as possible. These rules are explained to each individual alter as necessary and typically include the following:
   a. Self-abusive behavior is not tolerated on the unit. If a patient feels self-destructive, he or she is responsible for informing the staff and developing a plan to ensure safety. The multiple is allowed to determine and implement those steps that he or she feels would be most effective in promoting safety. This may include: interacting with other patients

in a "public" area; sitting at the nurses' station until a commitment to safety can be made; agreeing to periodic "sign-ins" at the nurses's station; using the quiet room as a refuge from the internal vigilance needed to ensure safety; reviewing positive affirmations that support life; seeking medication to moderate feelings of panic or anxiety; dissipating feelings of anger by beating pillows or sadness by crying; or simply talking one-on-one to share feelings with another patient or a staff member.

b. Consequences, should patients fail to maintain self-control, are clearly explained to the "system" by ward staff. The staff supports patients as necessary to ensure that safety and control are maintained in the least restrictive environment possible.

c. Patients are encouraged to participate in scheduled therapies, but can choose not to do so without recrimination.

d. A patient's relationship with his or her therapist is respected, and contact is allowed during emotionally stressful times as necessary.

3. Because the staff both accepts and understands MPD, it can assist the patient in developing effective coping mechanisms to manage troublesome symptoms. Switching, unless an alter intent on self-destruction emerges, is not perceived to be an undesirable symptom. Rather, staff can assist patients to understand when and why this occurs, and thus enable them to develop control over this process.

4. Experienced staff members honor a patient's alters, as well as memories, etc., that emerge while he or she is hospitalized.

Many group members who have been hospitalized were traumatized because their alters were not respected when staff members denied or ignored them, or attempted to control their "mood swings." As a result, positive benefits which could have been gained while an inpatient were lost. These included opportunities to learn about the patient's system, facilitate internal communication, develop worthwhile cooperation between alters, address safety issues using internal rather than external means, and address effective symptom-management techniques. Although the majority of group members described their experiences as primarily negative, a recognition was made that safety was maintained while hospitalized which, in most instances, was the precipitant for inpatient treatment.

The group decided to discuss this issue again at a later date.

SAFETY PLAN: MARCH 1994

I agree to follow this safety plan if I cannot maintain my physical safety, become uncontrollably angry, or fear that I will otherwise lose control of myself during the duration of my Safety Contract with _____ and Dr. _____. If, after following this plan, I cannot maintain my physical safety, I will page Dr. _____ to let him or her know and agree to keep myself safe until I have discussed the situation with him or her. I also agree to review and update this plan monthly as needed and provide Dr. _____ with copies of any revisions made.

1. Preventing uncontrollable suicidal ideation:
    a. I will pursue every means possible to prevent escalation of my suicidal feelings by recognizing early indicators that I am spiraling into a downward depression, and intervene to stop this cycle early:
       • Triggered
       • Become upset, anxious
       • React emotionally by crying and isolating myself
       • Become indecisive
       • Become overwhelmed by everything
       • Vegetate and find myself unable to do anything
       • Feel like a failure
       • Feel worthless
       • Feel hopeless
       • Act self-destructively in nonlethal ways
       • Become uncontrollably suicidal
    b. I will follow Dr. _____ orders as I agreed to do by identifying triggers that precipitate self-destructive behavior, and focusing my thoughts on positive affirmations of my self-worth every day. He or she will assist me by reviewing my triggers and helping me manage my symptoms early in the cycle.
    c. I recognize that my primary focus now is my recovery process, and expectations that I have for myself are unrealistic. _____ will assist me by identifying my unrealistic expectations and reviewing my calendar of activities each week to help me develop a schedule of achievable tasks.
       Before pursuing any activity I will ask myself, "Will this charge me or drain me?" If it will drain me, I will reevaluate the need to pursue the task, or will plan appropriately to offset the negative feelings that will result.
    d. I will discuss current or pending events that I find stressful with both _____ and Dr. _____ to explore healthy and appropri-

ate options to reduce the associated anxiety and resulting depression that may escalate my suicidal feelings.

e. If troubling symptoms, such as intrusive thoughts, nightmares, or insomnia, persist, I will try symptom-management techniques, or sensory awareness, recommended by both Dr. _____ and _____.

f. I will pursue activities with family members or friends to distract myself from self-destructive thoughts, especially those that give me enjoyment or bolster my sense of self-worth by enabling me to help others.

g. If I become virally ill, I will take additional measures to ensure my safety as directed by Dr. _____.

h. I will visit the cemetery no more than once monthly.

i. I will nurture myself like the good person that I am, by taking care of my physical needs appropriately, and indulging periodically in special treats.

j. When suicidal thoughts occur to me, I will try to put them out of my mind by reaffirming that "death is not an option" as Dr. _____ said, and that I *must* follow his orders. If necessary, I will progress to Section 3 of this plan to protect my physical safety. If, however, I successfully resist these thoughts and focus my attention on other alternatives to the triggering problem(s), I may reward myself weekly with fresh flowers.

2. Maintaining the safe room:

a. This room is to be maintained and treated with the respect of a hospital room to protect its sense of safety.

b. Neither this room, nor the adjacent bathroom may contain any sharps, unless requested and given to me by _____ for one-time use. Sharps that I may use if I give a safety commitment include my hair dryer, electric razor, mirror, tweezers, and nail scissors.

c. I must keep the room clear of clutter at all times to ensure its availability as a "safe room," and I will stock closet shelves with the following items:
   • Pad of legal paper or journal
   • Pen and pencil
   • Art pad
   • Colored pencils and magic markers
   • "Beauty and the Beast" coloring book
   • Airplane books
   • Harlequin romances
   • Current magazines and catalogues
   • "Safe" craft projects

- Bop bag
- "Safe plan" album

The bed is to be kept made at all times when the room is not in use, and the back rest and stuffed animals are to remain on the bed.

d. The bookshelf must be stocked with current reading material of interest to me, as well as the books given to me which affirm the value of life. In addition, albums containing cards and letters sent to me while hospitalized and positive affirmations that I have developed are to be housed on these shelves. Also, collages or albums with family pictures and photos of past vacations and special occasions are to be kept in the room.

e. No materials relating to pending litigation including past hospitalization records, work, or other identified stressors may be brought into this room at any time.

f. If a "Do Not Disturb Sign" is on the door it must be honored at all times by _____ or other people in the house (unless a fear for my safety exists). If the door is closed, anyone entering must first knock and be granted my permission to enter.

3. Using the safe room:

a. I will use the room whenever I cannot maintain my safety, and will first let either _____ or Dr. _____ know (by message) that I am unsafe and following my safety plan.

b. I agree to call Dr. _____ at least once every twenty-four hours and leave a message updating the status of my safety if my time in the room exceeds this period.

c. I, and others, are to consider and treat the room as if it is as safe as a hospital admission. Admission to the room, or unsupervised use of the adjacent bathroom, constitutes a commitment to safety on my part while in there, equal to that I would give to the nursing staff if actually hospitalized. In accordance herewith, I agree to treat the room with respect and express anger using only appropriate means as described in the following section.

d. If I do use the room to control my unsafe impulses, or angry feelings, I agree to allow _____ to perform "fifteen-minute checks" to ensure that I am following the plan as outlined and to provide me the opportunity to discuss issues of importance on a one-to-one basis. If I am acting unreasonably or respond to _____ in an angry manner, however, _____ will leave me alone and return in another fifteen minutes. This pattern will repeat until _____ considers me sufficiently calm to hold a reasonable discussion.

e. I will not be expected to answer the phone or the front door while in this room, and people who ask for me should be told that I am "unavailable," "away," or "hospitalized." Alternatively, the answering machine may record all calls.

f. I will not be expected to handle any routine responsibilities of life while using this room, including cooking, bill paying, etc., but I will be responsible to ensure that I eat, drink, and maintain my physical well-being, including managing my chronic medical conditions daily.

g. The room will be stocked with medication supplies for a twenty-four hour period, which will be updated by _____ daily as necessary. I agree to take all required medications while using the safe room, and will use valium or phenobarbital when I first feel that I am losing control of my physical safety.

h. I will list the reasons that I want to die and will review positive affirmations that I have written to reaffirm my sense of self-worth and understand that suicide is an irrational solution to a temporary problem. In addition, I may read positive, life-affirming books or magazine articles I may have.

i. I will review a list of my strengths and positive attributes, of which honoring my safety contract and following this plan is one.

j. I will review the journal detailing my daily goals and accomplishments to confirm that even though my actions may not be considered "great" by others, I do contribute each and every day in a positive way to someone's life.

k. I will review my positive accomplishments during my life to date, and update this with any that I perceive may not be listed. I may also review albums and scrapbooks containing mementos of special occasions and past events in my life.

l. I will peruse family photo albums and memorabilia related thereto, and focus on the pain that my suicide would cause the people that I love, and who care for me.

m. I will prepare a summary of future events to which I can look forward, particularly those that would bring me joy or allow me to make others happy.

n. I will pray for the strength to commit to life and to recognize the wonderful gift I have been given. I do not need to understand everything that happens along the way.

o. I will review my reasons for living, and update this list with at least two additional reasons to continue life at the present time.

p. If I am feeling so self-destructive that I feel that suicide is imminent and the above steps have not yet helped to mitigate my feelings, or I cannot add to the list in step "o," I will read the letters written to me by my family members during my first hospitalization detailing their reasons why I should live. I will then add two additional reasons for living to the list mentioned in step "o."

q. I will use art to express my feelings in a positive manner, using one of the following techniques:

- If my self-destructive urges are uncontrollable, I will use magic markers to draw these actions first on paper, and then in the form of cuts on my arm if drawing on paper for fifteen minutes does not alleviate some of the urgency.
- I may use artwork to express anger or rage, by drawing violent scenes or slashes in a quick, forceful manner to alleviate any internal tension that I may feel.
- Alternatively, I may draw a continuous border outlining a piece of art paper and depict my negative feelings "contained" inside, and then focus on the fact that the feelings cannot escape these borders.
- I may draw a "safe" scene depicting an image that relaxes me and imagine myself there for at least fifteen minutes.
- I will determine my three most predominant feelings during the past twenty-four hours, and rate them in order of severity. I will draw circles and color these circles to represent these feelings. If I express only self-destructive, angry, or hurtful feelings, I will draw three additional circles, and list these as the feelings that I deserve to have: happiness, a sense of peace, and self-worth.
- Alternatively, I will draw a bridge depicting at the left hand side the feelings I am experiencing now, and at the right positive feelings that I hope to attain. Along the bridge I will draw the steps that I must take to achieve these positive goals.
- Or, I may fold a piece of art paper and draw a castle in a wonderful country setting. Inside the castle (inside the folded paper) I will draw a picture window depicting three positive scenes— one from my past life, one from my current life, and one from my future life.
- I may also fold a piece of paper and draw a treasure chest at the bottom of a clear blue sea. When I open the chest (open the paper) I find the five objects which would be most helpful to me now to mitigate my feelings and reaffirm my sense of self-worth or interest in living. After drawing these objects, I must reflect on how I can obtain them or use substitutes to achieve my positive goals.

r. If I am feeling uncontrollably angry, I will use exercise to express my feelings, or release pent-up rage as necessary by using the punching bag kept in the closet. If this does not relieve the internal tension, and medication has not calmed me within thirty minutes, I will tear paper to shreds to release this tension. I agree that I will later clean up any mess I make when I am more in control, but it is understood that the paper shreds can remain scattered in the room as long as I need to see them to gain a sense of internal satisfaction.

s. If I am calm, but unsafe, I will attempt to quietly read a book or magazine of interest after completing each of the above steps, or I will work on a safe craft project.

t. If reading, or performing craft work does not mitigate my self-destructive feelings to a controllable level, I will attempt to sleep. If necessary, I will take further medication to allow me to do so.

u. If I feel myself "fading out" while in this room, I can remain unafraid and reassure myself that one of my alters, who only have my best interests at heart, is emerging. If I find colored pictures, or other evidence that they pursued activities during my "lost time," I will thank them for keeping me safe and honor them by keeping their artwork or other completed projects.

v. I will be fully informed, to the extent possible, by _____ or _____ in writing, of any activity that I pursue of which I might be unaware while in this safe room, as well as any activities that may have precipitated my self-destructive urges.

4. Additional steps to maintain safety if required:

a. If I have pursued the above steps and continue to feel uncontrollably suicidal, I will ask _____, my mother or father, _____, or _____, to speak with me or come to stay with me as necessary to avoid hospitalization.

b. As a last resort, I will contact Dr. _____ to arrange for hospitalization if I cannot otherwise remain safe, or discuss other possible alternatives.

STEPS TO FOLLOW IMMEDIATELY WHEN SUICIDAL

Death is not an option, and I must perform the following steps, which summarize my safety plan, in accordance with Dr. _____'s orders and my family's expectations for me:

1. Call _____ or Dr. _____ to let one of them know that I am implementing my safety plan.
2. Go into my safe room.
3. Take antianxiety medication as instructed by Dr. _____.
4. Read my safety contract and safety plan, if I am capable of doing so.
5. List the reasons that I want to die, and review positive affirmations to reaffirm my sense of self-worth and understand that there truly is no rational basis to my need to die.
6. Review my list of my strengths and positive attributes.
7. Review my past daily goals and accomplishments to confirm that my life has had value, and that I can continue to live productively.
8. Review albums and scrapbooks detailing special occasions in my past life, and depicting those people I love, and who care for me. Focus on the pain that my suicide would cause them.
9. Prepare a summary of future events to which I can look forward.
10. Review my list of reasons to live, and add two more.
11. Pray or meditate.
12. Use art techniques to control my negative feelings and bolster my sense of self-worth.
13. Vent my anger constructively.
14. Read quietly, perform "safe" craft work or sleep.
15. If I cannot maintain my safety after following the steps outlined in Section 3 of my safety plan, call someone to stay with me.
16. As a last resort, contact Dr. _____ to arrange a hospital admission.

CONTRACT FOR SAFETY ISSUES

Date: _____

I. General Provisions

I agree to not hurt myself or anybody else, human or animal, internal or external, now or in the future, accidentally or on purpose, until the date specified at 5:00 p.m., unless reasonably necessary to defend myself, my property, or my privacy.

II. Definition of "Hurt"

"Hurt" is defined as physically or emotionally damaging acts, whether painful or not. Physical hurt *specifically and emphatically precludes any attempt to kill myself or anybody else for any reason.* It does not include trivial harm such as bruises that result from bumping into furniture or minor cuts and scrapes which are not self-inflicted. Also, death or injury resulting from an accident or illness which I did not knowingly cause is excluded.

Emotional hurt is defined to include any action I knowingly undertake which harms another's emotional stability, hurts their feelings or damages their sense of self-respect. This includes destroying their property, spending their money without proper, prior authorization, insulting them or defaming them by calling them names or telling lies about them, screaming at them, or otherwise treating them in a disrespectful manner.

III. Control of Specific Suicidal Modality

I also agree to refrain from buying any pills or obtaining them from any source unless recommended by my physician(s), and I will take them only in the recommended dose. I will discuss any and all medications that I take during the course of this contract with Dr. _____.

In addition, I agree to refrain from obtaining any other devices or substances intended for self-harm and will discuss any lethal means that I consider using for self-destructive purposes with Dr. _____ prior to harming myself. I will inform him or her, as soon as it becomes known to me, if someone internally plans to take such action, and will immediately implement our agreed safety plan to preclude escalation of uncontrollable feelings and the potential need for hospitalization.

IV. Control of Fugue Episodes

I must remain in _____ unless I give prior notice to, and receive approval from, either _____ or Dr. _____. I also agree to relinquish control of vouchers I hold now, and any that I may receive during the duration of this contract, for frequent flier miles, free or discounted hotel rooms, and rental cars to _____.

V. Consequences

I agree to discuss any action taken that results in physical harm to myself or others, including animals, during my next scheduled therapy session to determine whether the specific act performed is permitted by the parameters of this contract. It is expressly understood that permitted acts *do not include killing myself.*

If I threaten suicide or attempt to take my life, Dr. _____ will discuss the need for hospitalization with me. If we both agree that this is necessary, I may voluntarily admit myself to avoid legal detention, unless extenuating circumstances exist, which in his or her opinion warrant detention. If Dr. _____ does determine that hospitalization is necessary, and I do not agree to voluntary admission, I may be detained. However, he or she expressly agrees that I will never, under circumstances that he or she can control, be detained in _____. If I am admitted to its psychiatric unit under circumstances outside of his or her control, he or she will act within his or her power to ensure that I am not held in a Quiet Room.

If I cut myself, or harm myself using other nonlethal means, I must extend the termination date of this contract by the number of days it requires the self-inflicted hurt to heal completely. I must discuss other violations of this contract with Dr. _____, and we will mutually agree on acceptable consequences which will subsequently be incorporated into this contract. I agree that the individual responsible for the self-destructive action will be the party to suffer the applicable consequence.

VI. Modifications

This contract replaces that dated _____, and will remain in full force and effect until the date and time specified unless modified in writing by both the Executor and the Witness. We will review this contract on a weekly basis to make needed modifications, if any. Unless a dissent is registered below, everyone internally agrees to abide by the terms of this contract as now written, as well as any modifications which may be made during its duration.

Date: _____   Signed: _____

Agreed and Witnessed: _____

Agreed and Witnessed: _____

Registered Dissent:

_____

_____

_____

_____

SAFETY CONTRACT

I and my parts agree not to attempt to kill myself nor to kill myself accidentally or on purpose, now or in the future. Before I ever again consider suicide I agree to the following safety plan:

1. Use escape routes such as sitting in my car, going to Dad's or Mom's, going to _____, browsing in a bookstore or library, or going to a restaurant.
2. Remember how sad and angry someone else's suicide attempts have made me; I don't want to do that to my family.
3. Think of the physical damage it could cause if it doesn't work, such as brain damage or liver damage.
4. Write a list of people who would be adversely affected by my suicide.
5. Look at pictures of any children and loved ones and remember the good times we've had and that I would miss them growing up and they would miss me.
6. Remember that things have been this bad before, and that with my support, they have gotten better.
7. Use my cognitive skills to better focus on the reality of the hopeless feelings.
8. Listen to the tapes my therapist made me.
9. Call friends.
10. Call my therapist or, if he or she is unavailable, call an alternative backup and say I am unsafe and need to talk.
11. Call physician and say I am unsafe and need to talk.
12. Call psychiatrist and say I am unsafe and need to be hospitalized.

I and my parts agree to have on hand only seven (7) days worth of the psychotropic medications that I take, and fourteen (14) days worth of all other prescription medications. Any excess medications will be kept in my doctor's office. Any medications that no longer are prescribed for me shall be destroyed. I and my parts agree to do no bodily harm, whether painful or not, which is self-inflicted. This includes scratching and cutting deep enough to bleed or to require sutures. If such actions occur, I will report it to my therapist and he or she has the right to suspend our sessions for 48 hours until such behavior stops. If more than two suspensions occur during one month, further action, which will be mutually agreed upon, will occur.

I understand that if I break this contract my psychiatrist (_____) and my therapist (_____) have the right to refuse to further treat me.

This contract will be in effect for the next 60 days. It can be amended only with both of our consent.

Signed by: _____ Date_____
Witnessed and agreed to by: _____ Date_____

REFERENCES

Barach, P. M. (1994). *ISSD guidelines for treating dissociative identity disorder (multiple personality disorder) in Adults.* Skokie, IL: ISSD.

Benjamin, L. R. and Benjamin, R. (1994a). A group for partners and parents of MPD clients. Part I: Process and format. *Dissociation,* VII(1), 35-43.

Benjamin, L. P. and Benjamin, R. (1994b). A group for partners and parents of MPD clients. Part II: Themes and Responses. *Dissociation,* VII(2), 104-112.

Benjamin, L. R. and Benjamin, R. (1994c). A group for partners and parents of MPD clients. Part III: Marital types and dynamics. *Dissociation,* VII(3), 191-196.

Briere, J. (1989). *Therapy for adults molested as children: Beyond survival.* New York: Springer Publishing Company.

Briere, J. (1992). Methodological issues in the study of sexual abuse affects. *Journal of Interpersonal Violence, 3,* 367-379.

Briere, J. and Runtz, M. (1988). Symptomatology associated with childhood sexual victimization in a nonclinical adult sample. *Child Abuse and Neglect, 12,* 51-59.

Brown, G. R. and Anderson, B. (1991). Psychiatric morbidity in adult inpatients with childhood histories of sexual and physical abuse. *American Journal of Psychiatry, 148,* 55-61.

Buchele, B. J. (1995). Group psychotherapy for persons with multiple personality and dissociative disorders. In J. G. Allen and W. H. Smith (Eds.), *Diagnosis and treatment of dissociative disorders* (pp. 85-94). Northvale, NJ: Jason Aronson, Inc.

Caul, D. (1984). Group and videotape techniques for multiple personality disorder. *Psychiatric Annals, 14,* 43-50.

Caul, D., Sachs, R. G., and Braun, B. G. (1986). Group therapy in treatment of multiple personality disorder. In B. G. Braun (Ed.), *Treatment of multiple personality disorder* (pp. 143-156). Washington, DC: American Psychiatric Press.

Chew, J. (1998). *Women survivors of childhood sexual abuse: Healing through group work: Beyond survival.* Binghamton, NY: The Haworth Press.

Chu, J. A. and Dill, D. L. (1990). Dissociative symptoms in relation to childhood physical and sexual abuse. *American Journal of Psychiatry, 147,* 887-892.

Coons, P. M. and Bradley, T. (1985). Group therapy with multiple personality patients. *Journal of Nervous and Mental Disease, 173*(9), 515-521.

Courtois, C. A. (1988). *Healing the incest wound.* New York: W. W. Norton.

Courtois, C. A. and Leehan, J. (1992). Group treatment for grownup abused children. *Personnel and Guidance Journal, 60,* 564-566.

Danieli, Y. (1994). Countertransference and trauma: Self-healing and training issues. In M. B. Williams and J. F. Sommer (Eds.), *Handbook of post-traumatic therapy* (pp. 540-550). Westport, CT: Greenwood Press.

Dolan, Y. M. (1985). *A path with a heart: Ericksonian utilization with resistant and chronic clients.* New York: Brunner/Mazel.

Donaldson, M. A. and Cordes-Green, S. (1994). *Group treatment of adult incest survivors.* Thousand Oaks, CA; Sage Publications.

Federle, N. and Harrington, E. (1990). Women's groups: How connections heal. Work in Progress, 57. Wellesley, MA: Stone Center Working Paper Series.

Feord, M. F. (1993). Session notes 4 and 5: Relationships. Falls Church, VA: MPD/DID Support Group at Dominion Hospital.

Feord, M. F. (1994). Process notes of the psychoeducational support group for DID/MPD. Falls Church, VA: MPD/DID Support Group at Dominion Hospital.

Grame, C. J. (1995). Internal containment in the treatment of patients with dissociative disorders. In J. G. Allen and W. H. Smith (Eds.), *Diagnosis and treatment of dissociative disorders* (pp. 77-83). Northvale, NJ: Jason Aronson, Inc.

Hogan, L. C. (1992). Managing persons with multiple personality disorder in a heterogeneous inpatient group. *Group, 16,* 247-256.

Horning, C. (November/December 1994). "Therapeutic boundaries with DID clients." *The Advocate,* p. 11.

International Society for the Study of Traumatic Stress Studies and Foy, D. W., Glynn, S. M., Schnurr, P. P., Weiss, D. S., Wattenberg, M. S., Marmar, C. R., Jankowski, M. K., and Gusman, F. D. (1999). *Group psychotherapy for posttraumatic stress disorder.* ISTSS treatment guidelines committee position paper. Northvale, IL: ISTSS.

Jehu, D. (1988). *Beyond sexual abuse: Therapy with women who were childhood victims.* New York: John Wiley and Sons.

Kluft, R. P. (1989). Treating the patient who has been sexually exploited by a previous therapist. *Psychiatric Clinics of North America, 12,* 483-500.

Kluft, R. P. (1993). Basic principles in conducting the psychotherapy of MPD. In R. P. Kluft and C. G. Fine (Eds.), *Clinical perspectives on MPD* (pp. 19-50). Washington, DC: American Psychiatric Press.

Linehan, M. M. (1993). *Skills training manual for treating BPD.* New York: Guilford Press.

McCann, I. L. and Pearlman, L. A. (1990a). *Psychological trauma and the adult survivor: Theory, therapy, and transformation.* New York: Brunner/Mazel.

McCann, I. L. and Pearlman, L. A. (1990b). Vicarious traumatization: A framework for understanding the psychological effects of working with victims. *Journal of Traumatic Stress, 3,* 131-149.

Miller, D. (1994). *Women who hurt themselves: A book of hope and understanding.* New York: Basic Books.

Overbeck, B. and Overbeck, J. (1995). *Starting/running support groups.* Dallas, TX: TLC Group Publications for Transition, Loss, and Change.

Pearlman, L. A. and Saakvitne, L. W. (1995). *Trauma and the therapist: Countertransference and vicarious traumatization in psychotherapy with incest survivors.* New York: W. W. Norton.

Putnam, F. W. (1989). *Diagnosis and treatment of multiple personality disorder.* New York: Guilford Press.

Riggan, W. (1998). Clinical and social issues related to dissociative identity disorder outpatient groups. *Treating Abuse Today, 8*(3), 19-21.

Rosenbloom, D. and Williams, M. B. (1999). *Life after trauma: A workbook for healing.* New York: Guilford Press.

Ross, C. A. and Gahan, P. (1988). Techniques in the treatment of multiple personality disorder. *American Journal of Psychotherapy, 47,* 103-112.

Roth, S. and Batson, R. (1997). *Naming the shadows: A new approach to individual and group psychotherapy for adult survivors of childhood incest.* New York: The Free Press.

Salston, M. and Baker, G. R. (1993). *Management of intrusion and arousal symptoms in post-traumatic stress disorder.* Los Angeles, CA: Workshop Handout.

Saunders, B., Villeponteaux, L., Lipovsky, J., Kilpatrick, D., and Veronen, L. J. (1992). Child sexual assault as a risk factor for mental disorders among women. *Journal of Interpersonal Violence, 7*(2), 189-204.

Simpson, M. A. (1995). Gullible's travels, or the importance of being multiple. In L. M. Cohen, J. N. Berzoff, and M. R. Elm (Eds.), *Dissociative identity disorder: Theoretical and treatment controversies* (pp. 87-135). Northvale, NJ: Jason Aronson, Inc.

Turkus, J. A. (1991). Psychotherapy and case management for MPD: Synthesis for continuity of care. *Psychiatric Clinics of North America, 14*(3), 649-660.

Turkus, J. A. and Courtois, C. A. (1994). *Group therapy with dissociative disorder clients.* Alexandria, VA: Eastern Regional Conference on Dissociative Disorders.

van der Kolk, B. A., Perry, J. C., and Herman, J. L. (1991). Childhood origins of self-destructive behavior. *American Journal of Psychiatry, 148,* 1665-1671.

Watson, D. E. (1994). *Surviving your crises, reviving your dreams.* Bedford, MA: Mills and Sanderson, Publishers.

Webb, L. P. and Leehan, J. (1996). *Group treatment for adult survivors of abuse: A manual for practitioners.* Thousand Oaks, CA: Sage Publications.

Williams, M. B. (1990). "Post-traumatic stress disorder and child sexual abuse: The enduring effects." Santa Barbara, CA: The Fielding Institute. Unpublished doctoral dissertation.

Williams, M. B. (1991). Clinical work with families of MPD patients: Assessment and issues for practice. *Dissociation, IV*(3), 92-98.

Williams, M. B. (1993a). Establishing safety in survivors of severe sexual abuse in posttraumatic stress therapy Part I. *Treating Abuse Today, 3*(1), 4-11.

Williams, M. B. (1993b). Establishing safety in survivors of severe sexual abuse in posttraumatic stress therapy, part II. *Treating Abuse Today, 3*(2), 13-16.

Williams, M. B. (1993c). Establishing safety in survivors of severe sexual abuse in posttraumatic stress therapy, part III. *Treating Abuse Today, 3*(3), 13-15.

Williams, M. B. (1995). Treating trauma in the family. In M. Harway (Ed.), *Treating the changing family: Handling normative and unusual events.* New York: John Wiley and Sons.

Williams, M. B. and Sommer, J. F. (1994). *Handbook of posttraumatic therapy.* Westport, CT: Greenwood Press.

Yalom, D. (1985). *The theory and practice of group psychotherapy* (Third edition). New York: Basic Books.

SECTION IV:
CHILDREN, STUDENTS, AND FAMILIES

Chapter 10

Treatment Strategies
for Traumatized Children

Mary W. Lindahl

In recent years, trauma has received a great deal of attention from psychologists and other mental health professionals. Most of the research, however, has been directed at adults rather than children. In the course of a thirty-year career, this author has found the techniques available to treat traumatized children inadequate to deal with the complexities of their situations and, thus, over the years, has been constantly confronted with the need to develop new approaches. This chapter, building on past research, presents new ideas and techniques that have worked to help children who have experienced many types of traumatic events, including those caused by human design (physical, sexual, and emotional abuse; domestic violence; witnessing a violent crime or the murder of a parent; parental death by suicide or sudden line-of-duty death in a law enforcement parent; kidnapping; and the deliberate terrorizing and attempted emotional destruction of the child) as well as those caused by nonhuman forces (fires, natural disasters, airplane and automobile accidents, death of a parent through illness or accident; necessary medical treatments, and discovering a mutilated body).

BRIEF OVERVIEW OF THE LITERATURE

Estimates of the percentage of children who develop PTSD after trauma vary considerably according to type of trauma, age and sex of the child, availability of family support, and strictness of criteria required to make the diagnosis (Vogel and Vernberg, 1993). A number of studies, using both qualitative and quantitative approaches, have examined the responses of children exposed to traumas of witnessing severe violence (Eth and Pynoos, 1985b; Malmquist, 1986; Nader et al., 1990; Schwartz and Kowalski, 1991; Zeanah and Burk, 1984); natural disasters (Galante and Foa, 1986; Garrison et al., 1995; Gould and Gould, 1991; Shaw et al., 1995); child abuse (Herman, 1992; van der Kolk, MacFarlane, and Weisaeth, 1996); being held hostage (Butler, Leitenberg, and Fuselier, 1995; Jessee, Strickland, and Ladewig, 1992); accidents resulting in physical injury (Jones and Peterson, 1993; MacLean, 1977); exposure to warfare (Arroyo and Eth, 1985; Garbarino, Kostelny, and Dubrow, 1991); and painful and frightening medical treatments (Nir, 1985).

Children who have experienced trauma are vulnerable to a wide variety of negative outcomes. An excellent literature review by Armsworth and Holaday (1993) documents the following effects of various kinds of traumas on children:

1. *Cognitive:* time distortions, development of omens, a foreshortened sense of future, memory impairment, decreased ability to learn, loss of academic skills, and impaired concentration
2. *Affective:* emotional reexperiencing, intrusive images and avoidance, depression, guilt and shame, feelings of helplessness and powerlessness, negative self-perceptions, and constricted emotions
3. *Behavioral:* increased aggression and disruptive behavior, withdrawal, regressive symptoms such as enuresis and encopresis, muteness, disturbances in attachment, repetitive play and reenactment including sexualized behavior, suicide attempts, chemical dependency, self-destructive and risky behaviors, and impaired social skills
4. *Physiological:* hypervigilance and nervous system changes (see also Famularo, Kinscherff, and Fenton, 1992; Finkelhor and Browne, 1985; Friedrich, 1993; Lewis et al., 1989; Green et al., 1991; Green, 1993; Payton and Krocker-Tuskan, 1988; Osofsky, 1995)

EVALUATION AND TREATMENT PLAN

A thorough evaluation resulting in a well-designed treatment plan is crucial to the effective treatment of potentially traumatized children (Brohl, 1996; Everstine and Everstine, 1989; Levin, 1993; McNally, 1991; Miller and Veltkamp, 1995; Putnam, 1996; Pynoos and Eth, 1986; Scheeringa et al., 1995; Viglione, 1990). Ideally, assessment begins with a broad range of psychological testing:

1. *Cognitive measures:* the Weschler Intelligence Scale for Children-Third Edition (WISC-III) (Wechsler, 1991); the Woodcock-Johnson Psychoeducational Battery-Revised (WJ-R) (Costenbader and Perry, 1990); and the Wide-Range Achievement Test-Revised (WRAT-R) (Reinehr, 1987)

2. *Projective tests:* the Rorschach Inkblot Technique (Rorschach, 1921); the House-Tree-Person Projective Drawing Technique (Buck, 1981); the Roberts Apperception Test (Roberts, 1982); and the Rotter Incomplete Sentence Blank (Rotter and Rafferty, 1950)
3. *Checklists:* Trauma Symptom Checklist for Children (TSCC) (Briere, 1996); the Children's Depression Inventory (CDI) (Kovacs, 1992); the Revised Children's Manifest Anxiety Scale (RCMAS) (Reynolds and Richmond, 1985); Devereux Scales of Mental Disorders (Naglieri, LeBuffe, and Pfeiffer, 1994); and the Child Behavior Checklist (CBCL) (Achenbach and Edelbrock, 1986)
4. *Structured interview formats* (to assess symptoms of PTSD): the Post-Traumatic Stress Disorder Reaction Index (PTSD-RI) (Pynoos et al., 1987); Children's Post-Traumatic Stress Disorder Inventory (CPTSDI) (Saigh, 1991); and the Children's Impact of Traumatic Events Scale (CITES) (Wolfe, Gentile, and Wolfe, 1989)

In addition to psychological testing, less formal interviews should be conducted with the child and family to gather as much information as possible about the events and circumstances surrounding the trauma.

Several interviews are usually needed with the child and parent or accompanying adult to complete the assessment and formulate a treatment plan. These interviews also educate about traumatic reactions, help the child tell the story of the trauma, target individual symptoms, evaluate the need for medication, encourage the expression and working through of feelings about the event(s), help the child's efforts to understand and find a meaning in the trauma, explore developmental and characterological issues and vulnerabilities, assess and strengthen family and social support, and refer to and collaborate with other sources such as group therapy or school support.

EDUCATING THE CHILD AND FAMILY ABOUT TRAUMA

Children tend to be fascinated by psychological information. They are intrigued to learn that the therapist has seen children with similar experiences before. Explaining the symptoms and naming the reaction (PTSD or depression, for example) brings them relief. It is helpful to give information to the child and then ask him or her to present that information to the parent. This retelling enables the therapist to see if the child understood the information and also helps her initiate a sense of control over the trauma.

In cases of sexual abuse, the social worker or therapist usually reassures the child: "Remember, it's not your fault; only the adult is responsible." To a child who has been groomed and entrapped in the abusive activity and who has internalized and come to share the cognitive distortions of the abuser, these words have no impact. Even very young children generally understand that, through sexual abuse, they have participated in acts that society and their parents say is wrong. Parents and prevention programs drum into children: "Don't 'let' anyone touch your private parts." This is *"bad* touch"; receiving that type of touch means they have done something *"bad,"* particularly when a child's body responded pleasurably during the abuse. It is not surprising that children do not tell what happened. Recent approaches, referring to "uncomfortable" or "confusing" touch are an improvement, but still may not effectively capture the child's experience.

Many offenders begin abuse with subtle and confusing preliminary touches that the child does not understand and thus does not protest. These touches may seem accidental or may occur in the context of ordinary activities such as bathing or roughhousing. By the time there is overt sexual touch, the child believes the rationalizations of the abuser who says, "It's your fault; why didn't you say anything before?" These children need to know the information that has been gained in interviews with convicted sex offenders as to how they entice and entrap children (Berliner and Conte, 1990; Burgess and Holmstrom, 1978; Conte, Wolf, and Smith, 1989; Elliott, Browne, and Kilcoyne, 1995; Singer, Hussey, and Strom, 1992).

When trauma takes the form of accidents, natural disasters, or acts inflicted by medical personnel in the course of necessary treatment, the therapist can explain, for example, the formation of the hurricane, the cause of the fire, automobile, or plane crash or the reason for a medical procedure. Explanation helps eliminate misunderstandings about causation and assists with mastery of the event.

THE ROLE OF PARENTS

Whenever appropriate, working with the parents of a traumatized child to support and strengthen the family system can be crucial to a child's recovery. Parents, to the greatest extent possible, should be cotherapists for the traumatized child. They can often recount the trauma more accurately, as well as explain the child's background and prior development. Moreover, researchers have reported that the child's reaction to trauma is heavily dependent on that of the parent (Foy, 1992).

Traumatized children need their parents to be involved closely in their treatment. Therefore, it is important to see them individually when necessary and, when practical, to include one or both parents in part of each session. At times, if the child is in crisis, it may be vital to bring a supportive parent into the session to hold or soothe the child. Of course, all too often, traumatized children do not have an available or supportive parent. For these children, a supportive adult, such as another family member or professional, can be helpful. Educating parents about children's reactions to trauma is also important. One way to educate them is to recommend a book such as *Children and Trauma: A Parent's Guide to Helping Children Heal* (Monahon, 1993). In addition, parents can serve as liaisons between therapists and teachers, as well as put the therapist's suggestions for ameliorating symptoms and promoting healing into practice between sessions. It is sometimes necessary to refer a sibling or parent, who may, for example, have been involved in the same accident or may simply be devastated by the suffering of the child, to another therapist or to a support group (Heft, 1993; Newberger et al., 1993).

TELLING THE STORY

Lenore Terr (1991) has differentiated between Type I and Type II traumatic events. Type I traumas are single, unexpected events that usually culminate in PTSD. They are often accompanied by detailed memories, omens, cognitive reappraisals, and misperceptions. Type II traumas are caused by long-term repetitive traumas (such as chronic child abuse) from which there is no escape. Victims tend to develop denial, psychic numbing, excessive dissociation, and characterological disturbances.

Regardless of the type of trauma, children often have an extremely difficult time telling the story of what happened. This recounting is perhaps the most difficult part of the treatment. Victims of Type I trauma are too frightened to tell; victims of Type II trauma tend to suffer memory problems and confusion. Sometimes the disclosure is accidental (for example, the child slips and tells a friend "a secret" or gives obvious clues through behavior) and other times purposeful (Sgroi, Blick, and Porter, 1982).

Currently, a wide range of controversy exists about the reliability or suggestibility of children's memories, particularly in allegations of sexual abuse (Ceci, Ross, and Toglia, 1989; Williams, 1995; Terr, 1988). Researchers have found that children's memories (as well as adults') can be distorted by a variety of factors, although children can be reliable historians and are more resistant to suggestion than was previously believed (Doris, 1976). It must be acknowledged, however, that there is a substantial difference between a trauma that is witnessed by many, such as a natural disaster, and one that occurs in private, such as sexual abuse, in which the child, often intentionally being confused by the perpetrator, tries to relate from memory an accurate account of the event.

Particularly in sexual abuse cases, it is important to acknowledge and to consider whether allegations are true or false. It is a difficult fact for therapists to admit that, ultimately, with the possible exception of situations in which there is an eyewitness to the trauma, it is not possible to discern the truth conclusively in spite of how credible the child's account may be. A child might make a false allegation because of developmental issues and/or misunderstanding of the event (for example, a parent touched the child non-sexually while applying medicine), indoctrination by an adult, suggestion by the interviewer, deliberate lying, and/or confabulation (Benedek and Schetky, 1987; Berliner and Conte, 1993; Bernet, 1993; Everson, 1997; Everson and Boat, 1989; Heiman, 1992). Paradoxically, the therapist must be totally committed to search for the truth while, at the same time, realizing that the full truth will probably never be known.

A credible allegation of sexual abuse does not necessarily result in protection of the child. Children also are at risk for psychological harm when false allegations are made. For example, a child may make a demonstrably false accusation of sexual abuse at the urging of a parent; the authorities determine that the charge is false, but the parent continues to press the allegation. The child may then be removed from therapy by the accusing parent, and be required to live as a sexual abuse victim when he or she may actually be a severe emotional abuse victim. Such experiences compromise the child's development of reality testing, accuracy of memory, trust of other people, and sense of morality.

Case Studies

Whether the trauma is public or private, younger children are usually never able to give a detailed chronology of the event. For example, Bryan was too young to communicate his traumatic event accurately. He was brought to therapy, dazed and virtually mute, three weeks before his third birthday and the day after his mother's funeral. He was the only witness to her murder by an intruder. Unable to give a coherent chronological story of what happened or a description of the murderer, he only referred to him as "the Big Man." He was never able to provide any information which could help the police, even with the use of a police drawing of the crime scene and pictures of possible suspects.

Children sometimes communicate about the traumatic event metaphorically because they are unable to understand what happened to them. Three-year-old Lisa communicated to the therapist through her terrifying obsession that Freddy Krueger (villain of the horror movie *A Nightmare on Elm Street*) was going to come in her bedroom to kill her while she was sleeping. Medical examination disclosed that she had been recently raped. Careful questioning of the child and family helped officials to conclude that she had probably been raped during a party. The perpetrator had exited out the back door of the bathroom directly into Lisa's bedroom, raped her while she slept, reentered the bathroom, and casually returned to the party.

Some children disclose in dissociative states or describe dissociating during the traumatic experience. Paula, age five, sexually abused in a painful and frightening way, was unable to sleep. She was also anxious, aggressive, and fearful, and it seemed as if all the joy had gone out of her life. One day she blurted out that she had not told her mother about the abuse "because I don't want to see any more cut-up bodies!" Urged to draw what was in her mind, Paula, eyes wide and teeth chattering, drew a series of bloody, violent, sexual pictures. It turned out that the abuser had replaced her bedtime story with a terrifying pornographic book. Although Paula maintained that there was no book, the disclosure enabled her to sleep again.

Two children treated by the author were able to describe and write stories about their sexual abuse in detail, including referring to the perpetrator by name, yet insisted that the character in the story was fictional. Many children, in order to distance themselves from overwhelming fear, initially disclose in fictional story form; eventually they are able to connect the story with their abuse. These children, however, were never able to connect their stories to the real incidents. They insisted that the abuse they described did not happen to them. For this reason, the authorities were never able to take any action, and the future of these children is unknown.

ADDRESSING THE SYMPTOMS

Children can be helped to reexperience the trauma emotionally in a safe environment one step removed, using drawing, story writing, and playing with toys. The therapist simultaneously helps the child express feelings of anger, fear, guilt, and/or helplessness in this safe environment. Emotions are labeled, explained, and worked through. If too directly confronted too early, children take strong steps to avoid the material. Some children simply ignore the questioner; others stick their fingers in their ears, hum, sing loudly, or scream, "I don't want to talk about it, and you can't make me!" At the other extreme, Terr (1990) has spoken of the need for the therapist to intervene when children are engaging in "posttraumatic play," i.e., repetitively and obsessively playing out the trauma with no resolution, by helping them change the ending of the story to achieve a more positive outcome. It is also necessary to address the issue of posttraumatic reenactments. For example, Donny, survivor of the crash of a large commercial airliner, gently fell and slightly broke both forearms several weeks later; he came to therapy with two tiny casts on his forearms.

Treating the physiological effects of trauma, such as extreme anxiety, sleep disturbances, and somatic problems, is vital to a child's recovery. Often these symptoms are diagnosed as attention deficit disorder and the child is treated with stimulants. More complete evaluation by the therapist may determine that the ADD-like symptoms actually represent the third cluster (physiological hyperarousal) of PTSD. The use of psychotropic medications to treat traumatized children is still in its infancy and some parents initially resist the idea of medication. However, several minor tranquilizers, beta-blockers, and antidepressants have been successfully used to relieve these symptoms (Everly, 1995; Terr, 1990).

Techniques of in vitro (in the office) and in vivo (outside the office) desensitization of fears and phobias secondary to the traumatic event help alleviate the symptoms of PTSD. Even after extensive desensitization activities, it is sometimes necessary for the child to leave the office and confront the terrifying memories more directly. Beginning in the office, aspects of the trauma may be remembered and symptoms alleviated by the use of toys and props specific to the event. For example, Donny, who survived the plane crash in which half of the passengers were killed, played out the crash many times in the office using bendable dolls and small metal scale models of airliners. Although he became an expert at identifying airplane types, read newspaper accounts, and saw the TV movie of the disaster, he continued to experience severe PTSD symptoms and was consumed with the image of rescuers spraying foam above the fire rather than onto screaming, dying passengers. Donny and the author visited the local airport several times, sat in the control tower, and "flew" the parked airplanes from the captain's seat. Finally, they were taken onto the runway where a foam truck was parked, and the firemen, explaining why the foam has to be aimed above the fire, turned the truck on. An exuberant Donny, dressed in a fireman's coat and helmet, was allowed to spray the foam around the runway. Thereafter, Donny decided to become a navigator and, within a year, had flown on the same model as the stricken airplane without a problem.

Some children develop psychophysiological symptoms in addition to extreme fears and phobias specific to the traumatic event. Three-year-old Anna, after an abuse report to Child Protective Services was determined to be unfounded, lost control of her bladder. She wet herself continually and was unaware that she was wet unless she felt her clothes with her fingers. Several painful examinations and tests looking for bladder or kidney problems were performed. It was eventually discovered in the therapy that she had developed a partial anesthesia for this part of her body because a male relative had frequently performed oral sex on her. The overstimulation had caused both sexual acting out and the need to block feeling in her genital area. Empowering her mother to supervise contact with the abuser, explaining to Anna the mechanism of the enuresis within developmental limits, and rewarding bladder control eliminated this symptom.

DOES TRAUMA HAVE MEANING?

Janoff-Bulman (1992) and others have described the devastating effect of traumatic events on a survivor's world (Hazzard, 1993; Lifton and Olson, 1976). Variously referred to as cognitive schemas, assumptive worlds, or themes (Janoff-Bulman, 1992; Newman, Riggs, and Roth, 1997), these assumptions are an individual's often unconscious but strongly held beliefs about the world and the place of human beings in it. Janoff-Bulman (1992) suggests that there are three fundamental or core assumptions: the world is benevolent, the world is meaningful, and the self is worthy (good, moral, etc.). People cling to these beliefs because they appear to be adaptive, even though a number of studies have found that they are not particularly grounded in reality (Salter, 1995). In fact, people who are more realistic about the world tend to be more depressed (Seligman, 1990).

Trauma shatters these assumptions and causes a crisis in the child victim (Janoff-Bulman, 1992). This crisis usually becomes evident after the initial symptoms are under control. Most children, through adequate early maternal care, have developed a belief that the world is safe and that they, therefore, are invulnerable to harm. This attitude protects them from excessive worry about the many real dangers of the world. When children experience a traumatic event, however, their sense of invulnerability is instantly crushed. They can no longer be confident that bad things only happen to other people or that they are immune. No matter how much an adult may wish to restore the illusion of control, the child's innocence is forever lost. Explaining the statistical unlikelihood that such a trauma will reoccur is useless. It does not matter if there is a 90 percent chance of rain; what is salient to the individual is that it did rain and he got soaked.

Eleven-year-old Maria developed severe PTSD symptoms when she was visiting a child in her class and heard a neighbor report that she could not find her husband. The child, sensing no danger, went outside to look around and happened to find the man's body. He had been thrown from his tractor, run over by it, and cut up into pieces. Maria developed severe symptoms of PTSD. For many months on leaving the therapy hour, she would ask the therapist if she thought there would be a dead body outside of the office. The therapist acknowledged that it was extremely unlikely but not impossible; for Maria, there was no certain safety ever again.

The issue of safety is especially complicated for abused children. With the vagaries of the court system, inaccurate decisions about protection of children will be made at times; thus it is not always possible to reassure children that abuse will not reoccur. Therefore, it is sometimes necessary to help children learn to protect themselves. For example, it is possible to teach children the warning signs that a parent is about to lose control and to help them learn to avoid situations that trigger impending physical violence. It is also possible to provide extensive education about the grooming process of sexual abuse to help children avoid future entrapment. Even very young children can be taught to protect themselves. The therapist educated the three-year-old girl with the bladder problem about the psychology of her offender, encouraging her to tell the therapist everything that happened on the visits to the abuser and to remind her mother that she needed supervision. The child watched *People's Court,* a nonthreatening TV program that presents the justice system with a sense of humor. She began to love this show and dressed up and played the role of the judge in her therapy sessions. This training enabled her to protect herself. Her offender stopped the abuse, and the child's symptoms ultimately resolved.

Many children, to combat a sense of powerlessness in the face of trauma, create intervention fantasies, a type of cognitive reworking. Children initially may embellish their role in the trauma by making statements such as "And then I kicked him and threw him out of the window," or "Then I helped the firemen put out the fire and saved my mother." Gradually, as children face and work through these feelings of utter helplessness, they revise and restructure the fantasy memory into a more realistic scenario. For over a year, the preschooler who witnessed his mother's murder maintained that he punched and kicked the murderer. Finally, with tears in his eyes, he told the therapist what he *wished* he had done: "When I was two, I tried to help my Mama. I couldn't help her because he was too mean. I would have took that knife out of his hand."

Most children have a strong but simplistic sense of right and wrong and believe in the inevitability of punishment for bad actions (Stage I of moral development) (Lickona, 1976). They firmly believe that bad things happen only to bad people. Traumatic events devastate this belief long before they begin to understand the subtleties of the human condition or the environment. Children who observe natural disasters and accidents are confused because they have no one to blame. Children who encounter trauma caused by human design learn that criminals and child abusers often are not caught, and if caught, they are rarely prosecuted, let alone punished. Recognizing this outcome can devastate a child's developing sense of morality, justice, and fundamental fairness. A child who testifies in court and is not believed is crushed. This occurrence turns on its head the child's faith in a safe and just world.

As stated earlier, many children do not disclose sexual abuse because they believe they are at fault. Salter (1995) describes the "interlocking thinking errors" between abuser and victim that occur when the child internalizes (introjects) the cognitive distortions and beliefs of the offender. Salter outlines a number of such interlocking errors. For example, the child might come to believe the abuse is his or her fault because he or she is an attractive child. If the child responded physically, he or she is responsible because he or she wanted it; if the child froze, he or she is responsible because he or she did not stop it. Or, it is not the offender's fault because he or she could not control himself or herself or the child is overreacting and needs to forget the abuse and move on with his or her life. Baumeister (1997) comments that "perpetrators tend to favor minimalist, distancing styles of thought . . . they do not wish to dwell on the victims' suffering; to do so would be disruptive to their work" (p. viii). Therefore, they need the victim to cooperate and to maintain these distortions. Explaining and disrupting the internalization process can extricate a child from this confusion.

Abuse by a trusted adult is confusing to children. For example, a neglected thirteen-year-old who was impregnated by her elderly stepfather commented, "He had put something in my hand—it was some money." When asked what she said, she responded, "I didn't say nothing to him. See money first; ask questions later!" When asked if she felt angry at him, she stated, "Basically I felt like going to the kitchen, getting a knife and cutting his guts out. I was a little blinded because he now and then acted like a real Dad. He took us to dinner; he took me and Mom out." Some children, trapped in a relationship of traumatic bonding with the parental figure (James, 1994; Shengold, 1989), are unable to achieve even this distance. Their therapy is extremely complex, especially concerning the issue of visitation with the abusing parent.

Eventually, the child's questions may reach a spiritual point beyond the limits of psychology. If the family is interested, it is often extremely helpful to bring in a member of the clergy to address issues of meaning, spiritual outcome to the abuser, and how the child can regain faith in God. For example, one young boy could not accept the fact that his abusing father killed himself and was buried in the garden of the family's church. His minister came to a therapy session, explained the church's reasoning for burying him in holy ground, and reaffirmed that such a burial did not mean that the harm done to the child was acceptable or even, necessarily, forgiven.

Children traumatized by human design eventually bring themselves and their therapist to confront the human capacity for evil. Traditionally, the problem of evil has remained in the province of theology and philosophy. From its inception, psychology has tried to remain morally neutral and analytical about human actions. Recently, however, a number of psychologists, reacting to the need to explain events such as the Holocaust, war crimes, and crimes against children, have begun to question this neutral approach (Doherty, 1995).

Some writers conceptualize evil as a situation wherein people delude themselves, as their actions become more and more severe, until they cross over the line into evil action (Peters, 1994). Others point to narcissism, the inability to empathize (Peck, 1983), the propensity of abusers to deny and rationalize their actions, and the need to draw the victim into the lie

(Baumeister, 1997; Salter, 1995). In discussing severe child abuse, Shengold (1989) described the process of "soul murder: the deliberate attempt to erad- icate or compromise the separate identity of another person" (p. 2). The child's need to deny unbearable suffering and crushed self-esteem and to live with the knowledge that the beloved parent wished to destroy him or her is maintained by the perpetrator's brainwashing, which consists of rational- ization, minimization, denial, and blaming the victim. The therapist needs to be aware of the ways people struggle to confront the problem of evil and, when appropriate, to work with the child in these areas. In addition, because confrontation with evil is complex and individual, having a representative of the child's faith involved in the therapy can be an indispensable aid.

ISSUES OF DEVELOPMENT

Psychological Development

The psychological development of traumatized children is incomplete. Evaluation and treatment planning is complicated and must take develop- mental stages into consideration. Furthermore, while treating the symptoms caused by the trauma, the therapist must address the danger that the child's development has been interrupted or distorted (Eth and Pynoos, 1985b; Newberger and DeVos, 1988). The therapist must consider preexisting vul- nerabilities. For example, a child's long-standing separation anxiety may be exacerbated after a traumatic event and become the focus of the sympto- matology. Children disclose and interpret the traumatic event in the light of their moral, social, intellectual, and sexual development, as well as the on- going influence of parental values and influences. Bearing this in mind, the therapist has to consider the advantages and disadvantages of correcting dis- tortions in the child's understanding. For example, when asked why the abuse occurred, young children, whose thinking is egocentric, often answer: "Because he hates me." Some children do not inform their mother of the abuse because, since mothers know everything, they believe their mother al- ready knew. When it is appropriate, the therapist can correct these misun- derstandings. Unfortunately, however, sometimes these beliefs are accurate. Other developmental distortions, particularly in the area of sexual knowl- edge, require the therapist to consider his or her response carefully. For ex- ample, two sexually abused sisters understood the incident quite differently. The seven-year-old told investigators that the offender had "peed" on her; her eleven-year-old sister decided he had a "wet dream." Although neither child's characterization was accurate, the therapist decided it would be more helpful to correct these distortions when the children matured.

Another important developmental issue is whether children are capable of mourning. Until recently, most researchers believed that children put off mourning until a later age because at the time of the trauma, the grief was too overwhelming (Furman, 1974). At the same time, parents avoided talking about grief because they believed that the child would simply forget about the trauma. This reasoning is not accurate. Children do mourn, although in short spurts and over a long time (Fitzgerald, 1994). Mourning is particularly complicated when the death being mourned occurred suddenly and traumatically, e.g., the line-of-duty death of a firefighter. The therapist must help the child mourn while at the same time treat the shattered assumptions and the posttraumatic symptoms. The therapist can encourage the child to talk about the lost person, to keep mementos and pictures, and can accompany the child to visit and place flowers on the grave.

Character Development

Herman (1992) and others (van der Kolk, MacFarlane, and Weisaeth, 1996) propose that chronic, abusive, Type II traumas foster development of a syndrome referred to variously as "complex PTSD" (Herman, 1992), and as "disorders of extreme stress not otherwise specified" (DESNOS). The working group for the *Diagnostic and Statistical Manual of Mental Disorders* is currently considering its inclusion in the next manual revision (Herman, 1992). The crucial issue is that prolonged trauma can create long-term characterological changes and distortions as well as alterations in affect regulation, consciousness, self-perception, perception of the perpetrator, relations with others, and systems of meaning (Herman, 1992). In addition, alterations in cognitive processes and achievement, and alterations in moral development can occur as well.

This diagnosis, while formulated for adults, has profound consequences for the treatment of traumatized children. Why wait to treat the syndrome if it is possible to locate these children, treat them early and prevent these profound and disabling alterations in character development from occurring? The author has treated a number of children who showed no obvious Axis I disorder (no PTSD, depression, or acting-out for example); yet, their character development was profoundly altered. For example, most perpetrators of child abuse rationalize and minimize their actions so as not to compromise their view of themselves as decent human beings. Most children strongly need to see their parents as good and loving. The clash between these two results in a form of brainwashing which has profound consequences upon the child's reality testing. As Shengold (1989) states, in referring to George Orwell's construction of the *1984* world, "Orwell's 'doublethink' is a system of vertical mind-splits that make it possible to believe that two plus two makes five" (p. 27). Sometimes these children show no overtly diagnosable disorders, yet they profoundly distrust people, expect betrayal, and lose faith that life holds any justice or meaning.

Another crucial issue is the impact of the trauma on the child's developing sense of morality and identifications. For example, one abused child may identify with the aggressor, thus making it more likely that he or she will become a future perpetrator, and perpetuating the "cycle of violence" (Caffaro, 1995). Another child may passively identify with the victim, possibly resulting in an adult more likely to be reabused. Children who have experienced a natural disaster and passively identify with the victim can continue to place themselves in the way of danger or grow up passively fearful and avoidant. Other children may take an active stance, working to master the trauma by seeking a career in that area. For example, the child who has suffered painful medical procedures may become a pediatrician; the child who has witnessed a fatal car crash may become a paramedic. A quite common response to private tragedies is for victims to determine to work publicly so that others do not have to suffer as they have. An effective advocacy group, Mothers Against Drunken Driving (MADD), was created by the mother of a child killed by a drunk driver. Moreover, many outstanding victim and child advocates, therapists, law enforcement officers, and cancer researchers suffered a particular trauma as children which led them to their careers.

FOLLOW-UP AND HEALING

Abused children often ask if they will grow up to abuse their own children. There are many factors besides the particular trauma which influence the future of a child. Some children seem to be particularly resistant to trauma, a factor first conceptualized as invulnerability and lately as resilience (Anthony and Cohler, 1987; Dugan and Coles, 1989). For example, one six-year-old child with a traumatic history of physical, sexual, and emotional abuse and some psychological scars, grew up to be an empathic, loving, productive adult. As a small child, she developed her own play therapy with many dolls. Each one had a different life story. The child lovingly talked to and cared for them, telling them daily that she would never do to her children what was happening to her.

Long-term follow-up care of these children of trauma is crucial. Unfortunately, there are rarely resources available to carry it out. Hopefully, education will help the general public to understand the cost-effectiveness of early treatment in terms of decreased rates of crime and adult mental illness, as well as the increased psychological well-being of the planet. In the meantime, if every therapist set aside one hour a week for some type of pro bono work, the added contribution to the public welfare would be substantial.

Re-treating the traumatized child for a period of time during a later stage of development can effectively address residual symptoms, developmental reappraisals of the events, and ongoing problems in character formation. It is important in the therapy process to keep careful notes of the sessions, as well as all of the child's writings and drawings. The therapist can show the folder early in treatment, indicating that it will be available whenever it is needed as the child gets older.

Healing takes place in many ways. The nature of the relationship between child and therapist can be critical in that process. Woznica and Shapiro (1990) discussed the phenomenon of the "expendable child," wherein the child feels like a burden and believes that the family would be better off without him or her. Rosenberg and McCullough (1981) discussed the importance of "mattering," the belief that I count, that I make a difference in someone's life, that I am important to someone. They found that adolescents who felt that they mattered little to their parents had lower self-esteem and were more likely to be anxious, depressed, and delinquent. Many traumatized children feel expendable and believe that they do not matter to anyone. The therapeutic relationship may be the one relationship in which they feel valued. This relationship can leave an indelible positive imprint on the child's life.

Often, it is helpful to refer the child to other types of help concurrent with individual therapy, such as group therapy, support groups, skills training, and involvement with school personnel. The therapist can encourage the child to participate in healthy activities such as scouting, religious exploration, social groups, meditation and relaxation, and physical exercise (which facilitates reclaiming the body). Recently, a number of ecologists and ecopsychologists have written about the healing powers of nature and the emotional bond between human beings and nature. The traumatized child may be nurtured, for example, by developing relationships with pets or planting a flower garden. Such activities decrease the child's sense of loneliness and increase the feeling of connection (Roszak, Gomes, and Kanner, 1995). A natural sanctuary can be a "restorative environment," with healing effects after even a brief encounter. Venolia (1988) writes about healing environments that bring nature inside, and addresses issues such as light, color, sound, indoor air quality, plants and gardens. The therapist can encourage such healing by growing plants in the office, taking the child outside to collect leaves, and educating the child and family about the healing effects of nature.

A traumatized child needs healthy touch to recover. Because of the current public sensitivity to sexual abuse issues and the possibility of false allegations, therapists and teachers have recently tended to avoid physical contact with children, thus depriving them of one of the most basic human needs. Many traumatized children previously found that touch was quite dangerous; many have had little access to healthy, nurturing touch. If used sensibly, touch by the therapist can be healing to a child: holding a small child in his or her lap while reading a book, allowing the child to hug him or her when leaving the office, or helping a parent to hold and soothe a child in crisis are examples.

James Pennebaker (1990) demonstrated the power of using writing to express emotions, thereby preventing physical illness and promoting healing from trauma. In another fascinating demonstration of healing, Campbell (1997) reported that music of many kinds masks unpleasant sounds and feelings; slows down and equalizes brain waves; positively affects respiration, heartbeat, pulse, blood pressure, and temperature; reduces tension and improves coordination; increases endorphin levels; reduces the level of stress hormones; boosts immune function; strengthens endurance, memory, and learning; changes perception of time and space; boosts productivity; and generates a feeling of well-being. Listening to music in a therapy session and encouraging parents to provide opportunities for the child to listen to and play music can contribute to healing.

CONCLUSIONS

Although all forms of trauma to children are distressing to therapists, children involved in war and terrorism or chronic child abuse are perhaps the most difficult to treat, for they require confronting almost unfathomable depths of cruelty. As Shengold (1989, p. 15) puts it:

> It isn't easy to peer into these pictures of childhood hell: The therapist who works with these children must be able to bear watching a child whose spirit, and sometimes body, is broken, whose life has been one of utter torment, and whose natural, exuberant, curious, and joyful spirit has been overwhelmed with helplessness and despair.

Therapists should try to prevent compassion fatigue (Figley, 1995) by acknowledging and working through these feelings, seeking support from coworkers, and maintaining adequate self-care.

In spite of the many possibilities for negative outcomes, there is also the potential for positive growth in the aftermath of traumatic experiences, both for the survivor and the therapist. Tedeschi and Calhoun (1995) wrote about a number of transformative outcomes, including enhanced spiritual development, deeper compassion and empathy for others, and the development of wisdom. In some individuals, the struggle with trauma will generate a life script, guiding a career path or a pattern of human relationships through which the individual will leave a legacy.

This chapter has described a number of approaches that the author has used to understand and treat traumatized children. A careful evaluation and treatment plan, developed in close collaboration with the parents, can help children tell the story in a therapeutic setting; resolve psychological symptoms; lessen the impact on emotional, social, and moral development; promote healing; and encourage transformative, and life-enhancing outcomes.

BIBLIOGRAPHY

Achenbach, T.A. and Edelbrock, C. (1986). *Manual for the Child Behavior Checklist*. Burlington, VT: Author.

American Psychiatric Association (1994). *Diagnostic and statistical manual of mental disorders* (Fourth edition). Washington, DC: Author.

Anthony, E.J. (1986). Terrorizing attacks on children by psychotic parents. *Journal of the American Academy of Child Psychiatry, 25*(3), 326-335.

Anthony, E.J. and Cohler, B.J. (Eds.) (1987). *The invulnerable child*. New York: Guilford.

Aptekar, L. and Boore, J.A. (1990). The emotional effects of disaster on children: A review of the literature. *International Journal of Mental Health, 19*(2), 77-90.

Armsworth, M.W. and Holaday, M. (1993). The effects of psychological trauma on children and adolescents. *Journal of Consulting and Development, 72,* 49-56.

Arroyo, W. and Eth, S. (1985). Children traumatized by Central American warfare. In Eth, S. and Pynoos, R.S., *Post-traumatic stress disorder in children*. Washington, DC: American Psychiatric Press.

Basson, M.D., Guinn, J.E., McElligott, J., Vitale, R., Brown, W., and Fielding, P. (1991). Behavioral disturbances in children after trauma. *The Journal of Trauma, 31*(10), 1363-1368.

Baumeister, R.F. (1997). *Evil: Inside human cruelty and violence*. New York: W.H. Freeman.

Benedek, E.P. and Schetky, D.H. (1987). Problems in validating allegations of sexual abuse, part 2: Clinical evaluation. *Journal of the American Academy of Child and Adolescent Psychiatry, 26*(6), 916-921.

Berliner, L. and Conte, J.R. (1990). The process of victimization: The victims' perspective. *Child Abuse and Neglect, 14,* 29-40.

Berliner, L. and Conte, J.R. (1993). Sexual abuse evaluations: Conceptual and empirical obstacles. *Child Abuse and Neglect, 17,* 111-125.

Bernet, W. (1993). False statements and the differential diagnosis of abuse allegations. *Journal of the American Academy of Child and Adolescent Psychiatry, 32*(5), 903-910.

Bloom, S. (1997). *Creating sanctuary: Toward the evolution of sane societies*. New York: Routledge.

Briere, J. (1996). *Manual for the Trauma Symptom Checklist for Children.* Odessa, FL: Psychological Assessment Resources, Inc.

Brohl, K. (1996). *Working with traumatized children.* Washington, DC: CWLA Press.

Buck, J. (1981). *The house-tree-person technique: A revised manual.* Los Angeles: Western Psychological Services.

Burgess, A.W. and Holmstrom, L.L. (1978). Accessory-to-sex: Pressure, sex, and secrecy. In Burgess, A.W., Groth, A.N., Holmstrom, L.L., and Sgroi, S.M. *Sexual assault of children and adolescents* (pp. 85-98). Lanham, MD: Lexington Books.

Butler, W.M., Leitenberg, H., and Fuselier, G.D. (1995). Child hostages: Incidence and outcome. *Journal of Interpersonal Violence, 10*(3), 378-383.

Caffaro, J.V. (1995). Identification and trauma: An integrative-developmental approach. *Journal of Family Violence, 10*(1), 23-41.

Campbell, D. (1997). *The Mozart effect: Tapping the power of music to heal the body, strengthen the mind, and unlock the creative spirit.* New York: Avon.

Carlson, E.B. (Ed.) (1996). *Trauma research methodology.* Lutherville, MD: Sidran.

Ceci, S.J., Ross, D.F., and Toglia, M.P. (1989). *Perspectives on child testimony.* New York: Springer-Verlag.

Cohen, J. and Mannarino, A. (1997, November). "Current controversies in the assessment of PTSD in children." Paper presented at the meeting of the International Society for Traumatic Stress Studies, Montreal, Canada.

Conte, J.R., Wolf, S., and Smith, T. (1989). What sexual offenders tell us about prevention strategies. *Child Abuse and Neglect, 13*, 293-301.

Costenbader, V.K. and Perry, C. (1990). Test review: The Woodcock-Johnson Psychoeducational battery—revised. *Journal of Psychoeducational Assessment, 8,* 180-184.

Csikszentmihalyi, M. and Beattie, O.V. (1979). Life themes: A theoretical and empirical exploration of their origins and effects. *Journal of Humanistic Psychology, 19*(1), 46-63.

deYoung, M. (1986). A conceptual model for judging the truthfullness of a young child's allegation of sexual abuse. *American Journal of Orthopsychiatry, 56*(4), 550-559.

deYoung, M. (1988). The indignant page: Techniques of neutralization in the publications of pedophile organizations. *Child Abuse and Neglect, 12*(4), 583-591.

Doherty, W.J. (1995). *Soul searching: Why psychotherapy must promote moral responsibility.* New York: Basic.

Doka, K.J. (Ed.) (1996). *Living with grief after sudden loss: Suicide, homicide, accident, heart attack, stroke.* Washington, DC: Hospice Foundation of America.

Doris, J. (Ed.) (1976). *The suggestibility of children's recollections.* Washington, DC: American Psychological Association.

Dugan, T.F. and Coles, R. (Eds.) (1989). *The child in our times: Studies in the development of resiliency.* New York: Brunner/Mazel.

Elliot, M., Browne, K., and Kilcoyne, J. (1995). Child sexual abuse prevention: What offenders tell us. *Child Abuse and Neglect,* 579-594.

Eth, S. and Pynoos, R.S. (1985a). Developmental perspective on psychic trauma in childhood. In Figley, C. (Ed.), *Trauma and its wake* (pp. 36-52). New York: Brunner/Mazel.

Eth, S. and Pynoos, R.S. (Eds.) (1985b). *Post-traumatic stress disorder in children.* Washington, DC: American Psychiatric Association.

Everly, G.S. and Lating, J.M. (Eds.) (1995). *Psychotraumatology: Key papers and core concepts in post-traumatic stress.* New York: Plenum.

Everson, M. (1997). Understanding bizarre, improbable, and fantastic elements in children's accounts of abuse. *Child Maltreatment, 2*(2), 134-149.

Everson, M. and Boat, B. (1989). False allegations of sexual abuse by children and adolescents. *Journal of the American Academy of Child and Adolescent Psychiatry, 28*(2), 230-235.

Everstine, D.S. and Everstine, L. (1989). *Sexual trauma in children and adolescents.* New York: Brunner/Mazel.

Faller, K.C. (1991). Possible explanations for child sexual abuse allegations in divorce. *American Journal of Orthopsychiatry, 61*(1), 86-90.

Famularo, R., Kinscherff, R., and Fenton, T. (1992). Psychiatric diagnosis of maltreated children: Preliminary findings. *Journal of the American Academy of Child and Adolescent Psychiatry, 31*(5), 863-867.

Figley, C.R. (1995). *Compassion fatigue: Coping with secondary traumatic stress in those who treat the traumatized.* New York: Brunner/Mazel.

Finkelhor, D. and Browne, A. (1985). The traumatic impact of child sexual abuse: A conceptualization. *American Journal of Orthopsychiatry, 55*(4), 530-539.

Fish-Murray, C.C., Koby, E.V., and van der Kolk, B.A. (1987). Evolving ideas: The effect of abuse on children's thought. In van der Kolk, B.A. (Ed.), *Psychological trauma.* Washington, DC: American Psychiatric Press.

Fitzgerald, H. (1994). *The mourning handbook.* New York: Simon and Schuster.

Ford, J.D., Thomas, J.E., Rogers, K.C., Racusin, R.J., Ellis, C.G., Schiffman, J.G. (1996, November). "Assessment of children's PTSD following abuse or accidental trauma." Paper presented at the meeting of the International Society for Traumatic Stress Studies, San Francisco, CA.

Foy, D.W. (Ed.) (1992). *Treating PTSD: Cognitive-behavioral strategies.* New York: Guilford.

Friedrich, W. (1993, January). Sexual behavior in sexually abused children. *Violence Update.*

Furman, E. (1974). *A child's parent dies: Studies in childhood bereavement.* New Haven, CT: Yale.

Galante, R. and Foa, D. (1986). An epidemiological study of psychic trauma and treatment effectiveness for children after a natural disaster. *Journal of the American Academy of Child Psychiatry, 25*(3), 357-363.

Garbarino, J., Kostelny, K., and Dubrow, N. (1991). *No place to be a child: Growing up in a war zone.* Lanham, MD: Lexington Books.

Garrison, C.Z., Bryant, E.S., Addy, C.L., Spurner, P.G., Freedy, J.R., and Kilpatrick, D.G. (1995). Posttraumatic stress disorder in adolescents after Hurricane Andrew. *Journal of the American Academy of Child and Adolescent Psychiatry, 34*(9), 1193-1201.

Gergen, K. (date unknown). The emerging crisis in theory of life-span development. Paper written at Swarthmore College, Swarthmore, PA.

Gislason, I.L. and Call, J.D. (1982). Dog bite in infancy: Trauma and personality development. *Journal of the American Academy of Child Psychiatry, 21*(2), 203-207.

Goenjian, A.K., Pynoos, R.S., Steinberg, A.M., Najarian, L.M., Asarnow, J.R., and Karayan, I. (1995). Psychiatric comorbidity in children after the 1988 earthquake in Armenia. *Journal of the American Academy of Child and Adolescent Psychiatry, 34*(9), 1174-1184.

Goodman, G.S. and Bottoms, B.L. (Eds.) (1993). *Child victims, child witnesses: Understanding and improving testimony.* New York: Guilford.

Goodman, G.S., Bottoms, B.L., Schwartz-Kenney, B.M, and Rudy, L. (1991). Children's testimony about a stressful event: Improving children's reports. *Journal of Narrative and Life History, 1*(1), 69-99.

Goodwin, J., Sahd, D., and Rada, R.T. (1993). Incest hoax: False accusations, false denials. *Bulletin of the American Academy of Psychiatry and the Law, 6*(3), 269-276.

Gould, B.B. and Gould, J.B. (1991). Young people's perception of the space shuttle disaster: Case study. *Adolescence, 26*(102), 295-303.

Green, A.H. (1993). Child sexual abuse: Immediate and long-term effects and intervention. *Journal of the American Academy of Child and Adolescent Psychiatry, 32*(5), 690-902.

Green, B.L., Korol, M., Grace, M.C., Vary, M.G., Leonard, A.C., and Gleser, G.C. (1991). Children and disaster: Age, gender and parental effects on PTSD symptoms. *Journal of the American Academy of Child and Adolescent Psychiatry. 30*(6), 945-951.

Greene, E., Flynn, M.S., and Loftus, E.F. (1982). Inducing resistance to misleading information. *Journal of Verbal Learning and Verbal Behavior, 21,* 207-219.

Hazzard, A. (1993). Trauma-related beliefs as mediators of sexual abuse impact in adult women survivors: A pilot study. *Journal of Child Sexual Abuse, 2*(3), 55-69.

Heft, L. (1993). Helping traumatized parents help their traumatized children: A protocol for running post-disaster parents groups. *Journal of Social Behavior and Personality, 8*(5), 149-154.

Heiman, M.L. (1992). Annotation: Putting the puzzle together: Validating allegations of child sexual abuse. *Journal of Child Psychiatry, 33*(2), 311-329.

Herman, J.L. (1992). *Trauma and recovery.* New York: Basic.

Howe, P.A. and Silvern, L.E. (1981). Behavioral observation of children during play therapy: Preliminary development of a research instrument. *Journal of Personality Assessment, 45*(2), 168-182.

Hughes, M. and Grieve, R. (1980). On asking children bizarre questions. *First Language,* 149-160.

James, B. (1989). *Treating traumatized children.* Boston: Lexington/Macmillan.

James, B. (1994). *Handbook for treatment of attachment-trauma problems in children.* New York: Lexington.

Janoff-Bulman, R. (1992). *Shattered assumptions: Toward a new psychology of trauma.* New York: Free Press.

Jessee, P.O., Strickland, M.P., and Ladewig, B.H. (1992). The aftereffects of a hostage situation on children's behavior. *American Journal of Orthopsychiatry, 62*(2), 309-312.

Jones, R.W. and Peterson, L.W. (1993). Post-traumatic stress disorder in a child following an automobile accident. *The Journal of Family Practice, 36*(2), 223-225.

Kellert, S.R. (1996). *The value of life: Biological diversity and human society.* Washington, DC: Island.

Kovacs, M. (1992). *Manual for the Children's Depression Inventory.* Tonawanda, NY: Multi-Health Systems.

Levin, P. (1993). Assessing posttraumatic stress disorder with the Rorschach projective technique. In Wilson, J.P. and Raphael, B. (Eds.), *International handbook of traumatic stress* (pp. 189-200). New York: Plenum.

Lewis, D.O., Lovely, R., Yeager, C., and Femina, D.D. (1989). Toward a theory of the genesis of violence: A follow-up study of delinquents. *Journal of the American Academy of Child and Adolescent Psychiatry, 28*(3), 431-436.

Libow, J.A. (1992). Traumatized children and the news media: Clinical considerations. *American Journal of Orthopsychiatry, 62*(3), 379-386.

Lickona, T. (Ed.) (1976). *Moral development and behavior.* New York: Holt, Rinehart and Winston.

Lifton, R.J. and Olson, E. (1976). The human meaning of total disaster. *Psychiatry, 39,* 1-18.

MacFarlane, K. and Waterman, J. (with Connerly, S., Damon, L., Durfee, M., and Long, S.) (1986). *Sexual abuse of young children.* New York: Guilford.

MacLean, G. (1977). Psychic trauma and traumatic neurosis: Play therapy with a four-year-old boy. *Canadian Psychiatric Association Journal, 22*(2), 71-75.

Malmquist, C.P. (1986). Children who witness parental murder: Posttraumatic aspects. *Journal of the American Academy of Child Psychiatry, 25*(3), 320-325.

McCann, I.L. and Pearlman, L.A. (1990). *Psychological trauma and the adult survivor.* New York: Brunner/Mazel.

McNally, R.J. (1991). Assessment of posttraumatic stress disorder in children. *Journal of Counseling and Consulting Psychology, 3*(4), 531-537.

Miller, T.W. and Veltkamp, L.J. (1995). Assessment of sexual abuse and trauma: Clinical measures. *Child Psychiatry and Human Development, 26*(1), 3-11.

Monahon, C. (1993). *Children and trauma: A parent's guide to helping children heal*. New York: Lexington.

Nader, K., Pynoos, R.S., Fairbanks, L., and Frederick, C. (1990). Children's PTSD reactions one year after a sniper attack at their school. *American Journal of Psychiatry, 147*(11), 1526-1530.

Naglieri, J.A., LeBuffe, P.A., and Pfeiffer, S.I. (1994). *Devereux Scales of Mental Disorders Manual*. San Antonio: The Psychological Corporation.

Newberger, C.M. and DeVos, E. (1988). Abuse and victimization: A life-span developmental perspective. *American Journal of Orthopsychiatry, 58*(4), 505-511.

Newberger, C.M., Gremy, I.M., Waternaux, C.M., and Newberger, E.H. (1993). Mothers of sexually abused children: Trauma and repair in longitudinal perspective. *American Journal of Orthopsychiatry, 63*(1), 92-102.

Newman, E., Riggs, D.S., and Roth, S. (1997). Thematic resolution, PTSD, and complex PTSD: The relationship between meaning and trauma-related diagnosis. *Journal of Traumatic Stress, 10*(2), 197-213.

Nir, Y. (1985). Post-traumatic stress disorder in children with cancer. In Eth, S. and Pynoos, R.S., *Post-traumatic stress disorder in children*. Washington, DC: American Psychiatric Press, Inc.

Ornstein, R. and Sobel, D. (1989). *Healthy pleasures*. Reading, MA: Addison-Wesley.

Osofsky, J.D. (1995). The effects of exposure to violence on young children. *American Psychologist, 50*(9), 782-788.

Payton, J.B. and Krocker-Tuskan, M. (1988). Children's reactions to loss of parent through violence. *Journal of the American Academy of Child and Adolescent Psychiatry, 27*(5), 563-566.

Peck, S. (1983). *People of the lie: The hope for healing human evil*. New York: Simon and Schuster.

Pennebaker, J.W. (1990). *Opening up: The healing power of expressing emotions*. New York: Guilford Press.

Peters, T. (1994). *Sin: Radical evil in soul and society*. Grand Rapids, MI: William B. Eerdmans.

Preston, S.H. (1984). Children and the elderly in the U.S. *Scientific American, 251*(6), 44-48.

Putnam, F.W. (1996). Special methods for trauma research with children. In Carlson, E.B. (Ed.), *Trauma research methodology* (pp. 153-173). Lutherville: Sidran.

Pynoos, R.S. (1993). Traumatic stress and developmental psychopathology in children and adolescents. In Oldham, J.M, Riba, M.B., and Tasman, A. (Eds.), *American psychiatric press review of psychiatry, Volume 12* (pp.205-238). Washington, DC: American Psychiatric Press.

Pynoos, R.S. and Eth, S. (1986). Witness to violence: The child interview. *Journal of the American Academy of Child Psychiatry, 25*(3), 306-319.

Pynoos, R.S., Frederick, C., Nader, K., Arroyo, W., Steinberg, A., and Eth, S. (1987). Life threat and posttraumatic stress disorder in school-age children. *Archives of General Psychiatry, 44,* 1057-1063.

Quinsey, V.L. and Lalumiere, M.L. (1996). *Assessment of sexual offenders against children.* Thousand Oaks, CA: Sage.

Reinehr, R.C. (1987). Wide-range achievement tests, 1984 edition. In Keyser, D.J. and Sweetland, R.C. (Eds.), *Test critiques compendium.* Kansas City: Test Corporation of America.

Reynolds, C. and Richmond, B. (1985). *Manual for the Revised Children's Manifest Anxiety Scale.* Los Angeles: Western Psychological Services.

Roberts, G. (1982). *Manual for the Roberts Apperception Test for Children.* Los Angeles: Western Psychological Services.

Rorschach, H. (1921). *Psychodiagnostik.* Berne: Birchen.

Rosenberg, M. and McCullough, B.C. (1981). Mattering: Inferred significance and mental health among adolescents. *Research in Community and Mental Health, 2,* 163-182.

Roszak, T., Gomes, M.E., and Kanner, A.D. (Eds.) (1995). *Ecopsychology: Restoring the earth, healing the mind.* San Francisco: Sierra Club.

Rotter, J.B. and Rafferty, J.E. (1950). *Manual for the Rotter Incomplete Sentences Blank.* New York: The Psychological Corporation.

Saigh, P. (1991). The development and validation of the Children's Post-traumatic Stress Disorder Inventory. *International Journal of Special Education, 4,* 75-84.

Salter, A.C. (1995). *Transforming trauma: A guide to understanding and treating adult survivors of child sexual abuse.* Thousand Oaks, CA: Sage.

Scheeringa, M.S. and Zeanah, C.H. (1995). Symptom expression and trauma variables in children under 48 months of age. *Infant Mental Health Journal, 16*(4), 259-270.

Scheeringa, M.S., Zeanah, C.H., Drell, M.J., and Larrieu, J.A. (1995). Two approaches to the diagnosis of posttraumatic stress disorder in infancy and early childhood. *Journal of the American Academy of Child and Adolescent Psychiatry, 34*(2), 191-200.

Schwarz, E. and Kowalski, J.M. (1991). Malignant memories: PTSD in children and adults after a school shooting. *Journal of the American Academy of Child and Adolescent Psychiatry, 30*(6), 936-944.

Schwarz, E. and Perry, B.D. (1994). The post-traumatic stress response in children and adolescents. *Psychiatric Clinics of North America, 17*(2), 311-326.

Schwarz, H. (1995). *Evil: A historical and theological perspective.* Minneapolis: Fortress Press.

Seligman, M.E. (1998). *Learned optimism: How to change your mind and your life.* New York: Pocket.

Sgroi, S., Blick, L., and Porter, F. (1982). A conceptual framework for child sexual abuse. In Sgroi, S. (Ed.), *Handbook of clinical intervention in child sexual abuse* (pp. 9-37). Lanham, MD: Lexington Books.

Shapiro, S.H. (1973). Preventive analysis following a trauma: A 4 1/2-year-old girl witnesses a stillbirth. *Psychoanalytic Study of the Child, 28,* 249-285.

Shaw, J.A., Applegate, B., Tanner, S., Perez, D., Rothe, E., and Campo-Bowen, A.E. (1995). Psychological effects of Hurricane Andrew on an elementary school population. *Journal of the American Academy of Child and Adolescent Psychiatry, 34*(9), 1185-1192.

Shengold, L. (1989). *Soul murder: The effects of childhood abuse and deprivation.* New Haven, CT: Yale.

Singer, M.I., Hussey, D., and Strom, K.J. (1992). Grooming the victim: An analysis of a perpetrator's seduction letter. *Child Abuse and Neglect, 16*(November-December, 6), 877-886.

Sorenson, T. and Snow, B. (1991). How children tell: The process of disclosure in child sexual abuse. *Child Welfare, 70*(1), 3-15.

Staub, E. (1989). *The roots of evil: The origins of genocide and other group violence.* New York: Cambridge.

Strauss, M. (1994). *Beating the devil out of them.* New York: Lexington Books.

Strentz, T. (1982). The stockholm syndrome: Law enforcement policy and hostage behavior. In Ochberg, F.M. and Soskis, D.A. (Eds.), *Victims of terrorism.* Boulder, CO: Westview.

Sugar, M. (1992). Toddlers' traumatic memories. *Infant Mental Health Journal, 13*(3), 245-251.

Summit, R.C. (1983). The child abuse accommodation syndrome. *Child Abuse and Neglect, 7,* 177-193.

Tedeschi, R.G. and Calhoun, L.G. (1995). *Trauma and transformation: Growing in the aftermath of suffering.* Thousand Oaks, CA: Sage.

Terr, L. (1983). Chowchilla revisited: The effects of psychic trauma four years after a school bus kidnapping. *American Journal of Psychiatry, 140*(12), 1543-1645.

Terr, L. (1985). Psychic trauma in children and adolescents. *Psychiatric Clinics of North America, 8*(4), 815-835.

Terr, L. (1988). What happens to early memories of trauma? A study of twenty children under age five at the time of documented traumatic events. *Journal of the American Academy of Child and Adolescent Psychiatry, 27*(1), 96-104.

Terr, L. (1990). *Too scared to cry.* New York: Harper and Row.

Terr. L. (1991). Childhood trauma: An outline and overview. *American Journal of Psychiatry, 148*(1), 10-17.

Terr, L. (1994). *Unchained memories: True stories of traumatic memories, lost and found.* New York: Basic Books.

Thompson, R.A. and Wilcox, B.L. (1995). Child maltreatment research: Federal support and policy issues. *American Psychologist, 50*(9), 789-793.

van der Kolk, B.A., McFarlane, A.C., and Weisaeth, L. (Eds.) (1996). *Traumatic stress: The effects of overwhelming experience on mind, body, and society.* New York: Guilford.

Venolia, C. (1988). *Healing environments.* Berkeley, CA: Celestial Arts.

Viglione, D.J. (1990). Severe disturbance or trauma-induced adaptive reaction: A Rorschach child case study. *Journal of Personality Assessment, 55*(1 and 2), 280-295.

Vogel, J.M. and Vernberg, E.M. (1993). Part I: Children's psychological responses to disasters. *Journal of Clinical Child Psychology, 22*(4), 464-484.

Wechsler, D. (1991). *Manual for the Wechsler Intelligence Scale for Children,* (Third edition). New York: Psychological Corporation.

Williams, L.M. (1995). Recovered memories of abuse in women with documented child sexual abuse victimization histories. *Journal of Traumatic Stress, 8*(4), 649-673.

Wolfe, V., Gentile, C., and Wolfe, D. (1989). The impact of sexual abuse on children: A PTSD formulation. *Behavior Therapy, 20,* 215-228.

Woznica, J.G. and Shapiro, J.R. (1990). An analysis of adolescent suicide attempts: The expendable child. *Journal of Pediatric Psychology, 15*(6), 789-796.

Zeanah, C.H. and Burk, G.S. (1984). A young child who witnessed her mother's murder: Therapeutic and legal considerations. *American Journal of Psychotherapy, 38*(1), 132-145.

Chapter 11

Provision of Trauma Services to School Populations and Faculty

J. Horenstein

INTRODUCTION

The increase of violence in developed countries and the use of the school system in the prevention of posttraumatic stress in countries at war, or during natural or accidental disasters has led to an evolution of mental health practices in the educational community. Mental health programs for children who have been involved in disasters that utilize the school system can be very effective. However, they must also reflect on the work of teachers in situations of crisis, on their participation in the prevention of PTSD, and on the specific hazards associated with working with traumatized children. In crisis situations, teachers play the same role as emergency service personnel, but without any recognition of their additional responsibilities.

The most sensitive subject for school professionals is the allegation of physical abuse brought against them by a student(s) or parent(s). Another issue is witnessing traumas experienced by students. The existence of psychological trauma arising from contact with a traumatized individual is increasingly admitted in the field of psychotraumatology. By cumulative effect, the more contacts, the more hazards. Headmasters (principals), in particular, are vulnerable to this type of trauma because of their leadership.

Prior Literature

Prior literature concerning post-traumatic stress disorder delineates the wide range of events that take place at school. Some early articles have been significant in the evolution of the PSTD concept (Blom, 1986; Dyregrov et al., 1994; Echterling, 1989; Hyman, Zelikoff, and Clarke, 1988; Klingman, 1989; Milgram et al., 1988; Mitchell, 1995; Nader et al., 1990; Pichene, 1995; Sack, 1986; Schwartz and Kowalski, 1991; Shelton and Sanders,

1973). PTSD literature examining the work of teachers in crisis situations reveals the complexity of the situation of these victims as compared to, for instance, victims of assault on a public highway. In the school setting, victim teachers are "victims' victims." Loss of professional identity often adds to the usual personal identity loss, which is characteristic of psychological trauma.

General Assumptions of Interventions

Preventive interventions in school systems differ, depending on whether they concern an individual, a group of teachers, an entire school, a school system, or the institution of national education itself. Table 11.1 describes these interventions.

The Interface Between Mental Health and National Education

This interface is meant to promote cooperation, provide mutual training, and encourage initiatives between the two institutions. Targets for future collaboration include communicating about actions in progress, developing of evaluation tools, examining of the relational and emotional climate inside schools and the impact of violence on the school community, evaluating the relevance of interventions, and stimulating research.

An example of this type of interface has existed in the Chicago, Illinois, area since 1982. The IEP (Interface between Education and Psychiatry, Inc.) has developed actions that mainly concern the special education of children with psychiatric handicaps. However, it could be considered as a model applicable to posttraumatic stress problems. In addition, the IEP organizes bi-

TABLE 11.1. Preventive Interventions

	Primary prevention	Secondary prevention	Tertiary prevention
Personnel	Education programs in psychological trauma	Victim support program	PTSD counseling
Group	Violence prevention training	Psychological debriefing	Supportive group
School	School crisis plan	Strategic group	Cumulative traumatic stress debriefing
Institution	Support network	Institutional narrative	Rehabilitation

annual seminars, including "The Impact of Death and Loss in an Educational Setting."

PRIMARY PREVENTION

Educational Programs

Various primary prevention programs can occur in schools. Training on psychological trauma and the school environment is a concern of mental health personnel as well as educational staff. However, experts on victimology do not necessarily know a particular school as an institution, and those who know the complexity of a school are not necessarily familiar with psychological trauma. Presently, schools do not seem to be viewed as natural sites of intervention for mental health professionals. However, child psychiatrists now identify them as the best environments for early recognition of developmental delays, psychological, or social problems (Berkovitz and Seliger, 1985).

Training of Educational Staff

Every available means should be used to circulate the psychological trauma concept to educators. Most initial training courses for students training to become teachers are more informative than active. They are aimed at students who are only interested in preparing for the entrance examination. In addition, self reports indicate a high proportion of teachers with over twenty years of experience are victims of physical abuse. Active training sessions based on real-life experiences, therefore, should be a matter of priority in the fields of initial and continuing education. Several subjects should be included in training to help teachers understand and cope with their experiences. Among them are traumatic situations of death and loss in the school environment, suicide, child abuse, risky behaviors (alcohol/drug use), intentional violence between students and against adults, parenting, anger and conflict management, and victims assistance programs (Futrell, 1996; Jenkin, 1994; Weeler and Baron, 1994; Wilson, 1995).

Mental Health Personnel Training

Schools should be available as sites of training courses for the continuing education of mental health staff. Prior to these sessions, a seminar should be organized on topics such as school environment and institutional practices, disciplinary practices, relations with community and other institutions, violence prevention, policies in the school environment, study group supervision, and work in partnership.

Mental Health Workers Consulting in the School Environment

The concept of vocational training for mental health workers employed in schools has faced many objections and hurdles by those who oppose the practice. Among these hurdles are the following:

- The school as a "free clinic" for emotionally disturbed children.
- The export of school problems into the psychiatric field. The goal is to integrate mental health workers in a multidisciplinary team focused mainly on school.
- "Medicalizing" violence problems. The goal is to deal with violence in a school setting according to the problems of the victims produced in this setting.
- The first and most frequent victims of violence at school, within families and society, are students. The best way to deal with their security is to take care of staff security.

How can staff be helped to manage emotional processes triggered at the workplace, while providing the most favorable outcome for students? Mental health workers in a school setting must make the transition from a therapeutic role to a preventive role. They must recognize that their first role is to take into account the legitimate needs and expectations of the educational staff and supply support without considering them as patients looking for therapy (APA, 1993). Mental health workers first must have knowledge of the functioning of schools before suggesting adequate solutions. In addition, one of the most useful functions of the mental health worker who consults at school is to detect individuals at risk after a traumatic event occurs and then refer them to a clinical environment. Interventions differ in the school and clinical environment. The cognitive approach, problem solving, discussion, and group analysis should occur at school. The more individual cathartic approach, including emotional and sensorial exploration, is more suitable to the clinical environment.

Staff Training in Violence Prevention

Group activities implemented within schools must be adapted to the specifics of the school concerned, using active methods to meet targets. Training will ensure that all school staff members are aware of potential security hazards and know how to protect themselves through established policies and procedures. Stress can be both a cause and an effect of workplace violence.

Providing services to faculty includes training in the management of violent situations and a full review of the school policy for providing support to personnel. Victims may have psychological injuries as well as physical injuries and social support can reduce the psychological trauma. Violence in the school setting, while expected, can be mitigated through preparation. Training should cover such topics as

- the kind of critical incidents faced by school personnel—direct or indirect victimization;
- policies and procedures for reporting and record keeping;
- school crisis contingency planning; and
- policies and procedures for obtaining critical-incident debriefing, posttrauma counseling, teachers' compensation, or legal assistance after a violent episode.

Training in Measures of Personal Safety

Because it is essential to have knowledge about fundamental principles of safety awareness, training provided should include the following:

1. Discussion of warning signs: behavioral signs of impending violence, environmental triggers, observation of environment and the development of vigilance beneficial to staff members. This type of training also includes discrimination between expressions of anger in a conflict situation and hostile or aggressive acts of violence.
2. Insight about patterns of behavior that trigger violence: an order, comment, accidental contact, infringement on property or privacy, confrontational behavior, control loss (Menninger, 1993).
3. The process of defusing hostility (Bacal, 1995) includes
    a. interaction control (strategies to avoid reactions to what the abuser says, in order to make the abuser react to what was said);
    b. active listening (accepting the idea that one has to take care of the emotional state of the individual before solving the problem); and
    c. problem solving (definition, providing information, finding alternatives, following up).
4. Stages in escalation include
    a. questions—"Why?";
    b. opposition—protest phase (the right thing to do, in this phase, is to defuse the process);
    c. nonverbal communication of anger emotions;
    d. attempts to intimidate—trespassing limits; and
    e. enacting (Dubé, 1993).
5. Verbal and physical maneuvers to defuse hostile situations: straightforward attitude, direct and structured, neither exceedingly friendly

nor too close; avoiding touching the person, making slow motions, respecting private space (three times larger for violent than for nonviolent individuals); noncritical listening, empathy, avoiding getting mixed up in a speech, not being in a hurry, not interrupting, maximizing the power of individuals to make alternative choices (violence represents a lack of alternatives); looking for a partly private space that is structurally open, leaving the option of a quick and separate exit for both parties, leaving doors open; and discarding objects which can be used in an assault.

6. Failures of defusing:
   a. planning procedures to refer to outside counseling or others,
   b. the disengagement tactic, and
   c. setting and enforcing limits.

7. Cognitive strategies and understanding about self-protective judgment. What one says to oneself in potentially violent situations can affect the outcome. The acceptability and taking into account of fear; becoming aware of personal reactions which can affect the consequences of a violent situation; taking unacceptable risks; reaction triggers; perception of signs of emotional overload and factors of modulation; personalization of hostility; recognizing that the most adequate person to protect the self against an assault is oneself; comprehension that everyone is responsible for personal security and that that responsibility cannot be delegated completely to others (Quarles, 1989).

Creating the School's Crisis Plan

Mental health professionals can help schools create intervention plans for crisis situations ranging from an assault against a teacher to disasters involving the whole community, including types of previously mentioned violence. In these plans, initial psychological support to children is provided by teachers while experts working with teachers provide debriefing and referrals. One target of a crisis plan is to anticipate the multiple tasks and responsibilities that arise due to an emergency to reduce the psychological impact on teachers and other school personnel. For this reason, a written plan defining the strategies and delineating an efficient communication network is necessary (Cox, 1991; Garza-Fuentes and Rose, 1995). According to Moriarty, Maeyama, and Fitzgerald (1993), a crisis checklist might include the following:

- Activation of strategic groups
- Plans for notification of police, emergency services, administrators
- Plans for notification of personnel
- Media relations

- Parent information plan
- Staff information meeting
- Segmentation of school space for parents, police, students, media
- Responsibility for telephone contacts
- Use of community resources
- Staff debriefing
- Provision of information to students
- Planning for memorials and anniversaries
- Follow-up plans and evaluation

The Staff Victim Support Network

Results of research and a review of international literature validates the importance of social support in limiting the psychological impact of violence in an educational setting, particularly in France, the primary focus of this chapter (Futrell, 1996). An incident report is the first essential link in this chain of social support.

The Incident Report

Incident reports of violent events taking place at school against staff should be differentiated from the reports (when there is one) of violence against students or property. Decision makers must accept the necessity of this double evaluation. The first report is a global incident report made through official channels (principal, headmaster, superintendent); the second report is a specific incident report for staff. This incident report is supposed to be followed by support. However, in France, for example, the *victim* has to ensure the coordination of the different institutions (for example, to get a refund of expenses): police, justice, and medical institutions.

Reparation

Victims are entitled to social reparation. They need an appropriate person in charge of the whole process to take initiative and coordinate what occurs. Testimonies of victims bear evidence that the usual tendency of institutions is to blame the victim as a form of crisis management policy. Furthermore, victims describe a bureaucratic process full of double and useless steps, contradictory or irrelevant information, and random rejection. These difficulties are evidence of the necessity of coordination centers. The School Safety Department of the United Federation of Teachers in New York City, and the Victim Support Program, have served as models. They receive all reports about staff incidents and contact every victim, assess each person's needs, and apply intervention strategies (United Federation of Teachers, 1995).

SECONDARY PREVENTION

Victim Support Program

Psychological trauma among teachers is exacerbated by some specific factors (Johnson, 1993). First, teachers feel the necessity to control a situation and assume a leadership role. They consider that an orderly, disciplined class exerts the most positive effect on student education. In the United States, since 1984, there has been a considerable increase in the number of teachers who feel this environment has a strongly positive effect (60 to 75 percent according to Harris, 1995). A traumatic event, however, leads to powerlessness and frustration. Next, the necessity for teachers to control emotions, as professionals, can come into conflict with the role of protecting children (caring). Expression of feelings (such as fear or sorrow) can be difficult (Rowling, 1994).

Third, teachers are questioning professional skills and the loss of professional credibility. Teachers may also experience a blurred balance between cognitive activities (instruction) and personal development. Society demands that they take charge of students' social relations as well as instruction. As a consequence, a blurred balance in the distribution of time between group and individual support activities generates the usual complaints: "We are neither psychologists nor social workers."

In addition, teachers may experience dysfunctional adjustment mechanisms such as isolation (deprivation of available resource) or overinvestment (inability to break away). Predictability and intelligibility are valued in pedagogy but are absent in a crisis situation. Teachers can be very affected and feel helpless in front of a child in mourning. Psychological impact of trauma can be lessened, at least partly, by the professional context, e.g., specific support processes inside the school community.

There are two types of models for staff support programs—centralized or decentralized (Johnson, 1993). The centralized model uses a team to serve all relevant schools. This model is useful for minor incidents and generates improved performance control by the administration. This model is dominant in France. The national hotline (SOS Violence) in the teachers' service, hotlines in district offices, and activities such as an audit and support unit in every division in the country provide immediate listening and support, individual interviews, and legal or professional advice. This model, however, leads to an inadequate use of resources outside the network. In a major crisis, services are unlikely to keep pace with the trauma.

The decentralized model mitigates these drawbacks. District offices promote, coordinate, and supervise small teams (crisis response teams) in every school. The advantage of this model is the optimal use of local resources, especially in the case of large scale crises. Ties made with mental health institutions during a crisis can be very useful. This model tends to strengthen the autonomy of a school and make the staff more responsible. The drawbacks of this model are linked to the difficulties of complex organizations, implying the institutionalization of links with noneducational organizations. The training effort of staff is more important and performance quality control is more difficult. In minor incidents, this model seems less efficient, probably because of uneasiness on the part of schools to request intervention from outside organizations.

Crisis Interventions

The evolution of concepts and practices concerning post-traumatic stress disorder since 1980 has led to raised awareness concerning the importance of prevention and efficient means to put prevention into place (Horenstein, 1994; Horenstein and Voyron-Lemaire, 1996; Horenstein et al., 1998). The negative impact of trauma on school performance, because of resultant concentration and confusion problems, and an incapacity to synthesize and regain speech coherence, should direct schools to take into account the psychological component in crisis management (Nader and Pynoos, 1993).

Communication in a Situation of Crisis: General Rules

Intervention teams clearly must assert the prevention perspective and avoid a clinical perspective. The communication style of the team must be adjusted to the target school staff, officials, school crisis team, parents, and age and developmental level of the school students. If possible, two different teams should provide intervention to children and to staff. As a means of action, supervision, rather than leadership, should be stressed: the role of mental health personnel in the school setting should be to support the efforts of the staff, not replace them (Yule and Gold, 1993).

Communication in Large Groups

The intervention begins with a forty- to fifty-minute conference held by the intervention team executive, which addresses the whole school community, presents the team and planned actions, provides information on mental health, and answers questions. This conference is not a public address announcement of the traumatic event. The announcement is the responsibility of the school crisis team in smaller groups. The conference describes and normalizes emotional and physical reactions usually felt in cases of loss or trauma (e.g., it is normal to react or not react) (Nader, 1995). It deals with themes specific to the situation (e.g., suicide) and encourages the expression of emotion. The team leader stimulates the discussion around adaptive behavior (how previous losses were overcome) and sets up a means to identify students at risk. At the conclusion of the conference, leaders outline expectations for the following days and give instructions for self-care (e.g., eat healthy, regular meals, exercise, relax, ask for help, etc.).

Communication for Parents and Teachers Assisting Children

It is important to give instructions to parents and teachers so that they feel supported as adults and so that they can provide emotional first aid to children. The following guidelines can be of help (Dyregrov, 1991):

- Avoid abstract explanations.
- Accept questions and conversations about the event, without avoidance.
- Do not hide personal emotions.
- Let children participate in rituals and ceremonies.
- Keep the memory of the lost one alive.
- Explain reactions in order to normalize them.
- Suggest ways to express reactions.

Psychological Debriefing

Psychological Debriefing of Students

Every school is different and every crisis varies in scope, therefore, flexibility is essential in a crisis. No one person will always manage a critical incident stress-debriefing group. Some people may think that the crisis justifies a professional intervention on the part of specialists who work outside the school (as is the case in France). Others may think that outside specialists should intervene with high school students while teachers should manage groups of younger children (Johnson, 1993).

Each crisis induces a different group segmentation of individuals more or less exposed to the trauma or with more or less risk factors. When most students from the same class are victims, the psychological debriefing should be organized inside the class, under the direction of teachers. Critical incident stress debriefing is education, not psychotherapy; group education is a matter for teachers to perform. Principles of continuity and familiarity (Omer and Alon, 1994) speak in favor of this orientation. Teachers need not feel a sense of losing control specific to situations of crisis because of the intervention of experts. However, it is very important to teach teachers how to refer children at risk and not to engage in individual advice.

The rules of debriefing follow the traditional pattern developed by Mitchell (1995). All classroom work implies order resulting from rules, procedures, and routines specific to classroom management. In general, the more loosely structured the process, the more likely that it will be difficult to talk about disturbing events. The academic achievement of the class is very closely linked to the cohesiveness of the group, but traumatic events destroy this cohesiveness. Thus, it is important to explain that one of the most important targets of debriefing is to promote cooperation and solidarity. If it is likely that this target cannot be met, other strategies should be used (individual debriefing or groups other than class groups).

When debriefing, teachers should first state facts of the tragedy (concrete information, identification of individuals most exposed to risk). Because rumors and misinterpretations of the event are especially frequent in a school setting, it is important for information to be as public and well-shared as is possible. During this phase, teachers may learn that some students have been confronted in an especially brutal way and need individual intervention. Debriefing in the classroom helps students to express thoughts, sensory impressions and reactions, it strengthens the expression of emotions and, at the same time, discards what could be interpreted as a coercion to speak, avoiding embarrassment of students. If very few people have experienced intense emotions, it is advisable to carry on this phase individually, not in the classroom.

Debriefers provide useful information to normalize reactions as students share reactions and support one another. They are given knowledge of the expected reactions during the acute phase of trauma and delayed reactions such as potential consequences on schoolwork and concentration, and memory problems which sometimes last the whole school year. While maintaining its traditional structure, debriefing in the school setting should be integrated into school schedules and activities within the time frame familiar to students. Educational methods currently used in classrooms (essay, poetry, narrative composition, drawing, music, theater) are very useful when projects are adapted to the nature of the event and to the nature of the loss. Educational strategies adapted to learning enable students to explore safety issues and community involvement. One such possibility is a class project as to how students might help families, school, or the community in the aftermath of tragedy.

Psychological Debriefing of Staff

The crisis team should also be available to staff members to help them break the news to students, and to manage classroom issues (e.g., balance between curriculum goals and class hours to express feelings). If the school so desires, psychological debriefing managed by individuals working outside the concerned school who belong to the staff support network, can offer counseling services and practical assistance to staff at a later time.

The place where staff debriefing occurs impacts the way it is conceptualized. Performing it at school or in an annex at the same time that students are working with the same team tends to put all victims on the same level and denies the specific part played by teachers in emergency situations. Performing debriefing in a mental health center can, without due consideration, aggravate the institutional tendency to blame victims. The responsibility of the school to protect staff is more clearly asserted when debriefing takes place in settings specifically identified for this use (integrated in a support network) and by staff foreign to school administration.

In view of the frequency of institutional conflicts in schools prior to the venue of a traumatic event, dividing staff into groups can be a delicate problem, solved satisfactorily only through preliminary knowledge of the educational team (during primary prevention actions). The principle of caution is essential: it is better to arrange individual meetings than to put staff into groups defined at random, where debriefing might have lasting aftereffects in team functioning. In the educational environment, more than in other fields, it is important to define targets clearly and to distinguish debriefing from worker's claim issues.

The orientation of debriefing is the mode of "debriefing the debriefers" (Talbot, Manton, and Dunn, 1992). This orientation minimizes the development of posttraumatic stress symptoms and the development of work problems through the integration of personal and professional experience. Its goal is to explore the impact of the event (personal integration), the impact on victim students (empathy management, response to staff victims [team interaction]), and staff response to students (professional integration). The distribution of work among staff, the crisis response team (district or school), and mental health personnel from outside the school should be negotiated beforehand.

In a staff debriefing, it is advisable to be very careful about the context of staff notification and participant expectations before confirming facts. Insist that staff discuss their thoughts about different roles and interactions between them and between them and other intervening parties, not just "what were you thinking about what happened?" The strategies and degree of elicitation of descriptions of body feelings should take the setting into account (whether clinical context or not) and the method (individual or group) without risk of aggravation of mastery loss. The expression of emotional reactions should concern direct confrontation to the event as well as vicarious reactions resulting from listening to student victims. Empathy management and its negative side effects should be treated with special care.

The normalization phase should provide information specific to debriefing and supervision. This is not a critical review of the school prevention plan (that is the task of the strategic group). Instead, it is a clarification of dynamics and issues between personnel, students and personnel, and staff personnel. After summarizing the salient facts of the crisis, debriefing should focus on expected stressors from contact with students and likely difficulties in the implementation of psychological debriefing in class. In a school environment, it is useful for staff to adjust the organization of debriefing sessions to the educational pace. Interventions are limited in general to six sessions to strengthen the educational model rather than promote a psychotherapeutic model. However, risky situations should be taken into account and sessions should be arranged in accordance with those risks: e.g., anniversary dates, memorial services, trials, and other events.

INTERVENTION STRATEGIES: A CASE ILLUSTRATION

On the day before Christmas vacation, a ten-year-old student died after falling out of a classroom window during the school day. (At the time of writing this chapter, nothing had been concluded as to whether this was a suicide or an accident.*) The school district delegated a school psychologist to arrange a very short discussion with the class and staff before school closed for the fifteen-day holiday period. After the holiday, the class then went away for five days for a "snow class" away from the setting of the event. Upon their return, the students were placed in a new classroom and the teacher was referred to the mental health center by a legal association belonging to our staff assistance network. This center is in a national psychiatric institution and was created by teachers for teachers and has a school violence prevention unit.

The teacher who witnessed the incident, a forty-three-year-old man without psychiatric medical history, presented with symptoms of PTSD, especially a ruminating activity on "How could she fall?" He questioned his own responsibility and had difficulties managing empathy and conflicts in class; he had feelings of neglect and problems making students work. He stated

---

*Approximately thirty deadly accidents per year take place in French schools (at the time this chapter was written). Among children under fifteen, death caused in an indeterminate way happens twice more frequently than among other age groups.

that he was unable to talk to students again for fear of losing emotional control and embarrassing himself and "providing students a hold on him." The second session at the clinic continued the debriefing process which began at school. The first session had neither interrupted the development of guilt nor avoidance behaviors. During the third session, the teacher explained that his father had died and that he was on sick leave because of this loss. A part of the session was devoted to making plans to start the new school term, to inform the children of his personal loss, and to associate his loss with the tragedy experienced by the class. He was given guidance on how to ask the children about personal loss, what they thought about their classmate's death, how they talked about the topic at home, and how they could help one another.

During the fourth session, he explained that he had planned daily time in class for free talk and took advantage of this activity to speak about the death of his father and the girl's death. The children proposed to write a condolence letter to the girl's parents, then volunteers read their letters (few volunteered). A student proposed to create a billboard in order for children to "write things." The teacher decided to continue this activity hourly every week. At this time, sessions were focused on the impact of the trauma on relatives and colleagues, with an objective of normalization and anticipation of risky situations. Reaching out to others became an important issue.

During the fifth session, the teacher told about how he carried on this work with the children. The children wrote sad stories in a creative writing workshop. During the voluntary presentation of stories the following week, one of the children expressed her guilt feelings. Classmates had accused her of pushing the victim out of the window. The teacher spoke about his own guilt and his actions to manage it. An eyewitness child stated what had happened. "A death silence had fallen on the class as if Sarah had died the day before." An outburst of sympathy for the eyewitness occurred. She spoke of a visit to a psychologist at the initiative of her parents. The teacher explained that he had also sought help. The class hung the stories on the billboard. Students wrote personal thoughts between sessions and the class prepared an article on the experience for the school newspaper. The teacher's last session at the center was devoted to a summary of the healing process and the teacher's progress as well as to organizing follow-up sessions.

TERTIARY PREVENTION

PTSD Counseling

Discussing prevention instead of treatment asserts the difference between educational intervention and usual psychotherapeutic approaches, even if it occurs in a clinical environment. In psychotherapy, individuals seek counseling in order to change; in a case of psychological trauma, the unfortunate change has already taken place and the goal is to contain, and to achieve closure (Müller, personal communication). The PTSD consultation is not focused on an individual as a whole, but also works with the trauma. The explicit goal is a return to the level of functioning, prior to the trauma, whatever this level was. After a limited amount of sessions (not over twelve, according to most specialists) and, after a period of a few months of observation, it is always possible to reassess problems and propose a new treatment. The limited amount of sessions forces the therapist and patient to focus on the trauma, and conveys the notion that it contributes, along with giving information, to the normalization of symptoms. Therapists should insist that these symptoms are a normal reaction to an abnormal event. The first goals in this type of therapy are to prevent chronicization of troubles by reducing negative emotions, to facilitate self-control and environmental control, to provide resources to manage these emotions, and to enable an adaptive mode of functioning. Information gathering, confrontation, and narrative restructuring are the tools used to meet these goals in ways that are less emotionally damaging.

Dysfunction

Unfortunately, schools sometime face not only a single crisis but, in certain cases, a succession of intense and complex crises. The frequency of crises makes resolution increasingly difficult. Each additional crisis adds up and the organization as a whole may become dysfunctional. Loss of the sense of a school mission, questioning of the leadership of the school and of the leader, developing of a collective sense of helplessness, defensive behavior, conflicts between individuals, and a division into interest groups are revealing symptoms of school dsyfunction (Johnson, 1993). Interventions centered on individuals may turn out to be inadequate and must be complemented with work on remediation of institutional dysfunction. The concept of vicarious traumatization explains the disintegration of educational teams through spreading. The well-prepared organization will take precautions to protect its own staff, taking into account these risks for educational staff confronted with traumas of their colleagues and students as well.

Cumulative Traumatic Stress Debriefings

Cumulative traumatic stress debriefings take into account the history of the educational team and its long-term cohesiveness. This makes it possible to structure an institutional intervention starting from the concept of vicarious traumatization. With this method, conflicts between staff can lead to supportive strategies (Johnson, 1993).

The choice of traumatic events previously experienced by the educational team that are dealt with during these debriefings provides an opportunity to detect the competitive or cooperative style of staff. Strategies for structuring group discussion can be used in this phase (personal list to establish priorities, master list and evaluation to reach consensus). The introduction phase, which sets the transformation of vicarious traumatization as a group goal, should promote the perception of complementary goals and limit the antagonistic perception of goals, specific to protest process. Because vicarious traumatization is a process rather than an event (Saakvitne and Pearlman, 1996), it is advisable to analyze repercussions of trauma over time, especially those on the organization of school and interpersonal relations. This delineation includes discussions about feelings and defenses against feelings.

Individual evaluation should lead to a collective distribution of reactions and an awareness of vicarious traumatization and its promoting factors (the silent witness exercise—sharing one's personal list of symptoms of vicarious traumatization in silence is a tool which should be used in this phase). The target of this intervention is to develop individual self-care and group support and to prevent risky situations. It is advisable to use cognitive strategies and stimulus materials rather than experiential exercises with school staff members to draw out ideas from their own experiences. Tasks that require interdependence (active listening, peer coaching, work in small groups about a topic being presented to a larger group, written tests, success stories, the ideal work situation) can be helpful. Utilization of a checklist of material, social, and institutional resources may also be helpful, as is the use of structured problem solving. In conclusion, these interventions solidify agreements by summarizing what individual and group changes were decided, giving a feeling of closure and accomplishment.

FINAL THOUGHTS

In France, in mental health practice, an evolution has occurred in the school community, including cooperation between schools and mental health organizations, creation of mental health clinics in schools, and the development of activities such as those found in this chapter (Fisher, Raundalen, and Dyregrov, 1993). These practices testify to a gradual development of responsibilities of the school system, though unfortunately, the development has not taken place everywhere. At present, mental health services for school populations and faculty are often limited to therapeutic measures for individuals and, often, consulting services for preventive approaches are not covered under health insurance. In spite of this, it is essential for the implementation of networks to structure the support of victim staff. When the individuals who are supposed to help, whether therapists or teachers, are traumatized in turn, additional suffering is likely to be imposed on them (Stamm, 1995).

BIBLIOGRAPHY

American Psychiatric Association (1993). *Psychiatric consultation in schools.* Washington, DC: American Psychiatric Association.

Bacal, R. (1995). *Defusing hostile and volatile situations: A guide for educational personnel.* Winnipeg, Manitoba: Bacal and Associates.

Berkovitz, I.H. and Seliger J.S (1985). *Expanding mental health interventions in schools.* Dubuque, IA: Kendall/Hunt.

Bloch, A.M. (1978). Combat neurosis in inner-city schools. *American Journal of Psychiatry, 135*(10): 1189-1192.

Blom, G.E. (1986). A school disaster. Intervention and research aspects. *Journal of the American Academy of Child Psychiatry, 25:* 336-345.

Coben, J.H., Weiss, H.B., Mulvey, E.P., and Dearwater, S.R. (1994). A primer on school violence prevention. *Journal of School Health, 64*(8): 309-313.

Cooke, G.J. (1996). Safe school for all. In Hoffman, A.M. (Ed.), *Schools, violence, and society* (pp. 135-145). Westport, CT: Praeger.

Cox, G. (1991). *Dealing with death and suicide in the school community.* Queensland, Australia: Guidance and Counselling Services, Department of Education.

Dubé, M. (1993). *La violence en milieu scolaire adulte.* Montreal, Canada: La Commission des Ecoles Catholiques de Montréal.

Dyregrov, A. (1991). *Grief in children: A handbook for adults.* London: Jessica Kingsley Publishers.

Dyregrov, A. (1993). School crisis contingency plan, First draft. Prepared for UNICEF, Mena Section. Unpublished paper.

Dyregrov, A., Matthiesen, S.B., Kristoffersen, J.I., and Mitchell, J.T. (1994). Gender differences in adolescents' reactions to the murder of their teacher. *Journal of Adolescent Research, 9:* 363-383.

Echterling, L.G. (1989). An ark of prevention: Preventing school absenteeism after a flood. *Journal of Primary Prevention, 9*(3):177-184.

Feder, J. (1989). Crime's aftermath. *School Safety,* Spring, 26-29.

Feder, J. (1992). Reducing the trauma of teacher victimization. *School Safety,* Fall, 7-9.

Fisher, N., Raundalen, M., and Dyregrov, A. (1993). "Reaching children through teachers: Investigating teachers' attitudes and their potential for communicating with children on sensitive issues." Paper presented at the third European conference on traumatic stress, Bergen, Norway, June 6-10.

Furlong, M. (1994). Evaluating school violence trends. *School Safety,* Winter, 23-27.

Furlong, M.J. and Morrison, G.M. (1994). Introduction to miniseries: School violence and safety in perspective. *School Psychology Review, 23*(2):139-150.

Futrell, M.H. (1996). Violence in the classroom: A teacher's perspective. In Hoffman, A.M. (Ed.), *Schools, violence, and society* (pp. 3-19). Westport, CT: Praeger.

Garza-Fuentes, F. and Rose, R.M. (1995). *Being prepared: The school emergency response plan handbook.* Boston: The Regional Laboratory for Educational Improvement of the Northeast and Islands.

Harris, L. (1995). *The Metropolitan Life survey of the American teacher 1984-1995: Old problems, new challenges.* New York: Metropolitan Life Insurance Company.

Horenstein, J.M. (1994). "Les enseignants victimes de la violence." Article presenté au congrés "Santé et droit de l'homme." Prague, Mai.

Horenstein, J.M. and Voyron-Lemaire, M.-Ch. (1996). *Les enseignants victimes de la violence.* Paris: Collection MGFN.

Horenstein, J.M., Voyron-Lemaire, M.-Ch., Reverzy, C., Lelievre, F., Kremer, N., and Faucheux, J. (1998). *Les pratiques du harcèlement en milieu éducatif.* Paris: Collection MGEN.

Hyman, I.A., Zelikoff, W., and Clarke, J. (1988). Psychological and physical abuse in the schools: A paradigm for understanding posttraumatic stress disorder in children and youth. *Journal of Traumatic Stress, 1:* 243-267.

Jenkin, J.B. (1994). Coping with violence in Australian schools. *School Safety,* Fall, 20-22.

Johnson, K. (1993). *School Crisis Management.* Alameda, CA: Hunter House.

Klingman, A. (1989). School-based emergency intervention following an adolescent's suicide. *Death Studies, 13*(3): 263-274.

Leymann, H. and Gustafsson, A. (1996). Mobbing at work and development of post-traumatic stress disorders. *European Journal of Work and Organizational Psychology, 5*(2): 251-275.

Menninger, W.W. (1993). Management of the aggressive and dangerous patient. *Bulletin of the Menninger Clinic, 57*(2): 208-217.

Milgram, N.A., Toubiana, Y.H., Klingman, A., and Raviv, A. (1988). Situational exposure and personal loss in children's acute and chronic stress reactions to a school bus disaster. *Journal of Traumatic Stress, 1:* 339-352.

Mitchell, J.T. (1995). "Coldenham, New York: Recovery from community trauma." Communication presenté au Quatrième Conference Europeènne sur le stress traumatique [Communication presented at the fourth European Conference on traumatic stress]. Paris: 7-Il Mai.

Moriarty, A., Maeyama, R.G., and Fitzgerald, P.J. (1993). A CLEAR plan for school crisis management. *NASSP Bulletin,* April, 17-22.

Morrison, G.M., Furlong, M.J., and Morrison, R.L. (1994). School violence to school safety: Reframing the issue for school psychologists. *School Psychology Review, 23*(2): 236-256.

Nader, K. (1995). Psychological first aid for trauma, grief and traumatic griefs a copyrighted document to assist school psychologists and mental health professionals in their work with parents and teachers.

Nader, K. and Pynoos, R. (1991). School disaster planning and initial interventions. *Journal of Social Behavior and Personality, 8,* 375-389.

Nader, K. and Pynoos, R. (1993). School disaster: Planning and initial interventions. *Journal of Social Behavior and Personality, 8*(5): 299-320.

Nader, K., Pynoos, R., Fairbanks, L., and Frederick, C. (1990). Children's PTSD reactions one year after a sniper attack at their school. *American Journal of Psychiatry, 147*(11): 1526-1530.

Omer, H. and Alon, N. (1994). The continuity principle: A unified approach to disaster and trauma. *American Journal of Community Psychology, 22:* 273-287.

Pichene, C. (1995). "Prise en charge psychiatrique des victimes de la catastrophe de Toul." Communication presenté au Quatrième Conference Europeènne sur le stress traumatique. Paris: 7-11 Mai.

Pitcher, G. and Poland, S. (1992). *Crisis intervention in the schools.* New York: Guilford.

Quarles, Ch.L. (1989). *School violence: A survival guide for school staff.* Washington, DC: National Education Association.

Rowling, L. (1994). "The hidden grief of teachers." Paper presented at the Fourth International Conference on Grief and Bereavement in Contemporary Society. Stockholm, Sweden, June 12-16.

Saakvitne, K.W. and Pearlman, L.A. (1996). *Transforming the pain: A workbook on vicarious traumatization.* New York: Norton.

Sack, W.H. (1986). The psychiatric effects of massive trauma on Cambodian children: II. The family, the home, and the school. *Journal of the American Academy of Child Psychiatry,* 377-383.

Schwarz, F. and Kowalski, J. (1991). Posttraumatic stress disorder after a school shooting: Effects of symptom threshold selection and diagnosis by DSM-III, DSM-III-R, or proposed DSM-IV. *American Journal of Psychiatry, 148*(5): 592-597.

Shelton, J.L. and Sanders, R.S. (1973). Mental health intervention in a campus homicide. *Journal of the American College Health Association, 21*(4): 346-350.

Stamm, H. (1995). *Secondary traumatic stress.* Lutherville, MD: Sidran Press.

Stephens, R.D. (1994). Planning for safer and better schools: School violence prevention and intervention strategies. *School Psychology Review, 23*(2): 204-215.

Talbot, A., Manton, M., and Dunn, P.J. (1992). Debriefing the debriefers: An intervention strategy to assist psychologists after a crisis. *Journal of Traumatic Stress, 5*(1), 45-62.

Terr, L.C. (1981). Psychic trauma in children: Observations following the Chowchilla school bus kidnapping. *American Journal of Psychiatry, 138,* 14-19.

United Federation of Teachers (1995). Report of the School Safety Department for the 1994-1995 school year. New York: Author.

Weeler, E.D. and Baron, A. (1994). *Violence in our schools, hospitals and public places.* Pathfinder Publishing of California.

Wilson, A. (1995). *Violence and traumatic stress in urban schools.* Boston: The Regional Laboratory for Educational Improvement of the Northeast and Islands.

Yule, W. and Gold, A. (1993). *Wise before the event: Coping with crises in schools.* London: Calouste Gulbenkian Foundation.

Chapter 12

Traumatic Stress in Family Systems

Chrys J. Harris

INTRODUCTION

Although the emotional consequences of a traumatic experience are usually enumerated in terms of an individual's response to the event, the outcome of the individual's demeanor on his or her family is of major concern to those who subscribe to systemic theory. According to Turnbull and McFarlane (1996, p. 483), "Trauma does not occur in a vacuum, and often a number of family members may be similarly traumatized." It follows that family members could experience trauma as a unit (all being victimized) or as Figley (1995) suggests, the family could be secondarily traumatized (secondary to a family member who experienced the trauma). Regardless of which effect trauma has, the entire family system may manifest emotional consequences.

This chapter presents a systemic orientation for assessing, treating, and preventing the traumatization that can occur in families. The assessment section is concerned with clinical interviews, evaluative measures, and other methods to assess trauma. The treatment section highlights some of the treatment paradigms presently being used and introduces innovative treatment models identified by The Subcommittee on Contemporary Approaches to Treating Trauma of the International Society for Traumatic Stress Studies the (ISTSS) Standards of Care Committee (acting for the Board of Directors of ISTSS). Finally, the prevention section focuses on several methodologies that have been successful in helping to prevent emotional trauma in individuals and in families. This chapter is not a "how-to" chapter, instead, it offers a conceptual framework for traumatized families. First, some insight into the archetype of systems theory is presented.

General Systems Theory

General systems theory has been around since the late 1940s and early 1950s, and was originally used in science and mathematics. In an effort to define organization in general, with systems specifically, von Bertalanffy (1968) adopted an organismic principle that stated that animals live together as organized entities and must be considered as such by science. The organismic principle established the groundwork needed to identify the family as a system and to perceive the family and its members in a social context. Furthermore, organization in the family system is regarded as different from that of an ad hoc group of individuals.

The thirteen years following the introduction of von Bertalanffy's organismic principle (between 1968 and 1981) were replete with general family systems theories and specific treatment paradigms—adding to the growth of family systems theory and practice. Finally, Gurman and Kniskern (1981) were able to conclude in their unique and innovative initial volume of the *Handbook of Family Therapy,* that the concept of the family as a system, at long last, had achieved a wide acceptance and recognition.

Nichols and Everett (1986) suggest that in general family systems theory, the whole (system) is not simply a summation of the individual parts. In fact, it is different and has heuristic value in and of itself. The concept of a change in one part of the system affecting the rest of the system is paramount in present-day family systems theory. Many family system therapeutic models are based on such change within the family system. These models are based on the belief that it is not the Freudian intrapsychic conflicts of the individual that are the focus of therapy, but the lack of homeostasis within the family system that is the preeminent treatment emphasis. This does not suggest that individual family members are not important; it suggests that the family system has value as well and is equally important. In fact, both are essential focal points for trauma therapy.

Nichols and Everett (1986) identified a primary form of a general system and represented it as follows: A system is

- a unified whole that consists of interrelated pals;
- the whole is different than the sum of its parts; and
- any change in one part affects the rest of the system.

Further, a system is concerned with

- identifying the functional and structural rules of the system; and
- identifying the attributes of the system, which include
    —the method of information processing,
    —adaptation to change circumstances,
    —self-organization,
    —self-maintenance, and
    —self-regulation (through communication).

There are a number of functional and structural rules to which systems in general subscribe. However—being concerned with families—this chapter explores systems by examining the family. Family systems advocate functional and structural rules that stem from family rituals, traditions, myths, customs, culture, heritage, conventions, and ceremonies. These rules establish parental dominance, sibling dominance, family member tolerance of a number of issues, family affection, abusiveness, cohesiveness, flexibility, and many other details that the family system requires to maintain itself.

Finally, systemic attributes are the crux of how one system truly differentiates itself from another. These attributes help to distinguish how a system processes information, adapts to change, organizes itself, maintains itself, and communicates to regulate itself. When these attributes are demystified—exposed to family members, say, in therapy—the system can be extremely susceptible to self-awareness and modification which can lead to an eventual abatement of traumatization.

The Family System

The earlier general systems representation devised by Nichols and Everett (1986) can now be rewritten to reflect a family system representation: A family system is

- a unified organization of individual family members;
- the family system is different than the sum of its family members; and
- any change in one family member affects the rest of the family system.

The family systems theory is concerned with

- identifying the functional and structural rules of the family system; and
- identifying the attributes of the family system, which include
  —family system methods of information processing,
  —family system methods of adaptation to change circumstances,
  —family system methods of self-organization,
  —family system methods of self-maintenance, and
  —family system methods of self-regulation though communication.

In his definitive work on traumatized families, Figley (1989, p. 12) suggests that family members have "a remarkable 'feel' for the normative behavior of fellow family members." By demystifying the family members' individual pre- and posttrauma behaviors and the family system's pre- and posttrauma behaviors, the family system can distinguish how their function, structure, and attributes have modified as a consequence of the traumatic event. These issues will be explored at greater length later in this chapter.

However, from this it can be inferred that there may be more than one way in which families are traumatized. Figley (1989) identifies four separate types of family system traumatization.

The first type is called *simultaneous effects,* in which a catastrophic event occurs to the entire family system. Examples of this include natural disasters, auto accidents, infectious diseases, and house fires. In these events, the family system, as a whole, is exposed to the traumatic event—*all* at the same time.

The second way a family system can be traumatized is through *vicarious effects.* Family members can be traumatized vicariously when they learn that another family member (or members) experienced a traumatic event. The most well-known traumatization of this type occurs when representatives of the military come to the family home to report that a family member has been wounded, taken prisoner, killed in action, or simply has been involved in some traumatic incident. Obviously, there are a number of other ways families can find out that their family members have been exposed to traumatic events. With the technology that exists today in television, radio, and satellite reporting, it is very easy for a family system to know about a traumatic event and a family member's potential involvement prior to being notified by the authorities. In fact, many individuals have reported symptoms indicative of vicarious traumatic responses as a result of hearing about, for example, floods in Iowa, tornadoes in Alabama, and fires in southern California—knowing they had family members in these areas.

The third method by which a family system can be traumatized is through what Kishur (1984) called the *chiasmal effects.* Chiasmal effects infect the family system. For example, when the traumatized family member relates his or her story to the rest of the family system, they can become secondarily traumatized or infected, as a product of their susceptibility. It should be noted that, in most cases, chiasmal effects are not intentionally produced. Harris (1995a, p. 101) defined these type of effects as "unintended, unexpected, and deleterious." They are emotional consequences that often appear regardless of the intention—in this case—of the family member telling the story.

The final way a family system can be traumatized is through *intrafamily trauma.* In this type, the family system comprises the necessary circumstance for the trauma (Figley, 1989). In these cases, family members create the traumatic event(s) and, thereby, cause the trauma (intrafamilial) for other family members. The most striking example of intrafamilial trauma is abuse—in which children or vulnerable adults are abused by other family members.

Based on this family systems representation, it can be rewritten to reflect a traumatized family system: A traumatized family system is

- a unified organization of family members in which one (or more) is traumatized;
- the traumatized family system is different than the sum of its traumatized family members; and
- any trauma experienced by one family member affects the rest of the family system.

The traumatized family systems theory is concerned with

- identifying the functional and structural rules of the pre- and post-trauma family system; and
- identifying the attributes of the pre- and post-trauma family system, which include
  —family system methods of information processing,
  —family system methods of adaptation to change circumstances,
  —family system methods of self-organization,
  —family system methods of self-maintenance, and
  —family system methods of self-regulation through communication.

This conception of systems theory is used throughout this chapter and is referred to it as the Traumatized Family Systems (TFS) Archetype.

ASSESSING FAMILY SYSTEM TRAUMA

As mentioned earlier, the emotional consequences of a traumatic experience are usually detailed in terms of an individual's response to the event. This is because such emotional consequences are idiosyncratic to the individual. French and Harris (1998) suggest that it is this idiosyncratic model of self and the world that determines how each of us will cope with the traumatic experience. Those who are successful in coping with the traumatic experience go on with their lives with few or no emotional consequences. However, those who are not successful in coping with their traumatic experience often develop post-traumatic stress disorder (PTSD) (see Chapter 1 for a detailed description of PTSD). To assess family system trauma we have to combine individual assessment and systemic assessment.

Litz and Weathers (1994) suggest three methods of assessing individuals for the consequences of a traumatic experience: the clinical interview, questionnaires or inventories, and psychophysiological techniques. Litz and Weathers state that all of these methods are important, but "the foundation of the PTSD assessment is the clinical interview" (p. 20).

The Clinical Interview

The clinical interview for traumatized families centers on two major themes: the individual (family member) response to the trauma and the family system response to the trauma. The individual response is dealt with by exploring the idiosyncratic response of each family member. The family system response focuses on the TFS Archetype features of the family's posttrauma functional and structural rules concurrent with the posttrauma family system attributes. These issues make the family system different than the sum of the responses of the individual family members.

Figley (1989) proposes that the family system assessment be taken with the entire family present. Inherent in such a proposal is a systemic philosophy that allows the entire family system to explore both the idiosyncratic trauma response of the individual family member(s) and the systemic trauma response of the family system. This exploration is basically an events-based approach (Greenberg, Heatherington, and Friedlander, 1996) in which specific circumstances described in the session encourage change (this will be discussed later in the prevention section). The assessment should include a pre- and posttrauma individual family member and family system history, details of the individual and systemic responses to the stressor, and an exploration of potential comorbid issues (other diagnosable disorders concurrent with the stress response).

Assessment for individual family members during the clinical interview involves allowing each to tell his or her story regarding his or her traumatic experience. Even though the TFS Archetype states that the family system is greater than the sum of its members, each member has value and therefore, each story has value.

Each individual family member presents a traumatic experience that is a unique and singularly individual response. Janoff-Bulman (1992, p. 5) proposes that all of us have a conceptual system that "developed over time, provides us with expectations about the world and ourselves." She asserts that we have a foundation of assumptions that provides the rudimentary basis for our beliefs about ourselves, our world, and the relationship between the two. It is from this conceptual system that individuals compose the idiosyncratic response to trauma (French and Harris, 1998).

The family system assessment helps to ascertain how well the family has integrated the individual stories—if they have even been shared—through the TFS Archetype posttrauma attributes. As these issues unfold, an assessment as to how the TFS Archetype pretrauma attributes have changed should become apparent.

The TFS Archetype pre- and posttrauma functional rules can be assessed by adapting some of the specific family system functions suggested by Figley (1989):

1. Does the family system have an apparent understanding and acceptance of the sources of stress affecting them?
2. Does the family system perceive their stress as a family problem or is one or more family members blamed?
3. Is/Was the family system solution-oriented or blame-oriented?
4. How do/did family members tolerate one another?
5. How committed are/were the family members to one another?
6. How much affection is/was there in the family system?
7. What is/was the quantity and quality of the family system communication?
8. Is/Was there evidence of family system violence?
9. Is/Was there evidence of family system substance dependence or abuse?

The TFS Archetype pre- and posttrauma structural rules can be assessed by adapting some of the structural needs of the family system also suggested by Figley (1989):

1. How cohesive is/was the family system?
2. How flexible is/was the family system in general?
3. How flexible are/were the family members in their family roles?
4. Does/Did the family system have and utilize resources outside the family?
5. Do/Did family members serve as resources for other family members?

In the assessment of the functional and structural rules for the family system, the distinctions between the family system's management during the pretrauma period can be directly contrasted with the family system's management during the posttrauma period. This highlights family system change directly attributed to effects of the traumatic event.

Assessing for the pre- and posttrauma attributes for the family system involves discussing the specific family system attributes listed in the TFS Archetype and contrasting the pretrauma period with the posttrauma period.

Questionnaires and Inventories

A number of psychometric questionnaires and inventories for assessing traumatic stress in individuals exist, but none appear to assess family systems. For further information on questionnaires and inventories, the reader is referred to Stamm' s compilation of psychometric tests and measures for trauma response, *Measurement of Trauma, Stress and Adaptation* (Stamm, 1996). Stamm recommends that the following measures be used on a regular basis: Life Status Review (quality of life); Stressful Life Experiences

Screening, Long Form; and Stressful Life Experiences Screening, Short Form.

Although there are no measures of stress response from a systems perspective, the *Family Adaptability and Cohesion Evaluation Scale (FACES)* (Olson, Russell, and Sprenkle, 1983) has proved helpful in this regard. Although this measure does not assess for systemic traumatic response, it does estimate the degree of adaptability and cohesion within a family system. The TFS Archetype identifies adaptability to change as one of the attributes of the pre- and posttrauma family system.

Psychophysiological Techniques

Litz and Weathers (1994) suggest that psychophysiological techniques are rarely used in the clinical assessment of PTSD. Regardless, there have been some studies which report that these methodologies may be of significant value to the assessment of individual trauma responses (cf, Blanchard et al., 1982).

Psychophysiological methods measure heart rate, blood pressure, and skin conductance and are used to calculate the degree of individual arousal. Other subjective measures include the Subjective Units of Distress Scale (SUDS) in which individuals rate distress on a scale from 0 (no stress at all) to 10 (the most stress ever experienced). Wylie (1996) suggests that practitioners who treat traumatic stress use the SUDS measure of arousal as an acceptable predictor of stress response, determining fluctuations along a continuum of treatment.

TREATING FAMILY SYSTEM TRAUMA

Although in most cases "the actual therapy will be relatively brief" (Figley, 1989, p. 60), brief is an arbitrary term and is operationally defined by some—including those in managed care—in many different ways. Brief therapy is not a term that is commonly associated with family therapy. However, with the onset of new treatment paradigms for individuals (detailed later), family therapy for traumatized families can be *briefer.*

Providing systemic therapy—especially for traumatized families—has always been a time-consuming process, when compared to individual therapy. As a result, any type of systemic intervention—as a useful treatment paradigm—has not been accepted by managed care and insurance companies. The primary reason for this appears to be the fact that systemic therapy does not customarily meet the establishment needs for specific remedial treatment such as brief (number of sessions) therapeutic intervention. However, research suggests systemic therapy is a successful form of therapy (cf., Gurman and Kniskern, 1991).

Treatment paradigms for emotional trauma remain focused on the individual. The only model that presently exists in the literature for treating traumatized family systems is Figley (1989).

The Figley (1989) model of treating traumatized families is a five-phased empowerment approach (encompassing both empowerment and prevention) derived from specific theories for crisis intervention, traumatic stress studies, cognitive psychology, behavioral therapy, and systems theory. The five phases of the Figley (1989) model are

1. building commitment to the therapeutic objectives;
2. framing the problem;
3. reframing the problem;
4. developing a healing theory; and
5. closure and preparedness.

These five phases are designed to achieve seven specific goals, which are

1. clarifying the therapist's role;
2. eliminating the unwanted consequences of trauma;
3. building family social supportiveness;
4. developing new rules and skills of family communication;
5. promoting self-disclosure;
6. recapitulating traumatic events; and
7. building a family healing theory.

Figley suggests that this model is designed to produce a positive therapeutic environment and to empower the family to heal themselves.

In analyzing Figley's (1989) goals in terms of the TFS Archetype's attributes, the attribute of information processing is inherent in all seven goals. The attribute of adaptation to change is specific to goal no. 2, goal no. 4, and goal no. 6. The attribute of self-organization is specific to goal no. 3, goal no. 4, goal no. 5, and goal no. 7. The attribute of self-maintenance is specific to goal no. 2, goal no. 3, goal no. 4, goal no. 5, goal no. 6, and goal no. 7. The attribute of self-regulation through communication is inherent in all seven goals.

The TFS Archetype helps identify the family's pre- and posttrauma attributes and sets a template for therapeutic intervention. In other words, by identifying family attributes to explore, and prescribing these attributes as targets for therapeutic change, goals for systemic intervention are established. The differences between pre- and posttrauma function in each attribute can help the family interpret its adaptation or maladaptation to the traumatic event, and determine courses of action in therapy.

Treating Individual Trauma

It has only been within the past five years that new PTSD treatment paradigms have come into use. The Subcommittee on Contemporary Approaches to Treating Trauma of the International Society for Traumatic Stress Studies (ISTSS) Standards of Care Committee (acting for the Board of Directors of ISTSS) has identified a number of contemporary therapeutic interventions for the treatment of PTSD (Dietrich et al., 2000). These current trauma therapies include Traumatic Incident Reduction (TIR), Eye Movement Desensitization and Reprocessing (EMDR), Thought Field Therapy (TFT), Time Limited Trauma Therapy (T-LTT), and Visual Kinesthetic Dissociation (VKD).

Each of these trauma therapies is viable in the treatment of individual stress response. TIR is used as an illustration for individual treatment for traumatization.

French and Harris (1998) suggest that the goal of treating PTSD in an individual is to move him or her from a chronic stage of victimization to an acute stage in which one assimilates and accommodates a traumatic incident. Gerbode (1995) advises that what must be successfully assimilated and accommodated is one's thoughts, sensations, feelings, and perceptions regarding the trauma and the traumatic event.

TIR helps the individual family member (referred to in TIR as a viewer) accommodate and assimilate through a methodical, sequentially directed number of recapitulations of the traumatic experience. During TIR, the therapist (referred to in TIR as a facilitator) helps the viewer to dissipate the emotional charge—trauma-induced—by reaching an end point where the viewer experiences an observable change in affect and new insight regarding the traumatic experience (French and Harris, 1998). TIR is unique in being highly focused, directive, and controlled; yet wholly person-centered, noninterpretive, and nonjudgmental.

Using TIR as the treatment of choice for the family member(s) when there is vicarious, chiasmal, or intrafamily trauma should allow the family therapist to treat the individual family member(s) in a relatively brief time. In the case of simultaneous family trauma, treating all family members independently could (1) obviate the need to treat the system entirely, or (2) result in a longer treatment time for individual family members and the family system. For a detailed explanation of TIR, see French and Harris (1998).

PREVENTING FAMILY SYSTEM TRAUMA

Critical Incident Stress Debriefing (CISD) is probably the most well-known *preventive* intervention for those who have been exposed to a traumatic incident. Although the research is not conclusive as to the efficacy of CISD (Dietrich et al., 2000), it remains a popular and commonly used intervention.

According to Harris (1995a) there are two major national models in the United States for CISD training: the National Organization for Victim Assistance (NOVA) model (Washington, DC), and the Critical Incident Stress Management (CISM) model of the International Critical Incident Stress Foundation (Ellicott City, MD). Harris (1995a) proposes a basic assumption of CISD centers on providing ventilation, validation, preparation, and education; and also notes that functions of CISD include

1. providing support after a critical incident;
2. providing referral sources for a number of needs;
3. providing follow-up service(s); and
4. offering education regarding the stress that follows a critical incident.

CISD is essentially sensory-based, commonly occurs forty-eight to seventy-two hours after the incident, is noninvasive (no therapeutic intervention), and generally lasts from one-and-a-half to two hours. The intervention is designed to help individuals organize their thoughts about the traumatic incident so that individual assimilation and accommodation of the incident is enhanced (Harris, 1995a). Although predominantly used in a group setting in which a number of individuals—usually in an ad hoc relationship—have experienced a common traumatic event, CISD appears to be rarely referred to in the systemic literature, if at all. Obviously, this oversight should be explored further—in research and therapy.

In their most recent publication, Crisis Management International, Inc. (1998) lists a number of psychological barriers that injured workers may face that tend to delay their return to the work environment. These same barriers can be applied to a family system that has been traumatized in some manner, and could account for delays in their ability to function properly, either independently or systemically. These barriers include the following:

- Anger
- Fear
- Outrage
- Immobilization
- Irrational beliefs
- Emotional numbing

- Traumatic stress
- Unrealistic expectations
- Desire to exploit
- Depression
- Vengeance
- Sense of entitlement
- Anxiety
- Strained relationships

Crisis Management International, Inc. (1998) offers three assumptions for debriefing traumatized workers. When systemically interpreted, they apply to families very well:

1. There are emotional barriers that complicate psychological readjustment and the return to a normal functioning, independently or systemically.
2. There is more to readjustment for individuals and systems than physical healing.
3. There is a need for the individual and the system to discharge the emotional residual of a traumatic experience.

Although the routine debriefing occurs within days of the event, it is not uncommon to debrief a family weeks or months after an event. It seems to be a viable method for moving the family into a more acute state in which the TFS Archetype can be utilized effectively. The assumption here is that the major work of assimilation and accommodation of the traumatic experience occurs in the acute stages of traumatic response rather than in chronic stages (Harris, 1995a).

Another method of preventing the onset of a traumatic stress disorder is to initiate family therapy as soon as possible following the event. As this is accomplished, it is difficult to gauge which of the family members are going to move through the acute stress disorder to develop a chronic stress disorder (if any do). As such, it is imperative that the therapist is not intrusive in a manner that will usurp the natural ability one might possess to assimilate and accommodate a traumatic event. In fact, the therapeutic intervention of choice here is more crisis intervention rather than advising.

A methodology for assuring that the clients' innate ability to integrate the stress response remains intact is to provide therapy from a least-intrusive therapeutic format. One example of this is the 3-E Formula (Harris, 1995b). The three Es are enhance, expunge, and engender.

This intervention is an events-based approach (Greenberg, Heatherington, and Friedlander, 1996) in which specific circumstances described in the session encourage change. In other words, as certain factors are disclosed, the family becomes empowered to initiate their own transformation from a traumatized family system to a surviving family system.

When providing the initial therapeutic interventions, the therapist should focus on enhancing all of the behaviors the family members are doing which contribute *positively* to a functional individual or system. In doing so, the therapist allows the family members to discuss what each is doing and to discover how it affects the family system attributes in the TFS Archetype. This type of intervention has been found—at times—to be enough to take the family members to a more functional place where they can continue their own work. In other words, enhancing what the family members and the system are doing correctly can allow them to end therapy and move ahead on their own.

However, if enhancing is not enough, then the therapist should judiciously use expunging and engendering. When working with families, there is usually a high tendency toward familial intrinsic resistance. This resistance is a result of the family's predisposition to homeostasis and natural propensity to counteract change. Because this inclination is frequently very strong, expunging behaviors can do more damage than help. However, expunging is often necessary when it becomes apparent that a behavior or set of behaviors is dysfunctional, nonproductive, and generally provides a barrier to emotional healing.

One tenet of the 3-E Formula is that nothing is expunged without engendering a replacement. As such, expunging a prevailing behavior should be followed immediately by engendering a replacement behavior. This reduces resistance and meets another tenet of the 3-E Formula, behaviors that persist serve a purpose and will be indisposed to being expunged.

Previously it was mentioned that expunging and engendering should be used judiciously. This is to allow the family's own healing ability to kick in (if it can) with as little intervention as possible.

CONCLUSIONS

Within this chapter, the words *victim* and *survivor* have been used to suggest negative and positive states of being. Figley (1983) has referred to a victim as one who is immobilized (suggesting a negative state) by a traumatic experience, while the survivor becomes mobile (suggesting a positive state) in spite of the traumatic experience. From this, one could easily recommend—and rightly so—that survivorship would be a worthy goal of therapy.

However, there are several states of being that Figley has not identified. First, numerous survivors of catastrophes who are functional—some marginally so—do not wish to be referred to as victims. As a matter of fact, they do not meet the Figley (1983) definition of either victim or survivor. They come together as members of special survivor groups which are oriented to their specific traumatic experience (e.g., survivors of childhood sexual abuse, survivors of suicide (family, relatives, and friends of the deceased), and families of victims of plane crashes such as Pan Am 103, TWA 800, or Swiss Air 111). As functional survivors, they participate in society—even if minimally—and consider themselves as enduring and persevering. Yet they also recognize that all is not well and their traumatic experience intrudes upon them continually.

Second, these functional survivors appear to have no place to move as a result of therapy—as victims move into survivorship. The proposal offered herein is to move functional survivors into a state of thriving.

To thrive, an individual must prosper, flourish, succeed, or advance in some manner. This implies more than becoming mobile in spite of the traumatic experience; it suggests that one prevails over the traumatic event. In doing so, one does not allow the traumatic experience to remain emotionally charged, nor is it allowed to be a barrier to everyday functioning. As such, the post-traumatic stress disorder can be essentially cured (Wylie, 1996).

As mentioned earlier in this chapter, "Trauma does not occur in a vacuum" (Turnbull and McFarlane, 1996, p. 483). The major focus of this chapter has been on the family as a system which can be and should be treated conjointly with individual family members. However, other systems should be considered (e.g., workplace, church, social group, etc.) as well. Those who do not treat trauma systemically should not ignore the potentially traumatized system from which the individuals came. Such unawareness could prove to be extremely unfavorable to the outcome of trauma therapy.

REFERENCES

Blanchard, E. B., Kolb, L. C., Pallmeyer, T. P., and Gerardi, R. J. (1982). The development of psychophysiological assessment procedure for post-traumatic stress disorder in Vietnam veterans. *Psychiatric Quarterly, 54*, 220-229.

Crisis Management International, Inc. (1998). *The crisis professional,* Vol. 1, No. 2. Atlanta: Crisis Management International, Inc.

Dietrich, A., Navarro, M. D., Gentry, J. E., Harris, C. J., Maxfield, L., and Figley, C. (2000). *A review of contemporary approaches in the treatment of post-traumatic disorders.* The Subcommittee on Contemporary Approaches to Treating Trauma of the International Society for Traumatic Stress Studies (ISTSS) Standards of Care Committee (acting for the Board of Directors of ISTSS).

Figley, C. R. (1983). Catastrophes: An overview of family reactions. In C. R. Figley and H. I. McCubbin (Eds.), *Stress and the family:* Volume II, *Coping with catastrophe.* New York: Brunner/Mazel.

Figley, C. R. (1989). *Helping traumatized families.* New York: Jossey Bass.

Figley, C. R. (1995). *Compassion fatigue: Coping with secondary traumatic stress disorder in those who treat the traumatized.* New York: Brunner/Mazel.

French, G. D. and Harris, C. J. (1998). *Traumatic incident reduction (TIR).* Boca Raton, FL: CRC Press.

Gerbode, F. A. (1995). *Beyond psychology: An introduction to metapsychology.* Menlo Park, CA: IRM Press.

Greenberg, L. S., Heatherington, L., and Friedlander, M. L. (1996). The events-based approach to couple and family therapy research. In D. H. Sprenkle and S. M. Moon (Eds.), *Research methods in family therapy* (pp. 429-443). New York: The Guilford Press.

Gurman, A. S. and Kniskern, D. P. (1981). *Handbook of family therapy.* New York: Brunner/Mazel.

Gurman, A. S. and Kniskern, D. P. (1991). *Handbook of family therapy,* Volume II. New York: Brunner/Mazel.

Harris, C. J. (1995a). Sensory-based therapy for crisis counselors. In C. R. Figley (Ed.), *Compassion fatigue: Coping with secondary traumatic stress disorder in those who treat the traumatized* (pp. 101-114). New York: Brunner/Mazel.

Harris, C. J. (1995b). "A statement of supervision philosophy." Unpublished manuscript submitted to the American Association for Marriage and Family Therapists in partial fulfillment of the requirements for certification as an AAMFT Approved Supervisor. Greenville, SC.

Janoff-Bulman, R. (1992). *Shattered assumptions.* New York: The Free Press.

Kishur, G. R. (1984). "Chiasmal effects of traumatic stressors: The emotional costs of support." Master's thesis. Purdue University, West Lafayette, IN.

Litz, B. T. and Weathers, F. W. (1994). The diagnosis and assessment of post-traumatic stress disorder in adults. In M. B. Williams and J. F. Sommer (Eds.), *Handbook of post-traumatic therapy* (pp. 19-37). Westport, CT: Greenwood Press.

Nichols, W. C. and Everett, C. A. (1986). *Systemic family therapy. An integrative approach.* New York: The Guilford Press.

Olson, D. H., Russell, C. S., and Sprenkle, D. H. (1983). Circumplex model VI: Theoretical update. *Family Process, 22,* 69-83.

Stamm, B. H. (Ed.) (1996). *Measurement of trauma, stress and adaptation.* Lutherville, MD: Sidran Press.

Turnbull, G. J. and McFarlane A. C. (1996). Acute treatments. In B. van der Kolk, A. McFarlane, and L. Weisaeth (Eds.), *Traumatic stress* (pp. 480-490). New York: The Guilford Press.

von Bertalanffy, L. (1968). *General systems theory.* New York: Braziller.

Wylie, M. S. (1996). Researching PTSD: Going for the cure. *The Family Therapy Networker,* July/August.

Chapter 13

Dealing with Trauma in the Classroom

Mitzi Mabe

Emotional dynamics in the classroom have everything to do with teaching, and in a society as violent as ours, it is inevitable that issues of trauma come to the attention of classmates and teachers. When dealing with these issues, teachers and administrators sometimes overlook surprisingly simple methods of response or instruction, despite the rich applicability of deeper, more meaningful education that accompanies them. Such oversight results from a perceived or actual lack of information, time, and confidence. Encouraging youth in the development of stable, healthy self-concepts is vital if those young people are to learn under optimal conditions and get the best return for their own investment of time. In a class that respects each student, each tends to feel freer to ask questions, to volunteer answers, and feels comfortable, or at least safe, to challenge the authority of the teacher and peers.

Faculty who find themselves doing less than they could to assist students toward being more responsible learners could indeed be victims themselves of a flawed educational system marked by fear and subsequent unhealthy coping mechanisms of the teachers themselves. Stephen Brookfield (1998), (MBA program, Human Resources Management, University of St. Thomas, Minneapolis, Minnesota) claims that too many teachers defend against their own vulnerablity inadvertently preventing themselves from being sensitive to the risks their students experience when learning. Universities must encourage faculty to acknowledge the humanness of both teacher and student and to respond to the student's need for psychological security as well as academic success. (For more discussion of higher education's obligation to become more student sensitive refer to C. Roland Christensen [1991], former professor at Harvard Business School, and Parker Palmer [1998], senior associate of American Association of Higher Education.)

SURVEYING THE SOCIAL LANDSCAPE

Based on the information that the U.S. Centers for Disease Control and Prevention (1998) has provided regarding students and violence, such as 18.3% having had a weapon in their possession while on school grounds in the preceding month, and 36.6% having had participated in a physical fight, one can easily surmise that many students recall the social disease of high school caused by unhappy peers, which has resulted in violent acts and other disruptive, dysfunctional behaviors.

Long before the devastating eruptions of guns fired upon students on school grounds in Colombine, Colorado, violence obviously had tentacled, stretched, and raced across the nation, manifesting itself in the lives of upset and dangerously armed individuals of all ages. These highly publicized horrendous student assaults reflect an interpersonal violence all too common in the U.S. culture. Given its ubiquitous reach into all strata of society, it is inescapable that such violence would occur to some degree in schools. Many students have lived with unrest and anxiety generated by the threat of "teenage terrorists" in the classroom. Gun-toting youngsters reach for a weapon largely out of a need, perceived or actual, to protect themselves from a highly aggressive society—to find power when none is experienced otherwise.

Although institutions everywhere must confront the disengagement and violence that affects each age group in the United States, colleges and universities are in a particularly strategic position. Students arrive on a campus from around a state, country, or even the world; they pool disparate experiences, and establish commonalities. If they are acknowledged, become "visible and heard," en masse, they have a powerful and much-needed healing influence on one another—and society. Also, the academic freedom found in college permits an ideal laboratory. College is a haven when compared to the typical high school.

The United States Centers for Disease Control and Prevention (1998) stated that, in 1997, almost one in twenty high school students (4 percent) had avoided school occasionally for fear of injury or death. Almost one in five (18.3 percent) had taken some type of weapon to school and about one in twenty (5.9 percent) had carried a gun onto school grounds. In fact, this national survey revealed that 7.4 percent had been threatened or hurt with a weapon on school property, 36.6 percent had been in a physical fight within the year prior to the report, and 3.5 percent of all students had received treatment from a doctor or nurse as a result of a fight.

The Children's Defense Fund (1997), in examining the world of students under age fifteen, revealed other disturbing realities of violence that American children encounter. According to the 1997 CDF yearbook, *The State of America's Children* (Children's Defense Fund, 1997), based on a comparative study conducted by the Centers for Disease Control and Prevention (1997), the American death rate for suicide and homicide for children under fifteen was over ten times higher than the rates of twenty-five other industrialized nations. Of all gun fatalities of children under age fifteen, the U.S. total comprised three out of every four homicides committed within the twenty-six countries. To add to this disturbing statistic, the Children's Defense Fund in 1997 emphasized that the United States ranks first in military technology, defense expenditures, and health technology, and highest in *not* "protecting . . . children against gun violence" (1997, p. xv). Furthermore, victims eighteen or younger constitute approximately 10 percent of all homicides in the United States (United States Department of Commerce, 1997).

Parents and teachers exert far too little positive influence in their communities to counteract such pronounced trends. The 1996 National Commission on Teaching and America's Future claimed that "by standards of . . . teacher education in other countries, U.S. teacher education has been historically thin, uneven, and poorly financed" (1996, cited in CDF, p. 77). As the CDF emphasizes, standards for veterinarians as to how to handle animals medically far surpass the attention paid to qualifications of teachers who handle children educationally. To exacerbate this problem, "1 in 4 U.S. teachers enter the field ill-prepared to meet the enormous responsibilities of teachers" (CDF, 1997, p. 77).

Such lack of preparation hardly helps teachers respond to the alarming trends demonstrated in students' emotional difficulties. In examining a national representative sample of over 16,000 high school students, the CDC (1998) indicated that in 1997 about one in five (20.5 percent) reported having seriously contemplated suicide within the previous year. The rate for females was 27.1 percent, males 15.1 percent, indicating more female self- and other disconnection. Moreover, approximately one in twelve (7.7 percent) high school students had actually attempted suicide within the preceding twelve months. That children would perceive their worth with so little regard broadcasts the extent of hurt experienced in such a system. Violence reported in the streets and in homes, if left unattended and unaddressed for too long, at some point overflows and naturally spills over into the schools.

Youth indeed suffer from epidemic acts of violence in the United States. When American youth (ages fifteen to twenty-four) were studied in contrast to youth of other countries, the United States ranked first in homicides. Among relatively stable, industrialized nations, only Colombia, Venezuela, Russia, and Estonia revealed higher percentages. In the United States, those aged fifteen to twenty-four are over twenty times as likely to be murdered as Europeans.

It should be stressed that while *all* schools need to receive community support to decrease the overwhelming degree of stress in children's lives, colleges could provide the genesis, as well as prepare the next generation of teachers for more student-sensitive work. The United States needs a strengthening of teacher-student rapport (as well as student-student and teacher-teacher rapport) at all levels of learners. Aggression, like depression, typifies a weakness in coping skills and/or articulation of emotion. Education needs to bring the human being—both the intellectual and emotional being—back into focus in the classroom. Too much harm is being done to too many young people by ignoring their needs for education in nontraditional subjects such as listening, conflict management, active development of civic skills, and democratic strength.

THE WAY OF LISTENING

Despite incredible technological advances or, perhaps, precisely because of them, many people, under pressure from persistent stress, have lost touch with much basic human awareness, including the "formula" for listening. Listening, the most available resource to improve relationship dynamics, is the most used and least taught communication skill in the formal education system, probably because most adults naively assume that they are good listeners (Adler et al., 1998).

The reality of youth's struggles with violence and destructive beliefs belies that assumption. The thoughts of adolescents and young adults frequently reveal unresolved issues and/or highly disturbing, traumatic realities. Sometimes these young people have watched friends or loved ones battle and sometimes succumb to disease, car accidents, sexual and other violent assaults, eating disorders, alcohol and other drug addictions. In the university setting, for example, away from their families and other moorings, often for the first time, these students often turn attention to issues of pain, loss, and grief not yet worked through.

Typically, as they head into adulthood, young people simply become more aware of that pain through encountering the self as more and more independent. One first-year college student described her thoughts in response to the self-destructive behaviors of three of her peers in high school (self-cutting, self-burning, and intentional overdose) by asking, "Why do my friends want to die?" She recognized the need to understand, and the relationship between impoverished thinking/painful experience and poor decision making.

STUDENT-DEFINED EDUCATION:
EMBRACING MATURE REALITIES

Naturally, young people wonder about life and reflect upon experiences. As Elisabeth Kübler-Ross declared (1989), when a person reaches adulthood, matters of spirituality and of meaning in life become central. For nearly a decade, at the University of Maryland, Baltimore County campus, many first-year students have responded to a writing assignment which asks them to describe their most educational experience, in or out of school. In response, the majority broach a deep emotional dimension within themselves, perhaps what Kübler-Ross would call spirituality. The choice of topic for the writing comes from the students' perception of what constitutes their definition of "educational."

For some, it suggests a kind of exciting opportunity given to them, such as having had a teacher or class provide incentive to decide on a career in chemistry or engineering, a summer camp position that convinced the student to work with children as a career, a coach that helped a young person believe in him or herself, or a travel experience in another country that broadened the student's life view. However, most of these young adults and adolescents relate events that were initially often extremely difficult to tolerate, but eventually yielded a more mature perspective of life, e.g., death or debilitating disease, date rape, violent relationship, or troubled home life.

Their selections acknowledge, in writing, the stirring of soul and psyche, often wrought by painful, traumatic events—including the loss of friends and diminishment of community via violent means. Many young people not only know of such brutal and senseless loss of life, but also have witnessed it, as one young man illustrates in his depiction of an all-too-common domestic war zone:

> If you grow up on the streets of New York as I did, death becomes an immediate and constant part of your life. The chalk outlines of fallen bodies are all around. The hellish nature of New York knows no shame and it never attempts to hide itself. So death was always there in my face; my young eyes and young mind had to take it as a fact of life, the way things were. As I got older and the availability of drugs and guns increased, the death became more frequent and a lot more violent. Some took place right before my eyes. As I grew up in the midst of this I never flinched once. I took it all in stride body by body and name by name. I took it like a trooper, cause I had to. (Isaac, as cited in Mabe, 1998, p. 42)

Isaac was eighteen when he developed the essay from which this excerpt is taken. Isaac's work later describes the eventual death of a youngster in his neighborhood, a death that finally "gets" to the toughened Isaac and makes him cry, a death that finally rips down his "trooper" stance—against his wishes, of course. Throughout the writing, Isaac uses the analogy of a weight lifter, taking on more and more weight—successfully—until after the psyche can take no more, a feather floats down on top of the barbell to make him, the powerful man, buckle and fall to his knees, defeated.

GIVING AUDIENCE TO PAIN: THE CIVIL BALM OF THE CLASSROOM

Writing gave this young man an opportunity to attempt to derive meaning from his experience, to reshape and redefine his world. The interaction that followed in the writing class, when he shared his work in a public forum, allowed more recognition and healing to take place. "Treatment" of the piece in class followed a simple, human approach: the class honored Isaac's voice. He read the essay aloud and, in so doing, revealed himself to a new, temporary community composed of classmates from around the world. Their response of silence was key. They showed reverence for the painful, poignant experience their classmate had endured and had managed to capture in words and in wisdom. They gave him acceptance and understanding of emotion—not of the particular experience per se, but of the feeling of being overwhelmed by change; of having too much happen too fast; of being finally forced to stop and take the emotional hit of pain, and deal with it. He read to them about a violence-filled world that would terrify most people, and of his vulnerability, his realness, and his human self.

Such connection among students helps form bonds within the writing class, and within the human community. Students find a safe place within which to offer their rendition of life experience and, wonderfully, find that they, inside, are very much like one another. Thus, they find the common ground of humanity. (In an argument-writing class, they might again find those things that make them seem different from one another, but, even then, they find that the winning argument is the one that acknowledges or honors part of the other's position and takes into account beliefs shared by both sides.)

Isaac wrote his essay for an assignment that asked him to discuss an experience with death in an advanced personal essay class called the writing workshop. Most students thrive on this opportunity to make their experiences known and thus become visible to the community, as long as the climate is a safe one in which the students trust that the teacher honors them and their experiences. Very quickly, students detect the same deep respect emanating from their peers. Much of that respect depends on modeling by the teacher, a commitment to the task of honoring connection in the community, and of affirming the role and status of emerging colleagues. It is surprising to see how much warmth and compassion arise in a group when the individuals see that it is "okay to be human while learning." Whether discussing topics before they begin writing, or sharing their finished products with some or all of the class later, students may become emotional. This engagement, the capacity to be touched by the richness of human experience, is an essential understanding if the students are to be very successful in their writing—and living. This success necessitates an uncompromised dealing with grief, fear, and other emotions ushered in by our current society. For example, some students have grieved the loss of friends through sudden death; the loss of parents through disease, divorce, alcohol, drugs, or jail; the loss of security through being robbed at gunpoint; and even the loss of connection in their lives shown through their own suicidal attempts. On the outside, these students may appear bright, untroubled, and well-adjusted. Inside, they may be grappling with something that tears at their peace. Writing helps make constructive use of the energy that is otherwise bound within self, coursing counterproductively.

Most teachers—truly, most people—would benefit from training and practice in profound listening, employing all elements as shown in the Chinese character which depicts listening: ears, eyes, and heart (Adler et al., 1998). The works of writers Rachel Remen (1996) and Carl Rogers (1980) might be explored by faculty and administrators wishing to promote development of communication skills. Indeed, it would be to the complete advantage of our country's long-term educational interests to turn a fuller audience to the troubles and traumas that our young people encounter, and too often face alone.

THE READ OUT:
ADDRESSING COMMUNITY IN THE ACADEMY

The Read Out, a successful teaching tool and community-building strategy, offers a way for students to examine and share their experiences with others in such a way that their "traumas" become secondary to their learning. Yet, by carefully *respecting* the trauma that has been instructive, the student develops a greater sense of calm or mastery over what once devastated them. In a Read Out, which reaches beyond the conventional classroom, two or more writing instructors converge their classes for a class period to present the strongest writings (preselected by the teachers) from their young essayists.

The Read Out not only showcases exemplary student writing, but also reveals aspects of students that they might not otherwise discover about themselves and one another—important, enlightening aspects. Many teachers have traditionally asked a student or two to read memorable work aloud to classmates. In the Read Out, the student moves beyond the "neighborhood" of the classroom into the larger world, when two or more classes assemble together as a merged group for the sole purpose of hearing the finest essays constructed by the students. Students develop a better appreciation for what teachers consider outstanding, or at least good academic work, and, more important, learn what constitutes effective writing and pick up, even through osmosis, ideas for strengthening their own crafting. However, the most profound feature of the Read Out is that it helps students perceive the world through the eyes and minds of others. They become more astute observers of the human experience. They learn about each other and respect grows. They learn about themselves and awareness builds. They become more motivated to share and they learn that it pays to take the time to craft their messages carefully, that they too might share winning insights with their peers. Planks of authentic collegial respect provide the foundation for their formative college years.

Ideally, planning a Read Out should begin early enough to influence class scheduling, so that collaborating teachers can find a large room, such as a lecture hall, in which to have their classes meet together occasionally throughout the semester. To design a rewarding team Read Out, collaborators need to establish a *safe audience* and *stage* for young writers to share with a large group, including strangers. To do so, two factors are important:

1. Selected essays (based upon thought-provoking assignments) should demonstrate strong, effective writing and hence serve as teaching models and help fellow students become more language-appreciative. A wide array of assignments could elicit thoughtful responses, such as topics that explore multicultural or multigenerational issues, environmental, political, or other social issues, admired individuals, and one's own desire for contributing to society.
2. Faculty should approach the presentation with respect and positive, warm regard—including providing a mechanism for prompt and meaningful feedback.

For teachers wanting to use this technique, the following tips can promote a successful exchange.

Tips for Hosting a Collegiate Read Out: How to Prepare

1. *Set an atmosphere of "honored seriousness."* You will be showcasing student skill in written presentation *and* student thought and feeling. Vul-

nerability *allows* the Read Out to be successful *but* that vulnerability *must* be honored. Teachers should prepare ahead of time either by knowing the specific essays to be read, so that they might anticipate any needed discussion, or by trusting the judgment and participation of fellow faculty to *keep the atmosphere a safe one for students* who might be risking more than they ever have to make a serious and public connection to peers and faculty. Preferably, the teacher should prepare and enlist the services of a team teacher in the event of a painful outburst. The Read Out, of course, promotes team interaction and provides intervention should a student need assistance while others engage with fellow classmates.

2. *Be assured of quality.* Carefully select the essays to be shared. Selections can be made by individual teachers and/or by class vote (following an in-class reading) before the Read Out date.

3. *Be sure that selected students want to share their work in a public forum.* Explain to those chosen students why others might want to hear their work. Help student readers see the importance of enlightening others in the community, of sharing experience and thought. (Faculty might coach students independently or as a group, as needed. Students could even coach one another to help with any stage fright.) *But* be sure to listen to any student who feels uncomfortable reading to his or her peers; never "push" anyone to the podium, no matter how "great" the essay. Self-disclosure is *always* the student's choice.

4. *Demonstrate an earnest interest in hearing students' work displayed in this fashion.* Tell the whole group why they're gathered—what the Read Out accomplishes.

5. *Model an involved, receptive audience member, grateful to hear of others' views.* (Practice being a good student.) Let yourself be absorbed in the happening.

6. *Guide discussion when needed.* Simply honor—through applause—the essays when honoring seems warranted. Provide feedback to each reader. A method that seems to work very well is to distribute two notecards to each student and ask that he or she respond to the two authors whose essays most affect him or her. The cards can be gathered and distributed to the students before they leave the Read Out.

7. *Trust students to steer themselves and to benefit in the sharing, in the shaping and growing of community that naturally results.*

8. *Trust yourself.*

9. *Seek and accept recommendations for improvement.*

10. *Most of all, enjoy the special opportunity to hear fellow humans speak with candor and insight about meaningful experience.* Appreciate the invitation to learn more deeply about students' realities.

After each exemplary essay is read to the audience, all should applaud. Although it might be constructive to have discussion following each essay, honoring the students primarily through applause creates a powerful community mood. Selected students appear awed. They seem to feel important and, of course, they are. This honoring is, above all, our message to students and our goal.

At the end of the Read Out, as stated, students pick the two essays that most touched them and respond to the authors on a note card. Each author receives the note cards as immediate feedback. This method also helps teachers see which essays appear most popular. In one case, Schonbachler (cited in Mabe, 1998), who read of her emotional growth following an abusive relationship (a situation a surprising number of students related to personally in their responses), received over forty responses from her peers out of a possible two hundred, or one-fifth of the total. (The remaining were divided among about ten other readers.)

Schonbachler read (Mabe, 1998) with great eagerness about how she emerged finally from an emotionally and physically abusive, three-year, high school relationship. This excerpt from her essay, titled "A Tough Education," began her response to an assignment that directed her to write of the most educational experience of her life:

> As I approach the parking lot, I see my ex-boyfriend waiting for me. . . . I know there is no real way to avoid him but I try to walk past as if he is not there. He reaches out, grabs my arm and says, "You're coming with me! We have to talk!" With my other arm I manage to grab hold of a nearby fence and pull myself away from his grasp. He wraps his arms around my waist and attempts to yank me free. The parking lot is full of other students in my [driver's education] class, so I start screaming for help. Some look at me and move on; others don't even stop to look. . . . By this time my ex-boyfriend is pulling so hard that the fence starts to cut into my palms. I realize that no wants to help me and that I can't hang on forever, so I give up and let him take me. He picks me up and throws me into the passenger seat of his Blazer. On the way in, I hit my head on the roof and am knocked unconscious. When I come to, I notice that we are already quite a distance away. I ask him why he always does this to me, and he answers, "I told you, you belong to me!" . . . For about six months after we broke up he stalked me, with an occasional kidnapping here and there. . . . Our relationship taught me about the people in the world around me and about myself." (Schonbachler, as cited in Mabe, 1998, pp. 48-49)

One response that Schonbachler received said, "I always thought that women who stay in abusive relationships were idiots, but after hearing your essay, I understand the struggle between love and hate that goes on within." In the Read Out, students become community teachers, what Alice Miller might call "enlightened witnesses" (Miller, 1990, p. 7).

Students need to talk about traumatic experiences to acknowledge the impact of happenings that have the capacity to unravel a soul. In the Read Out responses, it is not unusual to hear individuals compliment peers on how "real" their essays were. Students want to deal with the tough parts of their realities, in an atmosphere where it's okay to share their sense of self. It is the duty of their teachers to catch up to them and assist in the process.

Through the Read Out, educators shape and lead the "truth-telling process." In contrast, Dr. Sandra Bloom (1997) recognizes that patients may find a lack of full receptivity from largely "unknowing" and well-intentioned therapists and doctors an obstacle to the productive processing of healthier reintegration of trauma. Her inpatient clinic, "The Sanctuary," inspired by the profound safety needs that she recognized in patients, attempts to put into place a more effective climate for truth sharing (Bloom, 1997).

ULTIMATE DISENGAGEMENT, SUICIDAL IDEATION, AND THE HEALTH OF GRIEF

A tenth of the American population regularly battles depression, as well as sadness, fear, and anger that comprise the store of national *grief.* When asked to write a response to social issues or life goals, students often reflect upon the idea of their own deaths, and the topic of the ultimate grief testimony—suicide—even mentioning or describing their own attempts. In an essay titled "Contribution to Life," Doan shared her learning:

> Life is the most complicated word to define. Two years ago, I would have described it as cruel and unfair. It wouldn't have mattered if someone had stabbed me in the heart and left me to die. Sleeping became a way to escape from my problems. But problems don't usually resolve themselves. The longer I ignored them, the worse they became. (Doan, as cited in Mabe, 1998, p. 110)

After graphically describing her suicide attempt and the kind words of a teacher who responded to her articulation of pain in a journal, the student closed her essay with these words:

> I am still fighting each day to keep my head up and not to hide under a pillow. I do believe in myself. It's just that there are times when things will happen and my beliefs are cut short. Those are times that I really need someone who cares. I hope someday I can hold a little child's hand and let her know there are people who do care. And it will bring me joy to see that I can make a difference in someone else's life . . . I want to show the children and teenagers that they have the strength

and ability to choose how they want to live their lives. Life is a challenge that can be [met], even though it may seem impossible at times. No one should have to suffer what I have experienced, because life is not only about helping ourselves; it's about helping each other. (Doan, as cited in Mabe, 1998, p. 111)

Most suicides of college students occur within the first six weeks of their first semester, often in panicked reaction to a loss or change in a romantic relationship. Students also experience overwhelming change as they come to terms with the loss of known routines and subsequent difficulties of transitioning, as they work to establish new and satisfying connections in the goal to fit in, to belong. But not only the young student fresh out of high school is vulnerable. The following note, slipped under my office door about ten years ago by an older matriculating student, revealed a terrible awkwardness with transition:

I'm real lousy with words and I'm not to sure how to say this because it's my personal life. Saturday night I was taken to the hospital around 3:00 a.m. because I try [sic] to commit suicide. You see I don't want to live anymore and I am trying to cope with life. I need this class so I can hopefully gradate [sic] next May. I don't expect you to feel sorry for me I am just asking you to understand. I need to try to get through these next few classes hopefully with your support. I've been trying to tell you from the start of class but it just wouldn't come out and the only reason I wanted to know is in case something like this happen [sic] and if I run into some problem with this class. I want you to know I'm really trying but I just feel I have to be honest with you. This is all I wanted you to know. If you find any of this hard to believe you can call my psychiatrist. She is trying to help me pull myself together. (S., 1987)

Without a pause, "S." danced between suicidal contemplation and graduation in May. Moments of fantasy and moments of reality juxtaposed—one emotional, one physical—mingle, disconnect, engage.

To intervene more effectively through education, educators must do a better job of analyzing what it is young people need and then deliver it. Consumed by busy schedules and/or not accustomed to responding to students' most important needs, teachers and administrators risk becoming deaf to students' realities.

HOW TO DEVELOP A CLASS IN WRITING
THAT ACKNOWLEDGES THE IMPACT OF TRAUMA

During a Read Out in which a student might read an essay about a date rape, for example, faculty might want to review recommendations offered by McCammon (1995), who suggests posting faculty members by the doorway to intercept anyone who might leave the room in uncontrollable emotion. In nearly twenty years of teaching, only twice has a student abruptly left my class following the reading of an essay to a group of people. In these instances, a young athlete read of her mother's breast cancer and subsequent death, and an older, returning student read of a torturous, violent rape that nearly culminated in her death. In both instances, the remaining students continued the class until the distraught reader and I returned. The student was calmed by having "survived" a difficult and important disclosure, and "restored" to community with a short "time out" (or "time in") with me. Incidentally, even though the rape survivor bolted from the room as soon as she finished reading her essay, in the calm that followed, she reiterated her belief that she had been right to read the piece, and that it was important to her that younger peers knew of the dangers that lurk in society which threaten peace and sometimes life itself.

Sensitivities that grow in such a classroom spread so naturally that they can immediately fortify a poignant understanding and compassion for human suffering. One class witnessed a grown man remourn briefly the loss of his lifemate, his wife, to cancer. The tears that ran down his face while he stoically read his message, sang of the remarkable impact of a safe community, of sharing, and of bridges among human beings. It is not uncommon to see tears when students read of deeply moving events, but, in a writing class with the focus on structure and style of the message, perhaps an extra buffer against too much soul letting naturally forms. The class—the people—are real, okay, and can become safe. On a more basic level, for some, witnessing the tears of another helps them to understand healthy and natural emotional expression.

To encourage receptive submission of their works to a mature, sensitive audience, especially for shyer students, start by selecting an essay written by a former student, which typically yields both serious and spontaneous discussion (Mabe, 1998). This writing sample and conversation will help students frame their experiences and deliver a strong, thought-provoking essay. Sometimes, the class may discuss how a person's essay reminds individuals of similar experiences. Students may become involved at both cognitive and affective levels and ask meaningful questions of one another. Dialogue starts in this safe arena and continues because students want to communicate their realities and beliefs. The community that develops in this tightly formed writing class is a gift that offers reminders of the resilience and preciousness of the human being in everyone.

It is not automatically easy to get students to open up—but it is not necessarily difficult, either. It is an intuitive matter, really, that usually develops on its own. Everyone seeks acceptance and understanding. Perhaps a university writing class affords the opportunity to give testimony to human experience in such a way as to build resources in the communal bank of empathy. Saldinger (1998), in fact, remarks upon the manifold functions of such "bearing witness," based on her studies of Holocaust survivors.

Writing Class As Communication Enhancement for Students and Society

In the typically required writing class, first year composition, a tremendous potential exists to help students convey important thoughts and feelings. Through this course, they find that their ideas, their emotions, their experiences, and their realities matter. *They* matter. The university writing class can also provide an arena for young adults to discuss the inevitable emotions which arise following the tragic loss of other young people. Consider the following: fraternity drinking deaths (such as two first-year students at the Massachusetts Institute of Technology and Louisiana State University) ("When Students Die from Alcohol," 1998); drinking and driving deaths (such as five college students in Virginia, which prompted a strong state legislative response) (Levy, personal correspondence, 1998); or the loss of the University of Wyoming's Matthew Shepard in 1998 through violence fueled by hatred of sexual orientation differences.

Progress, Not Perfection: Steering Toward Health in Rocky Waters

Before instituting a writing curriculum that widely deals with trauma, teachers must receive training in the dynamics of intrapersonal and interpersonal conflict, trauma, and grief, so that they can be reliable helpers for their students. Although educators develop such courses, teachers can contribute with common sense and appreciative awareness of basic human nature: they need not be experts in psychology to help initiate and nurture the dialogue that young people are starving for. When writing teachers comfortably allow students to share their experiences, students can begin recounting stories of struggle. This recounting, in turn, helps others establish a sense of camaraderie that has proven helpful.

THE READ OUT AS A STRATEGY
TO CORRECT ABUSIVE RELATIONSHIPS

Students bring with them a great deal of invisible baggage. For example, when offered the opportunity, a surprising number write about domestic violence and date rape, as well as other highly sexualized and violent images. In one semester alone (fall 1998) at the university, three of twenty-five female students volunteered to me (first privately, then publicly) that, as young as fourteen, they had become involved with physically aggressive and emotionally and psychologically abusive boyfriends—(while under the alleged "protection" of their parents' roof). They wrote because these were realities they knew and because they were struggling to strengthen themselves and others.

University and college instructors have an extraordinary opportunity to model healthy interaction. They can show students how to be respectful not only of their minds—their own and each other's—but of their emotions as well. Teacher(s) and students together must create a necessary safe environment to enjoy the bounty of education. The writing classroom invites healthy student interaction and relationships and honest sharing and needed connection, including the relief of recognizing mutual emotional territories. To be successful, the writing classroom must have a sensitive, able leader and students willing to learn and to trust.

Interpersonal communication is another excellent course that can offer students the skills to gain valuable insight about being human and to build their communication skills. Good communication demands time. Without a commitment to spend time, as Schutz (1967) reminds us, we communicate poorly, if at all. *Understanding* is *not* automatically instantaneous and necessitates explanations, conversations, and questions. In an interpersonal communication course, students also cultivate a better understanding of intercultural and other perceptual differences, self-concepts, emotions, dynamics of relationships, and conflict management.

Two programs that actively inspire healthy thinking habits for students are the First-Year Experience, developed by John Gardner, Betsy Barefoot, Stuart Hunter and associates at the University of South Carolina, and On Course, designed by Skip Downing, formerly of the Community College of Baltimore.

A variation of this course, developed at the University of Maryland, Baltimore County, pairs administrators or faculty from other departments with writing teachers to help disperse damaging myths about language in the process. (Many students initially perceive "English class" as a necessary evil, a sort of obstacle on their path to a college degree.) Students emerge as more effective communicators, more connected, successful people. Writing teachers pair with faculty from other disciplines or administrators to present a model for teamwork, which is so crucial in communication, to demonstrate to the students the connections between academic course work and personal choices. The team teachers meet well in advance of the semester to begin planning and coordinating the schedules for their courses and sometimes visit one another's classes and share assignments. They develop a structure to discuss with greater clarity the concerns about specific students who might be experiencing distress during the first semester away from home or as learners in a new type of environment.

RECOGNIZING AND DISMANTLING OBSTACLES: SUPPORTING TEACHERS' WORK

Students perform at their best when they are open-minded and want to learn. It is easiest to do this when their leaders, the teachers and administrators, are themselves open-minded and committed to education. Professors must convince students of the benefits in wrestling with ideas—their own and others'—and experimenting with techniques to present thoughts successfully. Instructors must energize and motivate students. Once the students recognize that it is not only okay, but *desirable,* to think, the instructor can move forward. The teacher should encourage young-adult learners to observe with intent and interest the well-placed phrase, the cogent explanation, the insightful thesis, the indisputable, logical underpinning of a sound argument, the moving prose of a strongly crafted essay, the articulated emotion, and the experience that finds clarity in expression and more reward in response. It is the students' writing which reveals the depth—or lack of it— of their messages, analytical and critical thinking powers, and presentation skills. By reassessing the approach to teaching language, it will become easier to locate students in trouble and, in the process, will help them to develop a stronger sense of community, as they increase their skills in articulating expression of thought and feeling.

Building Student Esteem

Writing teachers typically set up comfortable discussion mechanisms in their classes by encouraging students to share their experiences and thoughts with others in the classroom. Sometimes, this interaction is reinforced by small group tasks, such as critiquing other students' essays. Because the ego is so often involved in writing, instructors know that students need both gentle encouragement and challenging standards. Getting students to relax enough to divine and communicate their ideas occurs only in an atmosphere of safety. One technique is to give constant attentiveness to the students' world, just as is promoted in the more public Read Out. This attention helps gauge where to set the classroom thermostat to promote a climate conducive to inviting free and thoughtful student expression.

Educational Intervention

Through fuller faculty development, schools could extend the influence of classes in which students learn to express thought, usually by writing essays. Promoting the work of these teachers is a challenge administrators must accept. Currently, most writing classes in colleges and universities are staffed by part-time instructors and other individuals regarded as lower-ranking within the existing university power structure (a structure which does not seem to place enormous emphasis on the importance of communication skill—written or otherwise). The current lack of resources for writing instruction at many universities hampers the acquisition of more effective communication skills for students. As classes are crowded, and poorly-paid teachers are burdened with work, the system reaps an unhappy crop: students whose voices cannot be heard because there are too many voices to be heard by one instructor, teachers who suffer burnout from dealing with an impossible situation of wanting to teach effectively with nearly intolerable work conditions, and of course, society, which must assimilate more individuals who have not had the opportunity to articulate what they would benefit from processing. (Incidentally, most high school and junior high school English classes are even more crowded than college classrooms. Traditionally, education has often been disregarded in terms of what teachers most need in order to do their jobs in a manner most helpful for young people). A healthy, responsive education system would help young citizens/future leaders process the realities of their lives. Administrators at all levels of education need to be more supportive of faculty in developing honest and healthy dialogue with and among all students.

CONCLUSION

Trauma exists in our nation's streets, neighborhoods, and homes. Traumatic events have invaded the lives of a significant number of Americans, young and old alike. Schools can help young citizens process human suffering and, particularly, of the type wrought by trauma—senseless violence that has become all too much a hallmark of the American way. When students have had too few models of healthy relationships in functional systems, teachers and administrators must champion the support of full intellectual growth of students by granting a gift of immeasurable service. Schools must help students recognize, honor, and harness the emotions that move and permit engagement of human beings with one another in significant ways. Universities can help steer society in a more positive direction; they take astonishly marvelous care of the minds—and hearts—of adolescents and young adults. Higher education should be compelled to consider the necessity of promoting healthy communication systems as the foundation of a viable democracy which reflects constructive recognition and articulation of natural emotion and logical thought.

REFERENCES

Adler, R.B., Rosenfeld, L.B., Towne, N., and Proctor II, R.F. (1998). *Interplay: The Process of Interpersonal Communication.* New York: Harcourt Brace College Publishers.

Bloom, S. (1997). *Creating Sanctuary: Toward an Evolution of Sane Societies.* New York: Routledge.

Brookfield, Stephen (1998). Plenary Session: "On the Certainty of Public Shaming: Working with Students 'Who Just Don't Get It'." Seventeenth Annual Freshman Year Experience Conference, Columbia, South Carolina, February 23.

Children's Defense Fund (1997). *The State of America's Children: Yearbook 1997.* Boston: Beacon Press.

Christensen, C.R. (1991). Every student teaches and every teacher learns: The reciprocal gift of discussion teaching. In J. Stewart (Ed.), *Bridges not walls,* eighth edition (pp. 621-639). New York: McGraw-Hill.

Kübler-Ross, E. (1989). "Life, Death, and Transition," Workshop, Authors Retreat Center, Front Royal, Virginia, May.

Mabe, M. (Ed.) (1998). *A Community of Writers.* Denton, TX: RonJon Publishers.

McCammon, S. (1995). "Painful Pedagogy: Trauma Survivors in Academic or Training Classes." American Psychological Association, 103rd Annual Conference, New York, August.

Miller, A. (1990). *Banished Knowledge: Facing Childhood Injuries.* New York: Doubleday.

National Center for the First-Year Experience and Students in Transition. Available online: <http://www.sc.edu.fye>.

Palmer, P. (1998). *The Courage to Teach: Exploring the Inner Landscapes of a Teacher's Life.* San Francisco: Jossey-Bass.

Remen, R. (1996). *Kitchen Table Wisdom: Stories That Heal.* New York: Riverhead Books.

Rogers, C. (1980). *A Way of Being.* Boston: Houghton-Mifflin.

Saldinger, A.G. (1998). "The Effect of Bearing Witness on the Witness: A Holocaust Study." Panelist on "The Rigors of Bearing Witness." *Ending Cycles of Violence: Integrating Research, Practice and Social Policy.* XIV Annual Meeting. The International Society for Traumatic Stress Studies, Washington, DC.

Schutz, W. (1967). *Joy: Expanding Human Awareness.* New York: Ballantine Books.

United States Centers for Disease Control and Prevention (1998, Aug. 14). "Youth Risk Behavior Surveillance—United States, 1997." Available online: <http://www.cdc.gov>.

United States Department of Commerce, Bureau of the Census (1997). *Statistical Abstracts of the United States,* 117th Edition. Washington, DC.

"When Students Die from Alcohol, Who Is to Blame?" (1998). *The Chronicle of Higher Education,* November 6, XLV(II), A57.

SECTION V:
SPECIAL POPULATIONS

Chapter 14

Police Hostage Situations

Lasse Nurmi

THE ROLE OF THE POLICE PSYCHOLOGIST IN HOSTAGE NEGOTIATIONS

In hostage negotiations, a psychologist employed by a police force or police academy/police college can play a variety of roles. One role is to act as consultant to hostage negotiators as was the author. In this role, the psychologist may attempt to recognize or interpret the feelings of the perpetrator and then suggest a concrete response or strategy for the negotiator. The psychologist may function as a profiler, advisor, or source of information (Baruth, 1988). McMains (1988) noted that the police psychologist functions in negotiations as a consultant on the emotional status of the hostage taker and also helps determine what strategies should be used.

Mohandie, Piersol, and Klyver (1995) noted that, during a critical incident involving hostage negotiations, the role of the psychologist includes the following duties:

1. To assess and evaluate the situation from a psychological perspective
2. To generate a profile of suspect and hostages if possible
3. To suggest strategies to the negotiators
4. To monitor and assess the processes of negotiation
5. To provide input to the negotiators, the management of the negotiations, and the command staff
6. To interface with mental health personnel who are involved in the negotiations
7. To debrief hostages after the incident
8. To debrief family members of the hostage taker and the hostages
9. To monitor the mental status of the hostages and the hostage taker
10. To monitor/assess and support the negotiators

After a hostage situation is resolved, it is the role of the police psychologist to debrief the hostage negotiators, the hostages, and to write an analysis of the incident.

Hostage negotiators in Finland are trained from basic training on in the techniques of negotiation. Police officers who want to be hostage negotiators receive special training and exercises in special courses. The courses range from two days to one week in length and include classroom theory, role plays, and critiques of the role plays. In addition, participants in the courses analyze cases. The case that is presented in this chapter is now a teaching case for the Police College of Finland.

CASE SETTING

The hostage taker, a man aged twenty-seven, had been serving a life prison sentence for the murder-for hire conviction in the death of a businessman. Finland does not have capital punishment and, in fact, the longest prison sentence for a capital crime is eleven to twelve years. This murderer, while in prison, met another inmate, and the two of them conceived a plan of escape. Somehow, this individual got a gun. In fact, after the shakedown of the prison occurred post escape, eight guns were discovered in the prison.

The individual took a female guard as a hostage, stole a car, and later released the guard and continued his escape with his fellow inmate. Approximately two weeks after his escape, an informant called the police and let them know that the escapee was in Lahti, Finland. Police intelligence had hints of his whereabouts prior to this time and had followed up on leads. However, wherever they went, the escaped prisoner had already left the location. During his escape, he robbed a bank and shot at a female teller. However, the bullet went through her hair without wounding her. Later, he said that he did not want to kill her.

Eventually, the two escapees did end up in Lahti, approximately 100 kilometers (60 miles) to the north of Helsinki (capital of Finland). One of the two knew the female member of a couple who took the two escapees into their apartment. Surveillance identified the second escapee (not the contract killer) to be in the apartment.

Officers from the local police department, using their own specially equipped officers (with shotguns and shields), got the key to the apartment building and went in. However, they did not know that the murderer was also there. The murderer had a magnum 44 and a 22-caliber pistol and began to shoot violently with both guns. The police asked for his surrender and, in turn, he shot one officer in the shield. The officer was lightly wounded by debris from the shield. The wounded officer was later debriefed by this author as police psychologist.

It was at this point that the SWAT team from the Helsinki Police Department was alerted and the police academy was notified of the situation. This author received a call and was asked to go to the situation. Because the police viewed the situation as a siege, they initiated tactics designed to resolve a siege situation. The "bad guys," however, viewed it as a hostage situation because the young couple, scared to death, soon were playing the role of hostages. Police, however, viewed all four individuals as criminals.

THE SITUATION

The Finnish police, in hostage negotiations, use the tactics and methods of hostage negotiation learned from a variety of police organizations including the German police, FBI, Scotland Yard, and the Swedish police. Numerous Finnish police officials have been sent to the United States to receive training by the FBI and have taken special hostage negotiations courses in various locations. This author, for example, has taken a course in Sweden and in Holland and has received training in Orange County, California.

This case was the first in Finland in which television and radio crews were on site. The situation became "big news" and the hostage taker was very talkative to the media. In addition, it was the first case in the country in which the hostage taker had an opportunity to have direct access to the media. In fact, the hostage taker gave interviews to the local radio station; the police warned the station that it would lose its license if it continued interviewing.

In this situation, the hostage taker told negotiators that he had approximately 100 pounds of C-4 military explosives with him. Law enforcement officials, in checking out his story, learned that some of these explosives had been stolen, and therefore, there was a possibility that he was telling the truth. Because of his threats, the police rented a room in the house near where he was barricaded and watched him with telescopes from outside. They also cleared out the surrounding area to protect inhabitants in case of an explosion. The situation could have become very lethal had the explosives existed and been detonated.

PURPOSES OF NEGOTIATION

Hostage negotiation has a variety of purposes. The first purpose is to solve the problem at hand and resolve the critical situation without causing harm or hurt to anyone who is involved. This is in agreement with Strentz (1995), who stated that the basis of hostage negotiation is the preservation of human life. The Finnish way of resolving hostage situations, historically, has been to use "speaking not shooting;" getting the hostage takers to capitulate and give up without bloodshed.

The second purpose of hostage negotiation is to buy time to allow members of the hostage negotiation team to develop tactical maneuvers that will allow them to capture the hostage taker, or develop attack plans and ways to set up a SWAT team. During this "buying time" process, another object is to tire out and exhaust the hostage taker so that he or she gives up. This is also in agreement with Strentz (1995), who noted that time is the most important ally of the negotiator. Time allows the opportunity to gather intelligence and improve tactical position while the perpetrator becomes fatigued.

The role of the police psychologist in Finnish negotiations is to help the hostage negotiators learn how to use time. Negotiators need to exhaust the hostage taker over an extended period of time; furthermore, talking and more talking may cause the hostage taker to get tired and frustrated. This author (together with his police psychologist colleague and two prison psychologists) had the task of trying to profile the hostage taker during the extended period of negotiation. In fact, when the hostage taker first talked about having a detonator and batteries to set it off, he gave the impression that he was going to put his plan into action. He was the type of individual who loved attention and wanted to give a demonstration of his power. However, when he seemed to lose his nerve, he started "shooting around." The advice of this negotiator was to ask him to demonstrate from the balcony what he could or could not do. When he only shot around without wounding anyone or without using explosives, it was concluded that he either did not have explosives or, if he did, not as much as he had first indicated.

Time played a very important role in these negotiations. During the extended time, negotiators got to know the hostage taker more intimately. They waited for him to get fatigued and become somewhat more rational over time. They also used time to their advantage to improve their tactical positions.

PHASES OF THE NEGOTIATION PROCESS

The process of negotiation has a variety of phases. The first phase is the Introductory Phase. Strentz (1995) calls this the Alarm Phase. In this phase, the hostage taker, hostages, and police try to consolidate initial positions while the hostage taker tries to gain some type of control over his or her situation. This stage can be very emotional, particularly prior to the initiating of contact. Eventually, the hostage negotiator, after learning about the critical incident, develops a contact with the hostage taker. The hostage taker then says "I want something." In this instance, it is the role of the negotiator to identify himself or herself and say "I am here to help you and solve the problem." The negotiator does not take an antagonistic view and negotiates from a cooperative stance. In fact, the hostage negotiator tries to develop some degree of trusting relationship between himself or herself and the hostage taker. It is at this point that the hostage negotiator tries to encourage the hostage taker to tell his or her story in great detail and become the central figure in the process.

In the Lahti situation, the hostage taker had specific demands. He ultimately wanted a car and a free escape without interference. However, he did not have the courage to come out of the building and take his chances with getting a car. As the negotiations proceeded, he wanted food. That food was given to him in a plastic bag. He also wanted fresh batteries for his portable phone which he used for communication; these were given to him every other hour because he kept the phone on all the time.

The hostage taker, in this situation, was on amphetamines. Therefore, he did not sleep and it was important to find any type of activity to keep him occupied. It was not until the morning of the third day of the situation that he slept.

This author was an advisor to the on-scene commander and to the chief negotiator, Pirrho Lahti, and was a member of a psychologist team. Another colleague, the hostage taker's therapist, was the second main negotiator. This author acted as a shuttle negotiator between the actual negotiators and the on-scene command. Information was gathered about the hostage taker and the other accomplice who had escaped from prison with him.

The second phase of negotiation is the Bargaining Phase. In this phase, the "bad guy" tries to blackmail his audience/negotiators. The police negotiator may respond in a particular way and tell the hostage taker that there are certain materials/things valuable to give. If (eventually) the hostage taker comes out alone, certain things may be done; however, alternative plans are available, should the hostage taker come out with hostages.

Strentz (1995) calls this the Accommodation Phase (his third phase of the model). It follows the crisis phase in which the hostage taker makes his or her initial demands. If communication is not established by this phase, the crisis often ends up with violence and bloodshed. The Accommodation Phase is generally the longest in the negotiation process. During this phase, the personality of the hostage taker becomes more apparent and the negotiators have more of an opportunity to profile him or her. During this phase, the author's job was to profile the hostage taker, particularly to determine if he had explosives or whether or not law enforcement officials should take his threats of having explosives seriously. The author contacted military authorities of the Finnish Armed Forces and asked if the hostage taker had had training in explosives. He had and, in fact, knew how to detonate explosives. When he said he needed a battery, however, his request led this author to believe that he did not truly have the materials to set off an explosion.

During this phase, the leadership team behind the scenes determined strategy and policy. This management team included police commanders and chiefs. One of the major considerations was what to do when and if the hostage taker left the building. If he came out holding a pistol to the head of the girl hostage, officials realized that snipers who were in place could not take a chance to try to shoot the hostage taker. In fact, they would have to let him go. Because of this situation, the leadership/management team determined that the best tactic was to "freeze out" the hostage taker rather than let him go. By freezing him out, he would get tired and then capitulate. However, because of his drug usage, he became more and more frustrated rather than tired.

During the third phase of negotiation, the hostage taker may have suicidal thoughts. The hostage taker, at some point, may find the situation to be impossible. In this situation, he may begin to think, for example, "If I am apprehended I will get ten more years in jail." The situation may become impossible to him and he may then believe that it is better to kill himself by exploding his (supposed) ammunition, "taking out" others in the process.

The final phase of the negotiation process is the Closing Phase or what Strentz (1995) calls the Resolution Phase. In this phase, the hostage taker is either almost ready to give up or wants to have a final solution to his situation. He may be tired and may want to have the situation resolved in a nonviolent way. He is told that if he decides to come out and surrender, the hostage negotiation team will "do all that it can do to protect him" from the media and, perhaps, the criminal justice system. He is reassured that he will not be "taken down" violently, and that his dignity will not be compromised. However, he is never promised something that cannot be given or fulfilled. It is in this phase, as Strentz (1995) says, that the outcome may be one of "trauma or tranquillity" (p. 144).

The Lahti situation ended tranquilly for the hostages when the three individuals were released. However, the hostage taker did not surrender. After hours of negotiating, he placed two pistols to his head (one in each hand) and fired. He died instantly.

To Reiterate: What Happened from a Hostage Perspective

A very dangerous criminal and another prisoner escaped and met up with a young couple who were drug users. They went to the couple's apartment as acquaintances. During the siege, the criminal said that he had taken his fellow escapee and the couple as hostages and demanded a car to get away. During the negotiation process, the hostage taker, his fellow escapee, and the couple talked with the police. The young couple begged the police, "Let us go before he kills us"; the girl, in particular, said that she was afraid that he would kill her. Thus, the three individuals were self-identified hostages in this situation.

In this hostage situation, the Alarm Stage lasted approximately two-and-a-half hours when the first officers tried to go into the apartment without knowing that the escapees were there. The actual situation began at approximately noon on a Wednesday and resolved itself with the freeing of the others in the apartment at 6 a.m. the following Friday morning, and the suicide of the escapee at 7:30 p.m. that Friday evening.

Contact between the escapee and negotiator(s) was initiated by the negotiation team. The most effective negotiator was a criminal investigator (a lieutenant) who was assisted by another lieutenant and a sergeant, as well as a police psychologist. The main negotiator, the lieutenant, was very good at handling problems as they arose and also was strong emotionally. The perpetrator trusted him and liked him best of the negotiators, although it is impossible to explain exactly why that trust developed. The hostage taker's therapist also came on site and had good contact with the escapee, although she did not assist a great deal in the actual negotiation process. The lieutenant was flexible, reacted according to the situation in a fluid manner, was quick to analyze and respond to changes in the emotions of the hostage taker as well as changes in the situation inside the stronghold.

This author had no direct contact with the hostage taker. My duties included: shuttling between the hostage site and the police department; consulting with the commander of that department, the on-scene commander, the negotiators, and the police psychologist on scene; helping in the intelligence arena; and gathering information from those who knew the perpetrators and from persons aware of the various aspects of the perpetrator's military service. I was moving all the time, motivating the police officers who were surrounding the area in case of the need for a siege, particularly when the situation was not immediately resolved and took a more extended length of time.

When the situation was resolved, no one from outside the police department debriefed the negotiators in any official manner. The team met after the situation to talk through the case and, in essence, debriefed themselves.

The model of negotiation used in this situation was a team model. One negotiator functioned as primary contact with the hostage taker while another kept the log. In this case, the main negotiator was a police lieutenant. The prison psychologist who had worked with the hostage taker served as a backup and resource.

WHAT MAKES A GOOD HOSTAGE NEGOTIATOR?

According to Getty and Elam (1988), negotiators should have certain characteristics. They should have verbal fluency and be outgoing and extroverted. They should have confidence, exhibit a positive self-image, be sensitive to others, and have a creative reasoning ability.

In the Lahti case, the following hostage negotiator characteristics were most important: flexibility, creativity, understanding the problems of this kind of criminal personality, understanding the criminal mind, being empathic, and trying to help the perpetrator resolve the situation without violence. The negotiator told the perpetrator that it was possible to find a solution to the situation and tried to find opportunities for negotiation so that it would not be necessary to use force. He tried to protect the hostage taker from the media and offered the perpetrator ways to "save face." This was the first negotiation this officer had done; he was new to this particular aspect of policing. Thus, he was seeking support.

Lanceley (1985) notes that police psychologists are professionals who realize that time is on the side of the negotiator. In fact, it is in the best interest of the negotiator to try to extend the time of negotiations. The longer the time, the greater the possibility that basic human needs (food, water, etc.) will become bargaining tools. As time goes on, hostage takers often become more rational and less anxious, and therefore less likely to use aggression against others. Also, there is a greater chance that the Stockholm Syndrome will occur and that hostages and hostage taker will bond. As time goes on, hostage negotiators learn more about the personality and life of the hostage taker; the more information that is gained, the greater the opportunity to make appropriate decisions and the less chance of making mistakes. It is also more probable that the hostage taker and negotiator will establish a rapport and the hostage taker will become more aware of the reality of the situation.

In hostage negotiations, the role of the police psychologist is often that of consultant. In this case, the police psychologist evaluated the personality of the hostage taker and the potential for dangerousness of the individual(s). "What is the likelihood of . . . ?" is a question that the police psychologist may be called upon to answer. For example, "Will the hostage taker harm his captives? Will he/she/they do damage or cause harm?" are frequently asked questions. As an observer, the police psychologist cannot rush into a premature assessment of the situation and must consider all the facts at hand.

LESSONS LEARNED

Police have learned that it is not an advantage for a hostage taker to have access to phone contact with the outside world. In the Lahti situation, the hostage taker had a portable phone that gave him access to a variety of persons. He gave interviews to the local radio station and contacted his brother, friends, the media, and police. As a consequence, the Finnish police have realized that it is important to have access to and utilize a portable phone instead. If this is the case, then hostage negotiations vans similar to those used in the United States (e.g., the Orange County [California] Police Department) need to be available. These vans have special equipment designed for hostage situations, including a portable (cellular) phone. On any type of phone, however, the only line available needs to be open to the police. Access to other individuals needs to be restricted.

A second lesson learned by the Finnish police was how to deal with the media in a situation of this magnitude. The radio stations in attendance began with a neutral and objective approach to the situation. However, they offered the public the opportunity to phone in and offer advice concerning how to resolve the hostage situation. The hostage taker, in this case, was listening to the broadcasts through a battery radio (since electricity had been switched off early in the siege). Law enforcement officials learned that it was impossible to tell the media to "go away" and that it was essential to provide media personnel with accurate information (as much as is possible). (This author provided information and served as media contact to television and radio and also asked the media for "fair play" in the situation.)

A third lesson learned was that the local law enforcement officials were not ready for a situation of this magnitude. The command post and negotiating post were conducted from the same place, from a car; however, these two posts needed to be in different places.

The fourth lesson learned was that police psychologists can perform an essential, positive role in negotiations. They can help in siege situations by providing information and also by giving law enforcement officials a chance to defuse, talk about what is going on, and express "black" humor.

The primary goal in law enforcement hostage negotiations is to use the minimum amount of force necessary to resolve a hostage situation. Although the Lahti situation resulted in the death of the hostage taker, that death was self-inflicted—not the result of police force. No innocent bystanders were killed, and no police officers were hurt, beyond the injury of the first officer who came to the apartment.

The organizational structure of hostage negotiations in this case was similar to that recommended by the U.S. FBI. The psychologist was consultant to the chief negotiator and was used to assess the mental status of the hostage taker, to provide suggestions to the negotiator, and to act as a shuttle between negotiating and tactical teams. In addition, the police psychologist offered debriefings postincident to the first patrol and to the special group of officers who first went in. When the bullet fired by the hostage taker hit the shield, a police officer was wounded in the leg. The author debriefed him privately. A tactical debriefing of the entire mission took place approximately two weeks postincident. All police officers, including the police psychologists and this author, were involved.

As Trompetter (1995) notes, a major role of the police psychologist is to monitor the negotiation process. In this instance, the author, as consultant and debriefer, was familiar with hostage negotiation techniques as well as with conflict resolution and crisis intervention. By monitoring the communication process between negotiator and hostage taker, the psychologist negotiator examined attempts at and successes with problem-solving activities, the ability of the hostage taker to delay gratification and/or compromise demands, and rapport-building with negotiators and the prison psychologist (Miron and Goldstein, 1979). Through this monitoring, the psychologist negotiator could evaluate the potential of the hostage taker for violent behavior and risk to those around him. A tactical response to this situation did not occur due to the death of the hostage taker from self-inflicted wounds; however, in other situations, a tactical end to the situation might have been necessary.

CONCLUSIONS

In looking back at the Lahti situation, it is hard to find ways that the actual negotiation could have been done differently. However, the involvement of the media was an embarrassment and showed the Finnish police departments and police college that there was a need to be prepared in a better fashion for such involvement.

The goal of utilizing a minimum amount of force was met in this case. The negotiation team functioned well with its primary negotiator (the lieutenant), secondary negotiators (other officers), consultants, and police psychologists. The team worked together with the tactical team that was ready to use force, should it have been necessary.

As a mental health and law enforcement professional, this author provided assessment of the perpetrator as well as postincident assistance. Responsibilities included assessment of the hostage taker's mental status and determination, within reasonable limits, of the risk of the hostage taker's use of imminent violence. There is no known way to predict this likelihood, although some markers have been documented (among them are an early conduct disorder diagnosis, military service which included the use of weapons, a history of criminal behavior, a history of assaultive behaviors, narcissism, absence of empathy, the ability to withstand a lack of sleep and food, the presence or absence of an audience (including the media) which provides an opportunity for "showing off."

Hostage negotiation is a challenge to resolve. This author was fortunate to be able to utilize a multitude of knowledge resources (knowledge of psychopathology, interpersonal dynamics, conflict resolution, forensics, crisis intervention, communications theory, problem solving, and others) in the Lahti situation. Saving life is the most important positive outcome of hostage negotiation. Even though the escapee took his own life, three others' lives were saved. The lessons learned through this situation will help future officers as they work toward saving the lives of countless other citizens.

REFERENCES

Baruth, C. L. (1988). Routine mental health checkups and activities for law enforcement personnel involved in dealing with hostage and terrorist incidents by psychologist trainer-consultant. In J. T. Reese and J. M. Horn, (Eds.), *Police psychology: Operational assistance,* (pp. 9-20). Washington, DC: U.S. Department of Justice.

Getty, V. S. and Elam, J. D. (1988). Identifying characteristics of hostage negotiators and using personality data to develop a selection model. In J. T. Reese and J. M. Horn, (Eds.), *Police psychology: Operational assistance,* (pp. 159-171). Washington, DC: U.S. Department of Justice.

Lanceley, F. (1985). *Hostage negotiations seminar.* Quantico, VA: FBI Academy.

McMains, M. J. (1988). Psychologists' roles in hostage negotiations. In J. T. Reese and J. M. Horn, (Eds.), *Police psychology: Operational assistance,* (pp. 281-309). Washington, DC: U.S. Department of Justice.

Miron, M. S. and Goldstein, A. P. (1979). *Hostage.* New York: Pergamon Press.

Mohandie, K., Piersol, F. E., and Klyver, N. (1995). Law enforcement turmoil and transitions and the evolving role of the police psychologist. In J. T. Reese and R. M. Solomon, (Eds.), *Organizational issues in law enforcement,* (pp. 383-396). Washington, DC: U.S. Department of Justice, Federal Bureau of Investigation.

Strentz, T. (1995). Crisis interventions and survival strategies for victims of hostage situations. In A. R. Roberts, (Ed.), *Crisis intervention and time-limited cognitive treatment,* (pp. 127-150). Thousand Oaks, CA: Sage Publications, Inc.

Trompetter, P. (1995). Determinants of imminent dangerousness: Exploratory psychological contributions to the incident command of a hostage event. In J. T. Reese and R. M. Solomon, (Eds.), *Organizational issues in law enforcement,* (pp. 267-278). Washington, DC: U.S. Department of Justice, Federal Bureau of Investigation.

Chapter 15

Law Enforcement and Trauma

James M. Horn

Law enforcement is one of the very few professions that drastically change a personality.

Guy Schiller

INTRODUCTION

Law enforcement is a paramilitary profession which includes uniforms, guns, individual and group tactics, and the responsibility to use deadly force if necessary. As in the military, there is pride, integrity, courage, loyalty to the cause (of justice), discipline, determination, dedication, toughness, and commitment. Many, if not most, police officers admit to closely resembling the personality profile of emergency service personnel postulated by Drs. Jeffrey T. Mitchell and George Everly (1999) of the International Critical Incident Stress Foundation, conceived as follows:

- Obsessive compulsive (do it right every time)
- Controller (of self, scene, and home)
- Action oriented
- Easily bored
- High need for stimulation (likes sky diving, motorcycles, etc.)
- Risk taker (with survival skills)
- Highly dedicated
- Strong need to be needed
- Difficulty saying "no"
- Rescue personality
- Family oriented (but will drop everything to respond to a call)
- Driven by internal motivation
- Generally high tolerance of stress and ambiguity

These traits help law enforcement personnel to be effective in their jobs, but they can also make them vulnerable to stress, because they may overload on their job responsibilities at the expense of their personal/family life. A need obviously exists for motivated and brave officers who can take charge of a situation and control the course of an incident as much as necessary or possible, but excessive dedication to duty at the expense of personal and social time may lead to exhaustion, burnout, or other undesirable outcomes.

Like everyone else, police officers may have to contend with trauma or crises in their personal lives, but their job insures that they will have to deal with trauma in other peoples' lives as well. If they succumb to these exposures with their own post-traumatic stress disorder (PTSD), then their families may become tertiary victims of the original precipitating trauma. Personality traits and training provide a solid foundation for dealing with society's crises and trauma with amazing resilience and stamina. It is not unusual to see officers perform with distinction while concurrently shouldering heavy personal stress loads. Many are indeed at their best when the chips are down. Their defensive armor can, on occasion, be penetrated by circumstances beyond their control, due to the fact that "the human response to trauma is universal" (van der Kolk, 1996, p. ix). Fifty percent of the approximately 200 police officers present at the San Ysidro McDonald's massacre in 1984, in which twenty-one people were killed and nineteen wounded, experienced some degree of PTSD. In fact, the four most common outcomes of untreated psychological trauma are anxiety disorders, depression, addictive behavior, and violence (Flannery, 1995).

A traumatic incident is an incident outside the normal range of experiences, which might be expected to produce a significant emotional response, and overwhelms or threatens to overwhelm the officer's normal coping mechanisms. It is often sudden and unexpected, and leaves the officer feeling out of control, vulnerable, or even helpless. It may result in a shattering of the officer's view of the world or of himself or herself.

THE NATURE OF TRAUMA

Incidents that may appear to be traumatic to ordinary citizens may be handled smoothly, professionally, and without noticeable effect by police officers time after time. However, everyone is vulnerable to some given set of circumstances. This vulnerability is influenced by many factors, including the following:

1. *Fantasy versus reality.* The incident may appear to pose a threatening set of circumstances even though the threat never physically materializes. Regardless, just the thoughts of the officer may create an immediate and compelling sense of danger, vulnerability, and/or mortality. The officer may

think about or visualize the worst possible outcome and then be witness to the best possible outcome. However, the damage may have already been done by the negative thoughts and beliefs. Believing that death or serious injury is imminent to one's self, partner, or an innocent party, may, by itself, traumatize an officer.

2. *Imagination.* Albert Einstein said imagination is more important than knowledge and Napoleon believed imagination rules the world. Sometimes a police officer's world can be very small and negatively affected by his or her own inaccurate imagination. For example, a police officer may imagine he or she, his or her partner, or hostages are dying or are dead even though that is not accurate. The damage may already be done by such an image. Such was the case when an experienced officer who had been involved in many traumatic incidents, including fatal shootings, described pulling a cover blanket off the body of a dead, believing for the first two seconds that the body was his own child's. He convincingly described that brief experience as the worst thing that had ever happened to him in his life, in spite of the fact that the worst scenario, the death of his own child, was only momentarily manufactured in his own imagination and perception, when it never occurred in reality. The lesson, of course, is that officers need to train themselves to control negative thoughts and machinations during traumatic incidents, less they make the impact of the event much worse than the facts support.

3. *Personalization.* Another factor affecting the impact an incident has on officers is perfectly demonstrated by the preceding anecdote. Isolating the affective response of a traumatic incident is easier if the officer does not personally know the victim(s). If the officer knows the victim or, as in this case, just imagines he knows the victim, the affective response is much more difficult to isolate because the event is now personalized. It will not be easy to leave the incident and its memory at the scene, not to think about it at home, or perhaps not to dream about it at night.

4. *Achilles heel.* Another significant variable which influences the amount of trauma an officer experiences during an incident is the Achilles heel factor (an area of vulnerability). Two of the more significant Achilles heels for officers are children and colleagues, especially partners. Most officers probably will never get to the point on the job when the child victims do not bother them, and that is good. To get to that chilling point of indifference, one would have to be brain dead or flat lined on the heart monitor. Of course, denial will also produce an appearance of immunity. If the children still bother an experienced detective, he is probably healthier than if they do not bother him anymore.

Dr. James D. Sewell surveyed hundreds of Florida officers and had them rank the worst things that happen to them on the job. The number one answer was the violent death of a partner in the line of duty (Sewell, 1981).

Such a loss is very personal and is an Achilles heel-type injury; it may even cripple the surviving partner, literally.

It is a genuine shame that the public often seems to have no real concept of the depth of the heart and the soul of police officers. The police have been stereotyped so mechanically and so negatively by the media since at least the mid-sixties, when Hollywood and the media put the white hats on the bad guys and the black hats on the good guys, that the public suffers from apparent brainwashing. The movie, *Bonnie and Clyde* was a classic example of Hollywood romanticizing, glamorizing, and dramatizing two of the worst murderers in U.S. history. In February 1997, a TV news anchorwoman reported an unsubstantiated story about Albuquerque, NM police using excessive force against an arrested accused criminal. She closed her broadcast saying, "It's getting harder and harder to tell the good guys from the bad guys." I have yet to work an officer-involved shooting that was accurately reported by the media. Thomas Jefferson noted the problem in 1807 when he said, "Nothing can now be believed which is seen in a newspaper." When journalists and reporters publicly display such bias and bigotry, they undermine the support of the public toward the men and women who put their lives on the line every day for America. Every year 130 to 180 of them give their lives while trying to serve and protect the citizens.

If imagination really rules the world, the media and Hollywood must become responsible and accountable again to truth and objectivity for the good of society, while there is still a society to inform and entertain. The challenging job of a police officer warrants the support of the public. Solomon and Horn (1986) report the significant value of support in reducing trauma. Attendees at the FBI Academy's Post-Critical Incident Seminars, which began in 1983, have listed peer support as their number one resource for helping them cope with trauma (Horn and Solomon, 1989). The United States learned the hard way of the value of support when it failed to support its returning veterans from Vietnam. It is not necessary to support a war or cause to support the warrior/officer. In his book about the black experience in Vietnam, Wallace Terry (1989) said the worst experience for any veteran is to be rejected by his or her society and nation. William James believed the most fundamental desire of human nature is the desire to be appreciated. Appreciation and support, at least for the sacrifice and effort, advance police officers' ability to constructively deal with the stress and trauma of the job.

Police officers accumulate many exposures to trauma during their careers. Some affect them, others do not. Prior trauma may sensitize or immunize officers to subsequent trauma, depending upon whether or not they worked through the earlier trauma. The degree of personality change experienced by an officer is certainly, in part, a factor of how well he or she has processed and integrated the traumatic experiences of the job. Working through the trauma is a process accomplished in various ways by different individuals. Each officer brings his or her own history, strengths, and potential vulnerabilities to the job. Each has his or her own coping mechanisms as well. Police officers who work for agencies with Critical Incident Stress Management (CISM) programs in place to deal with trauma will find support to address the effects of traumatic incidents. CISM programs provide education about traumatic stress, as well as resources and follow-up support to monitor progress and enhance the integration of traumatic experience into officers' lives.

Officer trauma can be extreme and can range from incidents involving as few as one adversary or even no adversaries, as in an officer's single car accident. The trauma can be understandably extreme. An example of this was the Oklahoma City bombing of April 19, 1995, which killed 168 people, physically wounded over 500 people, and emotionally/mentally wounded probably millions of Americans, especially Oklahomans and federal employees, many of whom understandably took the attack personally. Many people from every location in the United States have expressed their personal anguish over the Oklahoma City bombing. Thousands of lives and personalities were changed that day, forever. For thousands of victims and survivors, "the war is not over when the shooting stops." Hundreds of survivors put the healing process on hold until justice was served by the conviction and sentencing of Terry Nichols and Michael Fortier, and execution of Timothy McVeigh. Years later, many survivors felt as if the bombing was just a day behind them and could not get on with their lives until justice was served.

When thousands of volunteers responded to this disaster, the CISM resources were stretched beyond limits. When thousands of the volunteers returned to their homes from coast to coast, and from Canada to Mexico, many reported receiving debriefings and effective support resources back home; others reported isolation with no support.

FBI Chaplain Joe Williams of Oklahoma City, and Oklahoma City Police Department Chaplain Jack Poe solicited donations to fund critical incident workshops to assist the primary, secondary, and tertiary victims of the bombing. Three-day residential workshops were offered at no expense to the attendees. The workshops have been conducted monthly since April 1996 for groups numbering from seven to twenty participants. All room and board is provided at no cost to the participants; they spend an intense three days at a motel conference site from Tuesdays at 1:00 p.m. to Fridays at noon. The experienced staff consists of trauma specialists, who are facilitators, psychologists, peer supporters, and chaplains. In a confidential setting, the individuals are afforded an opportunity to express themselves fully and to put the experience into words with their individual stories. The workshop is conducted as an exercise in peer support wherein the emphasis is on sharing whatever is desired to a group of peers who will not judge and who will do their best to listen, understand, appreciate, acknowledge, accept, and validate the thoughts, feelings, and experiences of each participant.

In July 1998, Chaplain Joe Williams was honored by the International Conference of Police Chaplains (ICPC) as National Chaplain of the Year for his unending, selfless efforts to help, comfort, and heal the victims and survivors of the Oklahoma City bombing. He also received the FBI Director's Award for Excellence for Distinguished Service to the law Enforcement Community. Joe Williams was able to make remarkable contributions to help victims while simultaneously having to deal with his own family's grief at the loss of his newly wed son's father-in-law in the bombing. These awards are but a minute token of appreciation compared to the unbelievable amount of help Joe Williams, Jack Poe, Phyllis Poe, and dozens of other chaplains have provided since the bombing.

THE OKLAHOMA CITY MODEL

The efficacy of this model is largely based on the qualifications of the workshop staff who are specifically trained in CISM and are experienced police peer supporters, police psychologists, and police chaplains. This model is similar to the Post-Critical Incident Seminars (PCIS), which were previously run at the FBI Academy in Quantico, Virginia, from 1987 to 1994 by the author. Of the PCIS, FBI Employee Assistance Unit Chief Vince McNally wrote:

> Critical incident recovery can be a lengthy and complex process. Even after initial acceptance and resolution of an incident, negative reactions can resurface. Once individuals confront their vulnerability and mortality, they must learn to live with that reality. Going through a traumatic incident is like crossing a fence and losing one's naivete with no possibility of crossing back (Solomon 1995). To minimize long-term difficulties, follow-up contacts are made by the CISM team and Employee Assistance Unit personnel. Referrals for additional help are made on an as-needed basis.

> To promote resolution and to provide follow-up, the FBI initiated a Post-Critical Incident Seminar (PCIS). Agents and support personnel who have experienced a critical incident are invited to a four-day seminar to discuss their reactions in a safe, protective, and confidential environment. The PCIS is also open to spouses. Seminar size is usually between 15 and 25 people. Through sharing their incident with others, participants receive peer support, which enables normalization of re-

actions. Participants also learn about trauma and coping strategies to facilitate healing and recovery. A block of training on providing peer support enables participants to offer constructive interpersonal support to fellow employees who may experience critical incidents.

The PCIS enables the participant experiencing difficulty to access professional services in a safe environment. Participants have the opportunity [on a voluntary basis] to work one-on-one with clinicians who specialize in law enforcement issues, PTSD, and EMDR. The PCIS is often the vehicle which moves individuals who are "stuck" in resolving their incident, as the following example illustrates:

> One agent [who granted permission to disclose this example] who attended the PCIS was experiencing distress from a seemingly minor incident. He was following a drug dealer on a surveillance detail. The suspect, realizing he was being followed, drove at speeds in excess of 100 miles per hour. He eventually pulled over on the highway. He got out of his vehicle and approached the agent. The agent identified himself and the suspect surrendered upon command. Despite the positive outcome, the incident still bothered the agent. At the PCIS, the agent talked about this incident and realized his fear stemmed from the accumulation of several past incidents. These included Vietnam experiences, being on scene at two air disasters, and several hostage negotiation experiences. The agent recognized the connection between the surveillance and these other situations where he faced his own mortality. With EMDR, further discussion, and peer support, the cumulative stress issues were resolved. Follow-up has shown the gains to be stable over the past two years.

Issues of vulnerability, as illustrated in the above example, are commonly dealt with in the PCIS. The trauma of witnessing one's partner being shot, grief stemming from the sudden death of a loved one, guilt from having to use fatal force, the horror that comes with working mass casualties following a bombing or airline disaster, are other types of situations that have been dealt with in the PCIS.

Since 1983, the FBI has conducted 37 PCISs with 900 participants. Many of those who attend the PCIS volunteer to assist others who experience critical incidents. These agents, employees, and spouses are valuable resources who provide enlightened interpersonal support to their peers following traumatic events. The FBI believes that there is no better person to offer support than those individuals who have experienced, and emotionally worked through, a similar event. (Mc-Nally and Solomon, 1999)

The human response to trauma is universal (van der Kolk, 1996) and many critical incident workshop participants (as do the PCIS participants) come with multiple past episodes of trauma, in addition to the Oklahoma City bombing trauma. They are allowed and encouraged to articulate those stories as well. The bonding of the participants in each workshop is inspiring, to say the least. Some bombing victims have isolated themselves and come to the workshop with seemingly no friends, no one to talk to, no one who understands. Practically all participants seem to leave with a roomful of new friends who understand and agree to be there for each other if they are needed any time of the day or night. These new supporters are just a phone call, letter, or visit away. The bonding is such that, by noon on Friday, many of the participants are hesitant to conclude the workshop and extend it by going to lunch together prior to returning home. Many of the participants have reported that the workshop improved or even saved their jobs, marriages, and in some cases, their lives. They have reported that they returned home to loved ones who described them as being changed persons. A little appreciation and "V.I.P" treatment can go a long way toward helping people recover from or deal with horrendous experiences, even as monstrous as the Oklahoma City bombing.

The workshop even provides massage therapists who give brief neck and shoulder massage to all willing participants. Dozens of massage therapists showed up as volunteers in Oklahoma City after the bombing to provide their services free of charge to the rescue/recovery personnel and other workers. Some people who were unfamiliar with therapeutic massage had to be coaxed into trying it in Oklahoma City, but they only had to be coaxed once. They became some of the hundreds of new believers in the efficacy of this therapeutic art/science.

Eclectic, didactic comments and presentations are sprinkled throughout the workshop by the staff when times are judged to be right. Group meals are eaten at the conference center, and twice (one lunch, one supper) the group is treated to a nice meal out to promote further social bonding of the individuals and group.

One-on-one sessions are available to participants throughout the workshop and the participants can choose either a peer supporter, a chaplain, or a therapist who is a level 2 trained Eye Movement Desensitization and Reprocessing (EMDR) therapist for the sessions. The feedback from workshop participants about EMDR has been most impressive, including the author's personal experience. The Chief of the FBI's Employee Assistance Unit wrote of EMDR as follows:

EMDR is a component of the FBI's integrated response to a critical incident. EMDR is a therapeutic method that accelerates the treatment of trauma (Shapiro, 1997; Shapiro and Forrest, 1997; Shapiro and Solomon, 1995; Solomon and Shapiro, 1997). It is hypothesized that EMDR stimulates the brain's natural information processing mechanisms, allowing the "frozen" traumatic information to be processed normally and achieve integration (Shapiro, 1995). Research indicates that after three sessions of EMDR, 84 to 100 percent of people who had post-traumatic stress disorder (PTSD) due to a single traumatic episode no longer met the criteria for PTSD (Rothbaum, 1997; Wilson, et al., 1995; Marcus, et al., in press; Wilson, et al., in press; Sheck, et al., in press). Consistent with this research, the FBI has found EMDR to be effective when used with individuals exhibiting symptoms of posttraumatic stress stemming from a specific event. EMDR is administered only by mental health professionals. Where CISD and defusings are crisis intervention strategies, EMDR is considered treatment. It is important that the mental health professional have appropriate training in EMDR, as well as knowledge and experience in working with trauma. (McNally and Solomon, 1999)

There is an amazing difference in workshops of this nature when a chaplain is present than when a chaplain is not present. Although this author was the program manager of the FBI's Critical Incident Program, the positive impact was immediate when a chaplain was included in the FBI workshops beginning in 1991. Chaplains are permanent participants at the bombing workshops, and are there not to turn the workshops into religious services, but to facilitate a spontaneous inclusion of spiritual thoughts and matters. Usually this occurs for half of the participants or more when there is merely a chaplain present, who does not even have to speak. The chaplains call this phenomenon the ministry of presence, a concept the author understood as a U.S. Marine in 1969 near the demilitarized zone (DMZ) in South Vietnam when he approached a chaplain he had not even had a discussion with and said, "I couldn't deal with this if you weren't here," and then simply walked away.

> Never shall I forget those moments that murdered my God
> And my soul, and turned my dreams to dust.
>
> Eli Wiesel

Friday morning sessions of the Oklahoma workshops present positive, cognitive material, including inspiring examples of survivors. The process that the participants experienced during the workshop is explained and reinforced with emphasis placed on continuing the networking, and utilizing resources, including group peer support meetings of survivors, free counseling, available for example, from Project Heartland, and contacts with workshop staff as desired.

HELP TO LAW ENFORCEMENT THROUGH EAPs

Violence can disrupt our lives spiritually, physically, mentally, emotionally, and socially. Fortunately, employee assistance programs (EAPs) with comprehensive CISM programs are in place throughout the nation, benefiting hundreds of thousands of our police officers and their loved ones. For example, the FBI describes its program as follows:

> The FBI also has a responsibility to assist its employees in dealing constructively with and surviving the emotional aftermath [of trauma]. The FBI' s Employee Assistance Unit has developed a Critical Incident Stress Management (CISM) Program to better safeguard and promote the psychological well-being of its employees following a critical incident. Agents receive training, firearms, and bulletproof vests to equip them to physically survive critical incidents. The FBI is now providing agents with the tools to successfully survive the emotional aftermath of critical incidents. In June 1995, the FBI instituted four Critical Incident Response Teams. These teams are assigned to different regions of the United States to provide immediate response to critical incidents. The most commonly occurring incidents experienced in the line of duty include but are not limited to:
>
> Death of employee, spouse, or family member
> Violent traumatic injury to an employee
> Taking a life, or causing serious injury, in the line of duty
> Suicide of an employee, spouse, or family member
> Major natural disaster or man-made catastrophe (earthquake, bombing, etc.)
> Witnessing/handling multiple fatalities
> High speed pursuits that end in tragedy
> SWAT operations, where dangers are present
> Hostage taking/barricaded suspect negotiation
> Observing an act of corruption, bribery, or other illegal activity by a fellow worker
> Suspension and/or threat of dismissal

The goal of the FBI's CISM program is to provide FBI employees with a confidential program that will mitigate the adverse effects of the incident and promote positive resolution. Team members are drawn from the Employee Assistance Unit, FBI Chaplains, the FBI Peer Support Team and mental health professionals with expertise in police psychology and trauma. (McNally and Solomon, 1999, p. 24)

The use of trained and educated professionals who understand, appreciate, and support the police culture and its mission cannot be overstated. This does not mean that the occasional misconduct or wrong doing is condoned or excused. It does mean that when a resource person, be it peer, chaplain, or mental health professional argues with an officer during a post-shooting session about the ethics of shooting someone, even in the line of duty, that resource is likely doing harm, rather than good. The last thing officers need is a critic. Such a "resource" will likely not be used again and will be negatively branded by the grapevine.

Thousands of police departments with ten officers or less, and, perhaps, hundreds of thousands of officers and their loved ones, are still likely operating without the benefit of these important support/restorative resources. In spite of all the work and progress, obviously much remains to be done.

Because the four most common outcomes of untreated psychological trauma are anxiety disorders, depression, addictive behavior, and violence (Flannery, 1995), it is disconcerting to think of the police officers and other emergency workers who are still doing without CISM programs and technology. Police officers and their loved ones often pay an untold price for their service and dedication. During World War II, Winston Churchill reminded us that a nation of many can owe a great deal to a few, selfless public servants, i.e., the Royal Air Force. Such is the case of the United States toward law enforcement officers.

CONCLUSION

A final point pertinent to police and others who fit the emergency service providers personality profile is that the commonly stated cognitive, mental, emotional, and physical reactions to trauma may not be the biggest threat to the well-being of officers in and of themselves. Many traumatologists pronounce such abnormal reactions to abnormal events to be normal behavior, but unless officers understand and accept this, they may have life-threatening reactions to such normal reactions. Officers who consider themselves to be invincible, invulnerable, immortal, and "tough s.o.b.'s" may find that emotional reactions to trauma are especially unacceptable to their self-confidence. It may cause them to reevaluate totally their competence and ability to perform or return to work. It may threaten their self-image to the point of self-destruction. This author's professional experiences have included suicide interventions with officers who threatened or declared their intention to commit suicide, not because of their close brushes with death, but because their subsequent recurring emotional reactions, such as spontaneous uncontrolled crying, had shattered their self-image and confidence. They could not live with the perception that they had lost control of their emotions and had turned into "cry babies." With some effort, this "failing" was redefined as a normal and acceptable reaction to a brutal set of circumstances.

Police, perhaps more than any other profession in our society, encounter life's most tragic and brutal facts of life up close. If society expects them to confront these tragedies in a professional and competent way, it should, at the very least, afford them a reassuring level of support and appreciation. Such support *will make a difference* to the health and welfare of our police, and, consequentially, to their level of professional effectiveness. In spite of the media stereotypes, they are still just human beings.

More than anything else, the popular concept of community policing represents a concept of a cooperative citizen/police effort to maximize the safety of people while securing their liberties. A comprehensive CISM program available to all of America's law enforcement officers, including reasonable support from the public and the media, would be a major element in the constructive coping by law enforcement with the trauma inherent in their job.

REFERENCES

Everly, G. S. Jr. and Mitchell, J. T. (1999). *Critical Incident Stress Management: A New Era and Standard of Care in Crisis Intervention.* Ellicott City, MD: Chevron Press.

Flannery, R. B. Jr. (1995). *Violence in the Workplace.* New York: Crossroad Publishing.

Horn, J. M. and Solomon, R. M. (1989). Peer Support: A Key Element for Coping with Trauma. *Police Stress, 9*(1), 25-27.

McNally, V. and Solomon, R. M. (1999). The FBI's Critical Incident Stress Management Program. *FBI Law Enforcement Bulletin, 68*(2), 20-26.

Sewell, J. D. (1981). Police Stress. *FBI Law Enforcement Bulletin,* (4), 9.

Solomon, R. M. and Horn, J. M. (1986). Post Shooting Traumatic Reactions: A Pilot Study. In J. T. Reese and H. A. Goldstein (Eds.), *Psychological Services for Law Enforcement,* (pp. 383-394). Washington, DC: U.S. Government Printing Office.

Terry, W. (1989). *Bloods: An Oral History of the Vietnam War by Black Veterans.* New York: Ballantine Books.

van der Kolk, B. A. (1996). *Traumatic Stress.* In B. A. van der Kolk, A. C. McFarlane, and L. Weisaeth (Eds.) (p. ix). New York: Guilford Press.

Chapter 16

Trauma Services to War Veterans

Charles M. Flora

TREATING THE WAR VETERAN

First and foremost, a veteran's recovery from the psychological wounds of war is predicated on the idea that posttraumatic reactions have a natural history and are the consequence to previously well-functioning individuals exposed to the extreme life-and-death threatening stresses of war (Horowitz, 1986; Kardiner and Spiegel, 1947). In this regard, an important function of the therapist is to validate, appreciate, and understand the veteran's experiences in war. Starting at the point of initial contact, the veteran should be welcomed with an accepting attitude that conveys appreciation and respect for his or her military service. This function is advanced both by an informed understanding of the veteran's war as a large scale social event in the history of the nation, and by an empathic grasp of the veteran's particular war-related experiences and stressors. "The therapeutic process should be shaped by the therapists' deeply held belief in the reality of trauma and the understanding that traumatic residue shapes the survivors' current daily experience, including their experience of the therapeutic relationship" (Lebowitz, Harvey, and Herman, 1993, p. 382).

Gelsomino and Mackey (1988) also suggest that clinical interventions with veterans having traumatic stress reactions are more effective when guided by a theoretical framework that views clinicians not as treating a pathology, but rather as facilitating a normal stress recovery and postwar readjustment process. This treatment philosophy provides the veteran with a healthier recovery environment and validates the veteran's military service by recognizing combat as of the magnitude of stressful experiences that can cause such posttraumatic stress reactions in previously well-functioning individuals.

The preferred treatment for war trauma consists of helping the veteran tell his or her story of the significant events before, during, and after the traumatic war experiences (Horowitz, 1986). The veteran is gently encouraged to talk about the war in a safe and supportive setting. In casual conversation with the veteran, the outlines of the veteran's specific war experiences begin to take shape. Once a therapeutic relationship has been established, the counselor guides the veteran through a healing process by helping the veteran to recover and explore the roots of current traumatic reactions by systematically linking them to actual traumatic war experiences. The therapeutic relationship helps to anchor the veteran to traumatic war memories, a past that has often been defensively split off from everyday life, and facilitates a recovery environment, which is primarily embodied by the therapist whose authentic interest and empathy have been established. In time, the veteran is helped to embed his or her war experiences in widening circles of narrative significance, by placing them in the larger contexts of his or her life history and the history of his or her war.

COMMUNITY OUTREACH

Several interrelated factors make outreach in the community to locate, engage, and inform veterans about war stress, and available services, a desirable feature for serving war veterans. The single most important reason for inclusion of an outreach component for a veteran's war trauma program is the avoidance symptoms of PTSD. A core clinical feature of PTSD is a persistent avoidance of stimuli associated with the trauma and numbing of general responsiveness (not present before the trauma). Specific symptoms include avoidance of reminders of the trauma, amnesia for important aspects of the trauma, markedly diminished interest or participation in significant activities, detachment or estrangement from others, restricted range of affect, and a sense of a foreshortened future. Three or more avoidance symptoms are required for the diagnosis of PTSD (American Psychiatric Association, 1994).

The avoidance symptoms of PTSD comprise significant psychological barriers to care which may require the service provider to engage the veteran at or near to his home community to initiate trauma services. Given the reluctance by many veterans to seek help for war-related problems, it is often the case that other community service providers and/or emergency response workers may have first contact with a veteran in need. At times of emergent crises, for problems such as family or employment functioning, the connection to the veteran's military experience may appear to be remote and not immediately obvious. For this reason, it is strategic to provide education to community service providers on behalf of veterans, and to develop a functional professional network for referral purposes.

Due to the natural functioning of the avoidance symptoms of PTSD, many war veterans, upon their initial request for services, present with problems other than psychological war trauma. These include, but are not limited to questions about disability benefits, medical problems and/or employment concerns. For example, a veteran with heavy combat exposure in Vietnam developed painful intrusive recollections of his war experiences following a visit to the Vietnam Veterans Memorial in Washington, DC. Notwithstanding his own acute distress, he visited a local service agency after returning home to offer help to other veterans needing employment. As a local business owner, his interest was in providing job opportunities for needy veterans. He denied needing counseling assistance for himself.

Also, as Lindy (1985) has stated, survivors of a common catastrophe tend to bond together to form a group that functions to protect its members from the fear of reexperiencing the trauma and to exclude outsiders from access to the traumatic memories by creating a supportive internal environment. Given these natural tensions and survivor group dynamics, outreach to veterans can provide an important bridging function for reconnecting the veteran to needed parts of the civilian community. In this regard, an important service function on behalf of the veterans' needs is mediating with various community agents and service providers. Active intervention in the community to advocate for veterans and coordinate their efforts to access needed services and benefits may be necessary in some cases.

To promote a sense of healthful rehabilitation, trauma services should be provided as closely as possible to the veteran's actual living circumstances in the community. Gelsomino and Mackey (1988) have said that treatment in the community on an outpatient basis, which takes into account the individual's total life functioning, is, in most cases, the approach of choice for war veterans with PTSD. Treating the veteran as a whole person, closely coordinated to his immediate community setting, also promotes the cultural effectiveness of the services by focusing attention upon the veteran's specific social and economic circumstances. In addition to the clinical treatment of the psychological aftermath of war trauma, the veteran's postwar readjustment is enhanced by a social familiarity with the community to which the veteran has returned to live and work as a civilian. For this purpose, trauma service providers are well-advised to give careful attention to special cultural and socioeconomic circumstances characteristic of the veteran's local community.

Full postwar recovery for veterans may also involve an additional social/psychological dimension to the clinical treatment of war trauma per se. Veterans comprise an important status group in American society. As defenders of the Constitution, their contributions and sacrifices are duty-bound to their citizenship and associated with the nation's highest values. For their service as citizen soldiers, veterans are afforded a unique, achieved status and cultural significance. Helping traumatized veterans adopt a functional role as a veteran constitutes an important adjunct to clinical treatment with this population, taking the clinician out of the clinic and into the veteran's community. Helping veterans to effect values having to do with their citizenship and place in the civilian community often entails the resolution of postwar conflicts between the veteran and his or her social environment. This involves special attention to what Catherall (1989) refers to as the subsequent or secondary trauma (breakdown between the veteran and his or her postwar social milieu) in contrast to the initial or primary trauma (conflicts within the veteran's personality resulting from the traumatic war experiences per se).

In summary, the purpose of outreach is to intervene in the community to locate, inform, and engage veterans directly and/or engage significant others on their behalf. This serves to facilitate bringing veterans into contact with trauma counselors and/or other needed service providers and to effect other relevant social values on their behalf. Professional work in the community requires the acquisition of a relatively sophisticated understanding of the local social environment to include the major features of geography, demographic distributions, patterns of ethnicity and culture, and socioeconomic conditions. The professional social work "person-in-environment" paradigm is a useful perspective for organizing professional activities within the community (Hamilton, 1951; Perlman, 1957; Perlman, 1968). This perspective defines a psychosocial configuration that includes a complex interweaving of individual values, emotions, and actions with social institutions, and enhances an understanding of the veteran in his or her total life functioning. More of an exercise in applied social psychology than clinical service delivery, outreach strategies are attuned to the typical social situations and group relations that make up the local environment. Human groups and the social situations that reflect them can be thought of as organizations of mutually interacting (communicating) personalities (Mead, 1934; Warner and Lunt, 1941). As a component of the human group, its culture provides the conventional understandings that group members use to guide their actions and to make sense of their world (Shibutani, 1961). In terms of practical tasks, outreach involves (1) the investigation of functioning human groups in the local environment, and (2) purposeful intervention in social situations on behalf of veteran clients.

Mediating and Brokering a Referral: A Case of Community Intervention

Rick was referred to the author by a local police officer who had responded the night before to a report of domestic violence at Rick's home. Rick's twelve-year-old daughter, Sandy, had been taken into protective custody the previous evening following an outbreak of violence involving Sandy and her father. Sandy was placed in an emergency state foster home, pending the outcome of a hearing in juvenile court for alleged child abuse.

Sandy was Rick's child from a previous marriage, and his current wife, Mary, was not home at the time that the alleged violence occurred.

The police officer was himself a former U.S. Army infantry noncommissioned officer who had served a tour in Vietnam. He was aware that Rick also had served a tour in the infantry in Vietnam and that, since his return home, he had had domestic problems, couldn't hold a steady job, and had bouts of alcohol abuse. Due to these latter problems, the police officer thought that counseling would be of additional help to Rick in view of his current situation. An intake appointment was scheduled for Rick later the same day at the therapist's office.

Rick was on time for his appointment, but was rather noncommunicative and angrily abrupt in style. Regarding the police officer who referred him, Rick stated that "He was a f—— army lifer who didn't know s—— and didn't have any business messing in my life." Rick was dressed in a work shirt, Vietnam-style fatigue pants, and jungle boots. His person and his clothes were clean, and he had long red hair and a full beard. His mode of transportation was a Harley-Davidson motorcycle.

Rick was employed as a manual laborer with a local industry. His work was intermittent and allowed him time for "bike" trips either with a few friends or by himself. When on the road, Rick attired himself in a combination of biker and military gear to include a rucksack. During the time of the initial interview, the left side of Rick's face and his left forearm showed cuts and bruises from a recent mishap on his bike.

Regarding the presenting problem. Rick explained that he had not struck his daughter, but that he had become enraged because she had disobeyed him. As a result, he had taken out his rage on their home, destroying some of the furniture in the living room. Nonetheless, Sandy had been nicked in the forehead by a piece of broken chair thrown by her father, leaving a gash and a large bruise. Having become quite fearful, Sandy ran to the neighbors for help. The sound of Rick angrily tearing up his living room, in combination with the prevailing stigma about anger in Vietnam veterans, resulted in the neighbors calling the authorities.

Sandy's actions, which had triggered her father's rage, involved her "unauthorized" use of lipstick and makeup and her announcement that she was going to her girlfriend's house where they would also be meeting with some male classmates. Rick's fear was that Sandy would turn out "bad" like her mother, whom he had found living with another man when he returned from Vietnam in 1971.

Due to serious child neglect on the part of his former wife, after their divorce, Rick was awarded custody of his daughter. Rick's current wife was his second, and they had been married for five years. Between marriages, Rick had relied on his mother to help care for Sandy.

In mildly probing for a therapeutic foothold, the therapist suggested that it would be a good idea for Rick to stay in contact until the child abuse situation was resolved. Rick was doubtful about what could be accomplished, but agreed that he needed help and an opportunity to talk about what had happened. Rick knew that a hearing on the matter could reopen the question of Sandy's custody, allowing his former wife an opportunity to reenter the scene. When asked about what he did in Vietnam, Rick said that he did not see how Vietnam had anything to do with his problem.

As a result of the referring officer's interventions, the therapist was asked to accompany Rick and his family to a prehearing mediation meeting with the juvenile judge and the state child welfare authorities the following week. The therapist's role would be to mediate on Rick's behalf by providing expertise regarding combat trauma and its aftermath in veterans' behavior, and its possible relation to the domestic incident that had brought the family to the attention of the authorities. As a professional function, mediation can be defined as activities undertaken to effect reconciliation, settlement, and/or compromise between two conflicting parties when one of the parties is a war-veteran client and the other is a significant person or corporate entity in the veteran's social environment. In this case, the outcome was successful. The judge decided that Sandy could return home, given the understanding that Rick was planning to pursue professional counseling. Further particulars regarding Rick's case and the counseling services provided are presented in the next section.

PSYCHOTHERAPY FOR WAR TRAUMA

Individual Psychotherapy:
A Case of Intrusive Recollections

Bill appeared for his initial counseling appointment in a highly labile and agitated state. He alternated between grief-stricken emotional distress and angry, provocative threats directed toward the government. His demeanor was in sharp contrast to his usual easygoing and accommodating manner. He made it known that while he was in need of immediate assistance, he would have to be assured of absolute confidentiality and security because he feared he could be prosecuted for what he had done. Bill was accurately judged to be in the midst of a combat-related emotional crisis and was given the immediate attention and sense of safety his condition warranted.

Emergent crisis situations in veterans frequently involve the reexperiencing of their traumas through repetitive and intrusive recollections of troubling, war-related experiences. Horowitz states (1986) that most trauma survivors will seek professional assistance when they are overwhelmed and can no longer manage the unbidden intrusive ideas and emotions. The reexperiencing category of PTSD symptoms specifies the various ways in which a traumatic event is recurrently and persistently reexperienced. After initially working through the immediate crisis situation, Bill disclosed a traumatic event from his service in Vietnam, as well as elements from his life history before, during, and after his military experience. Bill was the oldest son in a family of four children, with two brothers and a sister. His father was a small construction business owner, noncollege educated, but had upward, mobile social aspirations for his children.

Bill had given up a college deferment to enlist in the U.S. Army and to volunteer for Vietnam because he thought it was his duty. He recalled, in retrospect, that he had been let down by his father's less than enthusiastic response to his decision to enlist when he had anticipated full support. Bill learned later that his father, a World War II veteran, was concerned for his son's safety and not convinced about the necessity for Americans to serve as combatants in the Vietnam War.

Bill arrived in-country in late 1968 and was assigned to an infantry unit operating in the central highlands. After several months of success as a rifleman, he was promoted to E-4 (sergeant) and took over the role of squad leader of a unit that had sustained a number of casualties in a recent fight. Bill took on his new job with the usual commitment and enthusiasm, but also with serious concerns about his ability to meet his new responsibilities.

A short time later, Bill's unit was on patrol moving through some rice paddies at the edge of a village suspected of enemy collaboration. A male figure clad in black leapt up some distance in front of the oncoming soldiers and ran for the nearest house in the village. When the running figure did not respond to their commands to stop, they began firing their weapons. As they approached the fallen figure, an excited, old Vietnamese man was seen running from the village, also toward the body. When Bill arrived on the scene, the old man was wailing over the torn body of his ten-year-old grandson.

Bill returned home from Vietnam in 1970. Feeling pressured to find gainful employment, he gave up his former ambition to finish a college education, and took instead a position with a large, local manufacturer. After two years on an assembly line, he was promoted to job foreman. As job supervisor, he complained that he felt caught between the needs of the workers and the deadlines and schedules imposed by the management. To a certain extent, Bill's discomfort with his current job responsibilities reflected a reenactment of his military role as squad leader, as well as his feeling of responsibility for the accidental death of the Vietnamese youth.

The previously described cyclic or biphasic nature of the human response to psychological trauma defines the longitudinal course of a natural recovery process and maps the direction for therapeutic interventions when counseling assistance is indicated (Horowitz, 1986). The central process of psychotherapy for PTSD, for all trauma as well as combat, consists of the systematic recovering and talking through of the traumatic memories of combat (Herman, 1992; Horowitz, 1986). The therapeutic talking through of traumatic memories is a progressive and emotionally controlled linking of the current PTSD symptoms (behaviors, thoughts, feelings, dreams, defenses, etc.) with actual traumatic experiences. Because the current behavioral derivatives of the original trauma may have undergone considerable elaboration and/or disguise, the therapist may have to function as a detective to interpret the connections. In this context, it is important to note that both the reexperiencing and avoidance symptoms of PTSD can occur at all levels of functioning, i.e., emotional conditions, visual perceptions, thoughts, behavioral reenactments, and/or physical or somatic disturbances (Blank, 1994).

In addition to helping the veteran retrieve and understand traumatic war memories, the therapist must also assist the veteran to contain, organize, and discharge potentially overwhelming trauma-related emotions (Lindy, 1985; Lindy, 1993a). The therapist's ability to hear and accept the trauma in tune with the veteran's natural recovery rate will enable the veteran to progressively review his or her war experiences. Psychotherapy will also help the veteran make sense of the traumatic experience by promoting the progressive integration of war memories with preexisting philosophical views and systems of belief (Horowitz, 1986; Lindy, 1993a).

The initial sessions of Bill's therapy provided him with a safe environment in which to tell his military story and guided him through a psychosocial assessment. The technical functions of his clinical assessment included

1. detecting the signs and symptoms of PTSD via the DSM-IV;
2. compiling and making intelligible the longitudinal history of the trauma and its aftermath;
3. distinguishing the effects of war trauma per se from other possibly associated disorders such as depression and/or substance abuse;
4. distinguishing the effects of adult war trauma from the possibly buried effects of earlier childhood trauma;
5. distinguishing the symptoms of war trauma from possibly preexisting personality disorders; and
6. assessing the level of functional impairment resulting to the veteran's work, family, and social life (Arnold, 1985; Blank, 1994).

During the assessment and throughout the course of the therapy, the therapist remained sensitive to the possible masking and/or misinterpretation of PTSD symptoms due to cultural differences between the therapist and the veteran. Differences in the cultural patterning of interpersonal communication, etiquette, deference, and demeanor, ideas about trauma and healing, and prohibitions against personal disclosures were all relevant in this regard.

Bill's therapy also involved a careful handling of the initial negative transference distortion of the therapist as a government prosecutor, facilitating a change to a transference based on the therapist as a fellow veteran. Facilitation of the latter transference was enhanced by the therapist's Vietnam veteran status. According to Lindy's psychodynamic conceptions, "Every facet of our appointment environment and every aspect of our personal interaction with the survivor is a potential starting point for the callback of traumatic memory" (Lindy, 1993b, p. 3). Identifying and understanding the specific, trauma-related landmarks in transference-bound reenactments is a main task of dynamic trauma therapy. The therapist and the veteran must work together to clarify how the current therapeutic situation, and the role of the therapist in the current situation, reflect the veteran's traumatic event.

Thus, further clarification of the meaning of Bill's traumatic reaction was revealed during a subsequent therapy session. The therapist noted that Bill was carrying a copy of the novel *Lord Jim* by Joseph Conrad. When asked how he liked the book, Bill said that it was one of his favorites and that he had read it three times since Vietnam. Further discussion revealed a parallel between Bill's Vietnam experience and the novel's main character. Like the story's hero, Bill also saw himself as an idealistic young soldier who had been misguided by his leaders and who had tragically abandoned his duty and failed those for whom he was responsible (his own men and the country he had joined the military to help). In addition, Bill was now drifting from port to port, engaging in menial tasks while trying to regain meaning and a redeeming sense of honor in his life.

Bill's experience of his role in the traumatic, tragic death of the young Vietnamese civilian induced an anguishing sense of shame related to what he perceived as an exposure of his inadequacy to lead in combat. Bill's prewar philosophy consisted of a rather rigid acceptance of the moral rightness of the world and an unquestioned sense of duty to serve its ideals and values. In this context, Bill experienced confusion after his father's less than full support of his enlisting in the army and volunteering for service in Vietnam. The core of Bill's trauma regarding this event consisted of his emotional and mental inability to encompass the dissonance between his prewar beliefs and expectations and the outcome of his actions on this particular occasion. Horowitz points out that stressful life events are, by definition, not in accord with a person's preexisting ideas of self and the world, and require integration through a process of successive comparisons with preexisting views (Horowitz, 1986).

After completion of Bill's planned brief psychotherapy, the therapeutic relationship was terminated by mutual consent. The therapeutic work in this case gave Bill the safety he needed to tell his story. Remembering and reconstructing its details entailed mourning the losses of the war, both American and Vietnamese, and led to acceptance of his own actions as a combatant. Finally, Bill was afforded the opportunity to incorporate his war experiences into his own life story. At the conclusion of the sessions, Bill was urged to take some time to work through further and digest what he had processed. He was also assured that he could return for additional sessions if and when he needed.

Individual Psychotherapy: A Case of Psychic Numbing

Joe was raised in a large, midwestern city by middle-class parents. He attended a state university and participated in the ROTC program during all four years of college. When he graduated in 1966, he was commissioned a second lieutenant in the U. S. Army. After attending the U. S. Army Infantry Branch School at Fort Benning, Georgia, he received orders for Vietnam. Joe served his first tour as an infantry platoon leader in the Mekong delta, and a second tour in 1971 as a Military Assistance for Command Vietnam (MACV) advisor to an Army of the Republic of Vietnam (ARVN) infantry unit. He recalled being pretty "gung-ho" about his first tour and thought seriously about a career in the army. However, he remembered a growing disillusionment which began about midway through his second tour. Joe was a highly decorated combat infantry officer when he returned home from his second tour, but he decided not to stay in the army.

Joe's presenting problem concerned his serious doubt about whether he would ever "feel human again" and he described himself as off in his own world watching others at a distance. He explained that his wife complained frequently about his lack of involvement with the family. In contrast to before the war, he did not feel connected to the everyday flow of social life and had lost hold of previously held expectations for family and career.

At a deeper, psychological level, Joe no longer had an adaptive sense of permanency and continuity about himself. He was experiencing fears about death which were associated with an intrusive visual image of a partially decayed human body lying face up on the earth in the bright sun. Exploring the Vietnam associations to this image, he recounted the following memories:

- Joe remembered the circumstances of his first view of a war casualty when he inspected several enemy soldiers who had been killed by Joe's platoon during an ambush the previous night. He recalled poignantly the bullet-ridden bodies, stiff limbs, and lifeless eyes. Feeling a nauseous sensation move up from his entrails, he heard himself say, "It's so final."

- During the latter part of his second tour, the ARVN unit Joe was assigned to as senior advisor was ordered to go out and retrieve a large number of enemy casualties for intelligence purposes. Joe and his ARVN counterparts had spent the previous two days in an engagement with several reinforced Viet Cong battalions. The fighting had been fierce and resulted in several hundred enemy dead. Lying where they had fallen in the field, the unburied enemy bodies were loaded on trucks and driven to regimental headquarters. There they were dumped onto the road until they could be examined for information. In addition, Joe had to help the ARVN soldiers disinter other bodies from shallow graves discovered from the air after the battle. The work was conducted under a hot tropical sun and many of the bodies were already black and bloated from exposure to the elements. Joe learned later that the ARVN command had ordered the bodies to be brought into the village for political reasons as well, i.e., as an example to local villagers of the fate of those who sympathized with the enemy.

Joe's fear of death was related to both the impact of his war experiences and to his postwar avoidance of normal family, career, and cultural activities, e.g., veteran-specific ceremonies such as Memorial and Veterans Day.

Although major depression and dysthymic disorder have some overlapping criteria with PTSD and are often comorbid with PTSD, what appears to be a depressed mood or attitude in veterans often, upon questioning, turns out to be trauma-related thoughts of existential despair or hopelessness about human nature and society. These thoughts result from a shattering of preexisting views about the basic rightness and/or transcendental permanency of life (Blank, 1994). In this context, Joe's war experiences shattered the psychological efficacy of his adaptive cultural symbols and exposed him to the raw realities of human death and finitude.

Joe's therapy focused on his fear of death, his loss of a personal sense of meaning, and his withdrawal from normal life activities. The therapist understood these difficulties to be various aspects of general social alienation and emotional constriction related to the avoidance symptoms of PTSD. Traumatized people tend to become withdrawn and distrustful; their sense of social reality diverges from that of the surrounding culture. The focus of Joe's therapy sessions paid special attention to what Herman refers to as the third phase of recovery, reconnecting the veteran with others in the veteran's environment (Herman, 1992). The goal of the work was to reestablish a functional connection between Joe, his community, and his culture. Achieving this goal also involved addressing Joe's trauma-distorted views through questioning and reexamining his assumptions about self, human nature, the meaning of life, and related issues. In therapy, Joe planned and accomplished the following social tasks:

- Visiting with his father to share and exchange military experiences and views about their respective wars
- Planning informal recreational activities with his wife and daughter
- Visiting the Vietnam Veterans Memorial with his wife
- Reading historical materials on the Vietnamese and the Vietnam war
- Investigating his own family history by visiting the graves of known ancestors and discussing the lives of deceased relatives with living relatives, with special attention paid to family members and ancestors who were veterans of wars in foreign lands

These tasks helped Joe reconnect to his historical context and reaffirm the significance of his own life.

Shortly before terminating his therapeutic relationship, Joe made a decision that had far-reaching consequences for his social functioning and involvement within the community. Joe joined the local post of a nationally chartered veterans organization. As an enthusiastic new member, he immediately became involved in the planning for a POW/MIA ceremonial parade and an all-night vigil at a local veterans memorial as part of the community's Veterans Day observances. Joe and his wife were instrumental in organizing the activities and galvanizing other members to participate. The therapist was also recruited to play a supportive role by being on hand for the parade and bringing coffee and food to those veterans and family members standing vigil through the night at the memorial. Without overly reflecting on the matter, Joe had become a veteran.

By the time he terminated therapy, Joe had gained a more adaptive adjustment to his social world by becoming more expressive of his ideas, more involved with his family and friends, and more interested in the affairs of the larger community. In addition, the counseling process gave Joe the time he needed to review his military experience, achieve a new understanding and appreciation of his service to his country, and to adopt his "veteran status" in a more meaningful way. Social ceremony and ritual gave cultural expression to the pain of war for Joe, while simultaneously recreating the anchors and connections which were necessary for providing his rites of passage to normal civilian human functioning (Warner, 1959). Culture provided Joe's mind with its coordinates in social space and historical time (Warner, 1959). Although the healing started in the clinic, Joe had to return to the arena of the social community for its full consummation.

The therapist used three global strategies to help Joe reconnect to his civilian social world:

1. Empathic repair of damaged self-identity
2. Guided reengagement in desired activities with family, friends, and community
3. Induced examination of cultural themes and values

These strategies were based on the perspective that human social reality consists of individual personalities, patterns of relationship combining personalities in various groups, and systems of socially significant ideas (culture) which give meaning to human action.

Joe's fear of death had become markedly attenuated as a result of supporting and facilitating his postwar reconnection to the normal social rhythms and cycles of the civilian community. The therapeutic equation for linking him to his traumatic memories also involved the empathic capacity of his therapist to grasp the psychological actuality of the traumatic experiences. Emotional comprehension of the existential horror related to grotesque human death in war was a main task for the therapeutic alliance. The culminating activity was Joe's visit to the Vietnam Veterans Memorial which assisted him in grieving his war losses and in making the transition to a veteran who was proud of his service.

Family Therapy: A Case of Alienation and Rebellion

Early on the morning following Rick's mediation session in juvenile court, his motorcycle was parked at the entrance to the therapist's office and Rick was slumped against the building. He had been drinking and was fighting back the tears. Very much afraid that other veterans would see him in an emotional condition, he was given refuge in the therapist's office. Socioeconomically, the community was predominately working class and there was a definite stigma attached to having psychological problems related to the war.

Rick related that he had been up all night with a loaded revolver as he walked the shoreline of a creek that ran behind his home. The thickly wooded area was situated between two bluffs that bordered the river into which the creek emptied. On warm summer evenings the area tended to became mist-filled, increasing its resemblance to the terrain in Vietnam.

Rick said that thinking about his daughter had overwhelmed him with anger and grief. Not knowing what to do, he secured his weapon and made his way to the creek to patrol the woods until dawn. Rick, at times, was openly emotional. The therapist interpreted this episode in the woods near Rick's home as a behavioral reenactment, reminiscent of his war trauma and triggered by his daughter's behavior, his own anger, and his subsequent fear of losing her.

After an initial period of working with the crisis situation, the therapist guided Rick through a brief military history and a retelling of a traumatic event that happened years earlier in Vietnam. Rick was the oldest of three and the only son in a rural, single-parent family. His father deserted the family when he was ten years old and his mother worked to support her children. Rick had been a dutiful son and had achieved good grades in school.

However, after his father's departure, his mother's dependence on him had become a problem. He thought that she was too strict, and at the same time, that she relied on him to keep the family together. Finally, as an older teenager, Rick rebelled against his mother's exacting demands and expectations by staying away from home whenever he could. After graduation from high school, he joined the army and volunteered for Vietnam.

While in military training, Rick met the young women who was to become his first wife. After she became pregnant, the couple was married just prior to his departure for Vietnam.

Rick arrived in Vietnam in early 1970 and was assigned to an infantry unit operating in the mountains in southern I Corps. He was promoted to NCO status after several months of successful performance in the field. Although he complained about the rigors of "orders" and "lifers" in the unit, Rick distinguished himself as an infantryman, enjoyed the excitement of patrolling, and often volunteered to walk point. During a routine patrol mission, the company commander ordered Rick's unit to move in support of another platoon held down by superior enemy fire on the opposite side of a dividing ridge line.

In carrying out these orders, Rick's platoon, the closest friendly element in the area, also came under heavy enemy fire, resulting in several wounded. Rick's best friend jumped out into the open to rescue the wounded, yelling to Rick to cover him with automatic weapon fire. Within feet of returning to safety, Rick's friend was decapitated by enemy automatic weapon rounds. By a twist of fate, Rick's weapon malfunctioned at the same time he witnessed his friend's death. Reacting in outrage and utter disbelief, he threw his weapon aside, stood up, and shouted curses at the enemy and was himself lightly wounded.

When he returned to duty after a brief hospitalization, he had lost his playfulness and easygoing attitude. He said that he had become quiet, serious, uncaring, and emotionally distant. Rick's view was that his own inadequacies were largely responsible for his friend's death and he could find no reasonable explanation for rationalizing this loss. The two had become friends early in the tour and their belief in each other and the omnipotence of their relationship had become rather magical. Superstitious about their mutual survival, each saw the other's survival as key to his own.

Returning from Vietnam in the spring of 1971 as a decorated combat veteran, Rick was anxious to get home to see his wife and baby daughter, born while he was in Vietnam. However, when he arrived, he found that his wife was living with another man and his daughter had been left in the care of neighbors. Rick said that he was ready to murder his wife and her boyfriend, but somehow found the strength to resist. Instead, with the help of his mother, he secured an attorney, sued for divorce, and won custody of his daughter based on a clear pattern of substance abuse and child neglect on the part of his ex-wife.

Subsequently, Rick moved to the community where his mother lived so that she could help him with parenting responsibilities. He rented an apartment and took a job as an industrial laborer. He had originally intended to maintain this employment only until he could settle on some sort of career direction. However, no such direction materialized and he started a rather itinerant lifestyle of going from one menial position to another. Underemployed, by comparison to his prewar interests and aptitudes, Rick was unable to stick with a job for long and was overly reactive to critical supervision.

To occupy himself between jobs, or when laid off, Rick bought himself the Harley-Davidson and began the routine of periodic bike trips. Rick's mother continued to help with his daughter and his closest associations were with a small group of male peers, some of whom were also veterans. Among his friends, Rick was known as a carefree and reckless independent spirit, not tied down and not afraid to take chances.

Rick's second marriage occurred after he met Mary. She was "not too pushy" and she understood and appreciated him. Also, she was a successful career woman and Rick admired her achievement, and he even thought that perhaps such a marriage could help him find some direction in life.

Although Rick presented in crisis with reexperiencing symptoms dominating the clinical picture at the time, his general postwar adjustment was primarily organized around PTSD symptoms of increased arousal and avoidance. Although Rick occupied himself with veteran-related activities and friends, he actively avoided thoughts and feelings associated with specific memories of his own combat experiences.

Rick was prone to exaggerated outbursts of anger at seemingly irrelevant occasions, subject to periods of sleeplessness, and had trouble focusing his attention on any one thing for very long. Mild feelings of confusion and uncertainty, lapses of memory, indecision, and inefficiency for tasks which were well-mastered before the war affected his ability to maintain gainful employment commensurate with his prewar potential.

He had lost hold of previously held goals for a higher education and a career in engineering. He described himself as feeling isolated and distant from normal people, "not fitting in with society." He experienced himself as inadequate, both as a father and a husband, because he could not seem to get his life together and could not show the attention and affection that his wife and child needed from him.

Rick's overall postwar social adjustment was a composite of several features. They included daring and reckless behavior such as impulsive fighting against unwinnable odds, irresponsible periods of social withdrawal and wandering, and provocative rebellion against authority figures. The first was a means to regain a sense of competence and mastery for dangerous undertakings; the latter two were a means to orient himself to a society toward which he felt ambivalent. Although provocative in appearance and demeanor, Rick's actions were actually passive, primarily designed to avoid any direct confrontations with authorities and control anger through distance. Rick resented his officers in Vietnam for their part in ordering his patrol into the situation which resulted in his friend's death. He no longer expected to experience a normal life of family and career, and disclosed that he felt far older than his thirty-four years, and that his hair and beard were "a means of hiding from himself."

In treatment, Rick agreed that more time was needed to talk through his Vietnam experiences, but said that he didn't feel free to do so until he resolved the pending difficulty with his daughter. In addition, he thought that his wife Mary should be involved, but he wasn't sure she would agree to help because she didn't get along with Sandy. The therapist instructed Rick to ask his wife to join him next time and added that, if he was unsuccessful, the therapist would call Mary and invite her to the session. When the therapist called Mary, she agreed to help her husband which, of course, was diagnostic about their marital relationship. Three sessions of introductory family therapy were planned to explore family relationships and to evaluate problems related to parenting Sandy.

According to Walsh (1983), clinical indication for family therapy requires adoption of a family relationship perspective, i.e., viewing individual problem behaviors as part of a system of mutually interacting personalities. This involves a shift of focus from the individual personality to family group structure and process, the social context in which the individual's behavior has function and meaning. "The symptom bearer, or identified patient, must be assessed in the family interactional context to understand what function the symptom may serve for the system" (Walsh, 1983, p. 471). The question of clinical indication, therefore, becomes a question of assessing the symptom-maintaining context of a specific problem. Wynne (1965) points out that family therapy should be considered for relationship difficulties to which each person in the family is contributing, either collusively or openly. Referring directly to the family relationships of Vietnam veterans, Haley (1984, p. 115) wrote, "as the time away from Vietnam lengthens, the stressful precipitants tend more and more to cluster around the interpersonal issues of closeness, marriage, and child rearing." The family therapist's task is complicated by the need to study family group structure and process simultaneously, in addition to the dynamic interplay of the beliefs and attitudes of each member in the family.

Thus, family treatment can be an important adjunct to direct treatment of the veteran to improve the clinical management of the effect of family relations on the course of the PTSD, as well as the impact of the veteran's PTSD on the quality of family relations. Family therapy was used to assist with Rick's postwar readjustment for the following reasons:

- A family problem was an integral component of the presenting problem.
- The presenting problem involved family violence directly related to the veteran's PTSD.
- Family relationships triggered a major posttrauma intrusive episode in the veteran.
- Rick requested family counseling to assist him in resolving current family problems prior to more intensive trauma work on his traumatic Vietnam experiences.
- Rick's traumatic war experiences were being reenacted in his nuclear family.
- Rick's PTSD avoidance symptoms were embedded in the structure of the family relationship system, and functioned to defensively contain and impede access to his psychological war trauma.

The family therapy was conducted in three sequential phases:

1. Preliminary exploration and assessment of family relationships with particular attention to the presenting problem
2. Restructuring of the marital relationship and the parental boundaries
3. Uncovering and overcoming traumatic memories

Three sessions were scheduled for assessment and preliminary exploration. Clinical assessment of the nuclear family is guided by the therapist's observation of family interactive patterns for signs of one or more possible categories of dysfunction:

1. Illness or social dysfunction in a spouse
2. Excessive and unproductive marital conflict
3. Impairment in one or more children (Kerr and Bowen, 1988)

The first session was conducted with all three family members and the latter two sessions were planned exclusively for the marital pair. The objective for the first session was to help elicit from each family member an understanding of the relationship system and how it related to the presenting problem and the veteran's PTSD.

The following family information was revealed in the family assessment interview:

1. Mary thought that Sandy and Rick were emotionally close to each other, but very distant toward her. Therefore, she felt shut out of their lives.

Mary said that Rick was not strong as a parent and that Sandy was disrespectful and needed more parental guidance. Mary added that she had tried by herself to guide the family, but felt like a single parent with two children.

2. According to Rick's view, his wife and daughter were always "at each other's throats" and he had to try continuously to settle things between them. When this often failed, he usually left on his bike until things cooled down. Rick added that he valued Mary's strength and abilities but thought that she was overly demanding and judgmental. He also stated that he was very worried that his daughter would leave home (as he had done). He wanted her to grow up to be a proper and accomplished young woman, but he was afraid "she would turn out bad" (like her own mother).

3. Sandy described a situation in which both parents were critical toward her. She said that she would like to have a better relationship with Mary, but that Mary was too busy and never listened to her. She felt guilty because she was not a better daughter to her father and more in compliance with his wishes. However, she said she was angry because her father did not listen to her side of things when she needed help or understanding.

The therapist's beginning assessment involved the following hypotheses about the structure of the relationship system:

1. Although it appeared harmonious and stable, the marital relationship was a rigid structure of inflexible boundaries, which kept the couple emotionally disengaged. In comparison to Mary's apparent overadequate functioning, Rick's social functioning was problematic, showing deficiencies for independent decision making and responsible leadership. This pattern of marital relationship has also been described for families with a depressed spouse (Feldman, 1976).

2. A second clinically significant feature of the family's organization was Sandy's apparent elevation into the parental hierarchy in covert alliance with her father against her stepmother. The boundary between parents and child was overly diffuse in this case, resulting in Sandy's having an enmeshed relationship with both parents. In relation to her father, this pattern included Sandy's functioning as a confidant and close ally. The relationship between Mary and Sandy took a different form and was punctuated with frequent episodes of conflict, often escalating into open fighting. These episodes could be triggered by either Mary's critical parenting or Sandy's provocative acting out, more characteristic of exchanges between two adults rather than between parent and child. Intergenerational blurring of boundaries and adolescent separation problems have been identified as common features in dysfunctional families (Lidz, 1963; Minuchin, 1974; Wynne, 1965).

3. Catherall (1997) notes that in families with a member with chronic PTSD, the afflicted member tends to reenact the trauma by pressing other family members into roles that re-create the relational aspects of the trau-

matic event. In relation to his Vietnam experiences, Rick's relationship to his daughter was a reenactment of the close attachment he had to his combat friend. In contrast, Rick's relationship with his wife more represented the attitude he maintained toward his commanding officers. The structure of the family system also functioned to serve Rick's posttraumatic avoidance tendencies. Structurally, the degree of emotional arousal and open fighting between Mary and Sandy allowed Rick to maintain a comfortable social distance. Dynamically, this interpersonal pattern allowed him to sustain denial about the impact of his war-related experiences, and contain intense trauma-related emotions of fear and rage. Thus, the presenting problem involved an episode of extreme emotional reactivity on Rick's part when Mary was not there to draw the emotional tension in her direction.

The last two sessions of this phase involved obtaining a detailed marital history from Rick and Mary, to gain a better understanding of the history and functioning of the marital relationship, and to shed light on other relevant areas of overlap between the current family system, the presenting problem, and Rick's PTSD symptoms. The following facts were revealed:

1. Rick admired Mary's competence, educational achievement, sense of direction, and take-charge attitude. He had thought that, through Mary's influence, he would be able to find direction in his own life.

2. Mary, on the other hand, was attracted to Rick's apparent easygoing, laissez-faire attitude, and his sense of daring and freedom. She anticipated that, by marrying Rick, she might learn how to relax.

3. However, in discussing their current relationship, Mary complained that she had to do everything because Rick took no responsibility. She felt as if she were the single mother of two children and, consequently, was lonely without a partner. Rick agreed that he couldn't seem to "get things together" and that he needed Mary to help "keep him in line". However, with some probing, he also revealed that he thought Mary was too critical and that she made decisions without taking his opinion into account. He wanted to enjoy the luxury of making mistakes without her judgmental critique.

4. Mary was the oldest responsible daughter in a family of three girls. Her mother was punitive and verbally abusive; her father was an alcoholic. Mary's mother tended to identify her with her alcoholic father saying, "You are just like him; you can't be trusted to do anything right." Mary was also the surrogate parental caretaker and grew up to be a rather typical rescuing adult child. However, in relation to her mother, she had identified with the aggressor and internalized rigid, perfectionist standards.

The second phase of the therapy included eight conjoint sessions. Drawing primarily on the structural family approaches of Minuchin (1974), the therapeutic goals were to increase the strength of the boundary around Rick and Mary, exclude Sandy from spousal transactions, and allow Rick to take on more of the parental functions. The therapist intervened to remove Sandy from inappropriate roles, enabled Rick and Mary to do their age-specific jobs, and assisted them as responsible adults to contain their mutual need satisfaction within their marital relationship (Catherall, 1997; Minuchin, 1974). It is interesting to note that Rick and Mary both functioned as parentified children in their respective families of origin. They each, however, adjusted to their roles by way of opposite defenses, i.e., Rick as a rebel and Mary as an overzealous caretaker.

Therapeutic family relationship work involves actively engaging both spouses in articulating and planning wished-for scripts and scenarios. The therapeutic setting also provides a safe environment for rehearsal of more mutually desirable behaviors on the part of both spouses, and an opportunity for negotiating the conditions under which each will agree to more permanently institute such behaviors.

Renewed hope and enhanced satisfaction provided the motivational impetus for these activities. Using the sessions as a safe forum, the therapist helped each partner (1) to express important needs and fears previously unexpressed, and (2) to listen to and respond to each other empathically. After planning, rehearsing, and contracting, Rick and Mary were mildly pressed toward independent performance, with a cautionary eye toward the vulnerabilities and worst fears of each partner. Helping them to stay focused and work collaboratively on problem solving during periods of emotional stress were major goals of the therapy.

Rick and Mary gained strength as a couple and improved their parenting skills. In addition, they made meaningful connections between Rick's Vietnam experience, the presenting problem, and his current family relationships. The therapist suggested that, perhaps, it was now a good time to resume talking about Rick's Vietnam experiences. The couple discussed this briefly, but weren't sure whether or not Rick should do this by himself. The therapist intervened and suggested that, perhaps, there was a way for the two of them to do this together, now that they had worked through some of their relationship problems.

The couple agreed to continue for five more sessions to work on uncovering and overcoming traumatic experiences from the past. Each two-hour session allowed both spouses sufficient time for psychological processing. The therapeutic focus shifted from the outside, the relationship system per se, to the inside, the traumatic experiences within each spouse's personality specific to their respective life experiences. These conjoint sessions further strengthened their marriage through the sharing of personal experiences and exchanging of empathic roles toward each other.

To this end, the sessions were split in half, each half devoted to one spouse's processing of traumatic memories with the therapist. The spouse not directly involved at the time was instructed not to intervene in any way, to listen attentively, and to record all salient thoughts and emotions in a notebook supplied by the therapist. At the beginning of the subsequent session, each spouse shared his or her recorded reactions from the previous session. The process was repeated five times.

The working-through phase for Rick focused on unresolved grief and annihilation anxiety related to the death of his combat friend, guilt and shame about the perceived inadequacy of his own actions in trying to save his friend's life, and anger at his superior officers as the responsible authorities. The working-through process with Mary focused on painful childhood experiences associated with having been the victim of abuse from one parent and the responsible caretaker of the other.

The relational aspects of Rick's traumatic combat experiences had become embedded within the structure of his current nuclear family. His family relationships functioned in the service of his avoidance symptoms to contain and deny painful combat memories. They also provided him with an arena in which to reenact an important, trauma-bound relationship with his tragically killed friend, a loss which he had not completely grieved. It was his daughter's disobedience that triggered his rage at authorities (whose orders he had not disobeyed in combat), and his fear of loss (related to the combat death of a valued friend engaged in carrying out orders). Rick's earlier, prewar life history also involved unresolved grief and anger. His father's abandonment of the family, and Rick's subsequent doubt about himself as the possible reason for his father's actions, continued to resonate in theme with his combat trauma and his current family relationships.

Within the year following his termination from counseling, Rick sold his Harley-Davidson so that he could spend more time with his family and enrolled for night courses in science and math at the local community college. He and Mary established a closer alliance and did more things together, and Sandy became increasingly involved with her peers, male as well as female.

SUMMARY AND CONCLUSIONS

These examples illustrate the process of psychotherapy for war-related PTSD: the telling of the story before, during, and after the traumatic event or events. During this process, the therapist helped the veterans to make connections between current symptoms and troubling behaviors and the actual events of war experiences. Important adjuncts to psychotherapy are understanding and intervening in the community on behalf of the veteran and engaging the veteran's family in the treatment process. Community and family are the social environments in which postwar functioning takes place. Also, veterans' roles as soldiers and as veterans are functions of citizenship in a democratic community. Trauma services for war veterans should not be provided in a psychological vacuum.

Psychotherapy outcomes are impacted by the therapist's use of self and relationship. Although war veterans may be eager to receive assistance to help them contain and process troubling reminders of their experiences, they will, nonetheless, remain fearful of, and resistant to, the emotional effects of remembering their trauma. Confiding in a therapist is a risk for the veteran; it entails trust in the therapist's motives and level of acceptance. The latter may even be more important than the veteran's confidence in the therapist's expert knowledge and credentials (Lindy, 1988). Professional credentials, although necessary to ensure the technical quality of the services provided, may ironically undermine the customer-satisfaction aspect of the therapeutic relationship. Overidentification by clinicians with professional credentials may set in motion a detrimental status hierarchy between the expert clinician and the veteran client. A kind of professional chauvinism can develop, exaggerating the in-group versus out-group distinctions between service providers and those they serve. When operative, this attitude will likely be transmitted to veteran consumers as dismissive arrogance. The therapist may have to proceed patiently, not pushing overly hard for trauma details, while possibly having to tolerate repeated testing of his or her reactions and motives by the veteran before a trusting working alliance can be established. As pointed out by Catherall and Lane (1992), one of the advantages of having a war-veteran therapist treat a war-veteran client is the increased potential for developing rapport and a more ready engagement of the veteran in treatment.

E. H. Erikson (1945), a nonphysician lay analyst, spent much of his clinical practice during World War II seeing combat returnees at the Veterans Rehabilitation Clinic of Mount Zion Hospital in San Francisco. He used his clinical work with war veterans to reintroduce environmental factors (to include traumatic experiences) into the psychological equation for understanding adult adjustment. Erikson's comments from his work with war veterans validate the importance of a relatively informal, trusting therapeutic relationship, and of the value of veterans treating veterans:

> The administration of the help given should be locally centralized so that the veteran will not feel "pushed around" and "up against red tape" when asking for a little assistance. The assistance should be handled, not by the impersonal representatives of organizations, but by specially selected people who have a direct, informed, and resourceful approach and preferably are themselves veterans of this or the First World War. (Erikson, 1945, p. 121)

REFERENCES

American Psychiatric Association (1994). *Diagnostic and statistical manual of mental disorders,* Fourth edition. Washington, DC: American Psychiatric Association.

Arnold, A. L. (1985). Diagnosis of post-traumatic stress disorder in Vietnam veterans. In S. Sonnenburg et al. (Eds.), *The trauma of war: Stress and recovery in Vietnam veterans,* 101-123. Washington, DC: American Psychiatric Press.

Blank, A. S. (1994). Clinical detection, diagnosis, and differential diagnosis of post-traumatic stress disorder. In D. A. Tomb (Ed.), *The psychiatric clinics of North America,* 351-383. Philadelphia: W.B. Saunders.

Catherall, D. R. (1989). Differentiating intervention strategies for primary and secondary trauma in post-traumatic stress disorder: The example of Vietnam veterans. *Journal of Traumatic Stress, 2*(3), 289-304.

Catherall, D. R. (1997). Family treatment when a member has PTSD. *Department of Veterans Affairs National Center for Post-Traumatic Stress Disorder Clinical Quarterly, 7*(2), 17-21.

Catherall, D. R. and C. Lane (1992). Warrior therapist: Vets treating vets. *Journal of Traumatic Stress, 5*(1), 19-36.

Erikson, E. H. (1945). Plans for the returning veteran with symptoms of instability. In L. Wirth (Ed.), *Community planning for peacetime living,* (pp. 120-125). Stanford: Stanford University Press.

Feldman, L. B. (1976). Depression and marital interaction. *Family Process,* 15, 389-395.

Gelsomino, J. and D. W. Mackey (1988). Clinical interventions in emergencies: War-related events. In M. Lystad (Ed.), *Mental health responses to mass emergencies,* 211-238. New York: Brunner/Mazel.

Haley, S. A. (1984). The Vietnam veteran and his preschool child: Child rearing as a delayed stress in combat veterans. *Journal of Contemporary Psychotherapy, 14*(1), 114-121.

Hamilton, G. (1951). *Theory and practice of social casework.* New York: Columbia University Press.

Herman, J. L. (1992). *Trauma and recovery.* New York: Basic Books.

Horowitz, M. J. (1986). *Stress response syndromes.* New York: Jason Aronson.

Kardiner, A. and H. Spiegel (1947). *War stress and neurotic illness.* New York: Hoeber.

Kerr, M. and M. Bowen (1988). *Family evaluation.* New York: Norton.

Lebowitz, L., M. R. Harvey, and J. L. Herman (1993). A stage-by-dimension model of recovery from sexual trauma. *Journal of Interpersonal Violence, 8*(3), 378-391.

Lidz, T. (1963). *The family and human adaptation.* New York: International Universities Press.

Lindy, J. D. (1985). The trauma membrane and other clinical concepts derived from psychotherapeutic work with survivors of natural disasters. *Psychiatric Annals, 15*(3), 153-160.

Lindy, J. D. (1988). *Vietnam: A casebook.* New York: Brunner/Mazel.

Lindy, J. D. (1993a). Focal psychoanalytic psychotherapy of post-traumatic stress disorder. In J. P. Wilson (Ed.), *International handbook of traumatic stress syndromes.* New York: Plenum Press.

Lindy, J. D. (1993b). PTSD and transference. *Department of Veterans Affairs National Center for Post-Traumatic Stress Disorder Clinical Quarterly, 3*(2), 1-4.

Mead, G. H. (1934). *Mind, self and society.* Chicago: University of Chicago Press.

Minuchin, S. (1974). *Families and family therapy.* Cambridge: Harvard University Press.

Perlman, H. H. (1957). *Social casework: A problem solving process.* Chicago: University of Chicago Press.

Perlman, H. H. (1968). *Persona: Social role and personality.* Chicago: University of Chicago Press.

Shibutani, T. (1961). *Society and personality.* Englewood Cliffs, NJ: Prentice-Hall.

Walsh, F. (1983). Family therapy: A systematic orientation to treatment. In A. Rosenblatt and D. Waldfogel (Eds.), *Handbook of clinical social work,* 466-489. San Francisco: Jossey-Bass.

Warner, W.L. (1959). *The living and the dead: A study of the symbolic life of Americans.* New Haven: Yale University Press.

Warner, W. L. and P. S. Lunt (1941). *The social life of a modern community.* New Haven: Yale University Press.

Wynne, L. C. (1965). Some indications and contraindications for exploratory family therapy. In I. Boszormenyi-Nagy and J. L. Framo (Eds.), *Intensive family therapy: Theoretical and practical aspects,* 289-322. New York: Harper and Row.

SECTION VI:
MEDIA ISSUES

Chapter 17

A Primer on Interviewing Victims

Frank Ochberg

INTRODUCTION

Whenever a reporter meets a survivor of traumatic events, there is a chance that the journalist will witness—and may even precipitate—posttraumatic stress disorder. Therefore, it is important that working journalists (including grizzled veterans) anticipate PTSD, recognize it, and report it, while earning the respect of the public and those interviewed. The recognition of PTSD and related conditions enhances not only a reporter's professionalism, but also the reporter's humanitarianism.

What Is PTSD?

PTSD is three reactions at one time, all caused by an event that terrifies, horrifies, or renders one helpless. The triad of disabling responses is

1. recurring intrusive recollections;
2. emotional numbing and constriction of life activity; and
3. a physiological shift in the fear threshold, affecting sleep, concentration, and sense of security.

This syndrome must last at least a month before PTSD can be diagnosed. Furthermore, a severe trauma must be evident and causally related to the cluster of symptoms. Some people are fearful, withdrawn, and plagued by episodes of vague, troubling sensations, but they cannot identify a specific traumatic precipitant. PTSD should only be diagnosed when an event of major dimension—a searing, stunning, haunting event—has clearly occurred and is relived, despite strenuous attempts to avoid the memory.

A version of this chapter appeared in *Nieman Reports,* Fall 1996, 1(3), pp. 21-26, published by The Nieman Foundation at Harvard University.

Intrusive Recollections

The core feature of PTSD, which distinguishes the condition from anxiety or depression, is the unavoidable echo of the event, often vivid, occasionally so real that it is called a flashback or hallucination. The survivor of a plane crash feels a falling sensation, revisualizes the moment of impact, then fears going crazy because his or her mind and body return uncontrollably to that harrowing scene. A victim of the "cooler bandit," whose modus operandi was to rob urban convenience stores at gunpoint and force the clerks into refrigerated storage rooms, had nightmares for more than a year.

Emotional Anesthesia Constricting Life Activity

Numbing may protect a person from overwhelming distress between memories, but it also robs a person of joy and love and hope. Numbing and avoidance are less prominent, less visible, and less frequent than the more dramatic memories and anxieties. Early on, most survivors of trauma will consciously avoid reminders and change familiar patterns to prevent an unwanted recollection. Numbing and avoidance are adaptive to a point, then become a serious impediment to recovery. They can also mislead an interviewer of a survivor into seriously underestimating the severity of a traumatic event. Popular belief suggests that victims of rape, kidnapping, and other violent crimes should be full of feeling, tearful, shuddering, even hysterical, after the assailant leaves. When feelings are muted, frozen, or numb, the survivor may not be believed. When testimony in court is mechanical and unembroidered, jurors may assume that damages were minimal or never inflicted.

This dimension of PTSD includes psychogenic amnesia. Along with the loss of emotional tone and limited life pursuits, are holes in the fiber of recollection. For example, an opera singer, battered by her husband, could not recall the most serious beatings. She was finally ready to divorce and needed to testify in court at a settlement hearing. After several supportive sessions, she remembered his choking, almost strangling her. Eventually, all the memories returned and she could joke, "He not only threatened my life but my livelihood. No wonder I put that out of my mind."

Lowered Threshold

This response is physiological. Unexpected noises cause the traumatized person to shudder or jump. The response is automatic and not necessarily related to stimuli associated with the original trauma. It is as though the alarm mechanism that warns of danger is on a hair trigger, easily and erroneously set off. A traumatized person lives with so many false alarms that he or she cannot concentrate, cannot sleep restfully, and becomes irritable or re-clusive. A normal sex life is difficult with such apprehension. PTSD there-fore impairs the enjoyment of intimacy, and this, in turn, isolates the sufferer from loved ones—the ideal human source of reassurance and respect.

Often, anxiety takes familiar shape: panic and agoraphobia. Panic is a sudden, intense state of fear, frequently with no obvious trigger, in which the heart beats rapidly, respirations quicken and are shallow, and fingertips tingle. Light-headedness occurs. Sensations of choking or smothering may be experienced and the person may feel that he or she is dying or going crazy or both. After a few panic attacks, a person will often suffer agoraphobia, avoiding places such as shopping malls and supermarkets, where an attack would be particularly embarrassing.

PTSD not only has a variety of dimensions and components, but has vastly different effects and implications. Some trauma survivors are contin-ually reminded of their victimization and experience relief when they tell the details to others. Some survivors are humiliated by their dehumanization or laden with guilt for harming another person and may refuse to discuss de-tails. Some are dazed, moving in and out of trancelike states. Some are full of fear, hypervigilant, easily started, unable to concentrate, wary of strang-ers. The syndrome may be evident soon after the trauma, or may emerge years later.

Who Gets PTSD?

Most current research shows that the intensity and duration of traumatic events correlates positively with the occurrence of PTSD. However, individ-uals exposed to the same extreme stress will vary in their responses. Hered-ity could play an important role. Just as some children are born shy and oth-ers exhibit a bolder temperament, some individuals are born with the brain pattern that keeps horror alive, while others quickly recover. As a varied, in-terdependent human species, human beings benefit from these differences. Those with daring temperaments fight the tigers. Those with PTSD preserve the impact of cruelty for the rest. There is nothing abnormal about those who suffer; anyone could develop PTSD given enough trauma.

A GUIDE TO INTERVIEWING

An understanding of post-traumatic stress disorder is vital to journalists in their coverage of the way in which victims experience emotional wounds, particularly wounds that are deliberately and cruelly inflicted. A relatively new area of clinical science, traumatic stress studies, teaches that victims of violence have several distinguishable patterns of emotional response. These patterns are easily recognized once their outlines are understood. Seeing the logic in a set of psychological consequences rehumanizes and dignifies a person who may feel dehumanized and robbed of dignity. A sensitive explanation of the traumatic stress response aids recovery. Journalists can report on victims, help victims as multidimensional human beings, and possibly, just possibly, reduce the impulse toward vengeance in the process.

Timing

When reporters seek a trauma survivor's comments soon after the event, they have a high likelihood of encountering one or more of the emotional states mentioned. As time passes, there is a greater possibility of emotional composure. But, there is also a possibility of distorted recollection, selective memory, and competition from many other interviewers, each with a different agenda, each raising new questions in the mind of the person interviewed. Therefore, even from a psychiatric point of view, there is no formula for setting the ideal time for a posttraumatic interview.

For example, a reporter has access to a clerk who was robbed at gunpoint an hour ago. She appears uninjured. The reporter begins, "Have you had a chance to discuss this with anyone else?" The response will tell the reporter where the interview is in the predictable sequence of police investigations, insurance and management inquiries, and conversations with family, friends, and others, including other reporters. It also allows the reporter to follow up with questions about those discussions, if they occurred. An interviewee reveals a lot about conversational preferences when given the chance. For example, he or she might indicate a desire to talk at length, to be brief and to the point, to learn about the incident from the reporter, or to get away from the scene—all in response to an open-ended question such as, "How was the previous discussion for you?"

The reporter then can set the stage for the interview, having assessed the subject's attitude and emotional state before he or she regards the reporter as being responsible for his or her feelings. One technique for the reporter is to have subjects focus on how someone else made them feel.

A very different interview would occur on the one-year anniversary of a major catastrophe, such as the Oklahoma City bombing. In this instance, the reporter is assigned to interview a survivor who now lives outside Oklahoma in the reporter's small town. The reporter telephones to arrange a meeting. This story, a year, rather than an hour later, deals with emotions throughout that year and on this anniversary date. The incident is now less important than the impact of the incident on one individual through time. The interview may—probably will—cause vivid recollections. Should the reporter mention this impact over the phone? Or does the reporter assume that a willingness to be interviewed signifies a willingness to revisit painful memories?

A feature story, in contrast to a news story, gives the reporter more flexibility to arrange the time and place and to decide to meet once or on several occasions. Still, the journalist may be the cause of emotional injury, since this person was exposed to major traumatic stress and has reached some new adjustment state that the interview may (will) disrupt. In a way, this is a more delicate, difficult situation.

Setting the Stage

Setting the stage is important regardless of the timing of the interview. A trauma survivor should be approached with respect, neither gingerly nor casually. This person has witnessed and lived through a newsworthy event outside normal experience and has something to share with the community. This person will undertake some reexposure to traumatic memories by talking with the reporter. If the reporter conveys respect for this situation, then he or she is off to a good start.

Consider the possibility that a survivor might be more comfortable at home or might want to be out of the family circle. Some might feel more secure with a friend or relative. The clerk robbed at gunpoint probably would be encountered first at the convenience store. But, if she had the authority to leave, to be joined by a friend, the reporter might get more details and more spontaneity than if that reporter stayed at the scene of the crime. Of course, a deadline might preclude taking the extra hour to learn about the emotional impact of the robbery on the witness/victim. Obviously, removing someone to a comfortable, secluded place, enhances concentration and reduces the chance of interruption.

Interviewing people as a Red Cross volunteer at disaster sites is more like the field conditions journalists encounter. When serving in that capacity, the reporter should set the stage as best as he or she can, and try to assess quickly whether a person wants privacy or the proximity of others and whether the comfort level is greater with the door open or closed. One woman preferred to sit on the floor, surrounded by her soggy belongings, as she sought help at a shelter after the 1994 northern California floods. This woman was agoraphobic before the floods, more so afterward, and her trust was earned by bringing social workers and small business loan specialists to her, rather than have her join the crowd in a busy service center.

When setting the stage for an interview, a reporter should remember that the person may be in a daze, numb, easily startled, hypervigilant, or confused. The victim can usually tell the reporter the setting that will suit him or her best. This may require a companion, an open door, and several breaks for self-composure.

Eliciting Emotion

As an interviewer, the reporter can either elicit or avoid emotion. Does the reporter want to see and hear a person's emotional state or does he or she want the individual to describe his or her feelings without displaying them? A person can say, "I was very upset, crying all the time, unable to work," or that individual can sob as he or she speaks.

Most reporters would prefer to have their interviewees describe rather than display strong emotions (TV talk-show hosts excepted) in initial interviews with trauma survivors. The ultimate objective is to help the survivor master uncontrolled feelings. Therefore, the reporter may say, for example, "We can, if possible, defer dealing with the full impact of the event until we know each other better, until some progress has been made."

At other times, for example, when debriefing Red Cross volunteers, the debriefer will want to see strong feelings, if they are present, to get them talked out before the volunteers have gone home (and to show respect for the person and for his or her emotions). That is the point of the debriefing. But, journalists are not PTSD therapists or after-incident crisis debriefers. They are interviewing a witness who will become the subject of a story.

From an ethical point of view, the reporter should afford the interviewee as much control and foreknowledge as possible. This can be done by explaining the journalistic objectives. For example, the reporter might begin, "I'm really interested in the facts of the robbery. I know this may be upsetting right after it happened, but I won't be reporting on how he made you feel." However, if the reporter's intention is otherwise, he or she could say, ". . . and I am interested in how he made you feel, then and now. Readers need to know what kind of impact these events have and I thank you for being willing to describe them."

It is not uncommon for tears to flow during the telling of an emotional event. Therapists usually offer tissues and say, "I'm accustomed to hearing people while they are crying, so don't worry about me." This neither urges nor discourages someone from continuing to talk, but does try to normalize the situation. Thus, reporters, as well, should bring tissues if a tearful interview is anticipated.

When survivors cry during interviews, they are not necessarily reluctant to continue. They may have difficulty communicating, but they often want to tell their stories. Interrupting them may be experienced as patronizing and as denying an opportunity to testify. Remember, terminating an interview unilaterally, because the reporter finds it upsetting or because the reporter incorrectly assumes that the subject wants to stop, may revictimize the victim.

Some people who have suffered greatly—for example, political torture victims in Chile—have benefited psychologically from the opportunity to provide testimonials; those testimonials have been substantiated by research. Members of the Michigan Victim Alliance, who serve as interviewees for the journalism students at Michigan State University, reported some PTSD symptoms (anxiety and intrusive recollections for one or two days), and an overall increase in self-esteem after an interview because their stories had been heard. The facts had been told with considerable depth of feeling. The issue is not about the journalist attempting to control subjects' emotions but, rather, how can that journalist best facilitate a factual, full report, while giving the interviewee a sense of respect throughout.

Informed Consent

Should journalists offer the equivalent of a Miranda warning? "You have a right to remain silent. Anything you say can and will (especially if it is provocative or embarrassing to somebody important) be used on the front page."

That approach would not work. However, the medical model of informed consent could be adapted for interviews with trauma victims. The reporter might explain, "This procedure—interview and article—has benefits for the community and may benefit you. Remembering, however, may be painful for you. And your name will be used. You might have some unwanted recollections after talking and after the story appears. In the long run, telling your story should be a positive thing. Any questions before we begin?"

STAGES OF RESPONSE

The first set of responses after shocking events involves the pathways of the autonomic nervous system, connecting the brain, the pituitary gland, the adrenal gland, and various organs of the body. Blood is shunted from the gut to the large muscles. The pupils dilate. The pulse accelerates and the stroke volume of the heart increases. These physiological changes, shared by all mammals, prepare us for fight or flight. It puts us in a state of readiness for dealing with the threats that our ancestors faced on the great plains of Africa: wild beasts, sudden storms, deadly enemies. Humans are not adapted for fine motor movements, nor for deep, conscious thought. The surge of adrenaline and pounding heart experienced when the car skids on an icy highway does not help to maneuver that piece of machinery. Humans' danger biochemistry is atavistic. Humans have to fight their bodily changes as they respond to modern mechanical dangers, such as a high-speed skid.

Perceptual changes occur as well. The focus on a source of danger, be it a wild beast or a pointed pistol, is intensified. Objects in peripheral vision begin to blur, a function not only of the organs of perception, but the result of how impulses are received, recorded, and analyzed in the brain. Detectives, doctors, and journalists all know the implications of this phenomenon: details are notoriously distorted, except for a few central features, when eyewitnesses report from incidents of threat and sudden danger.

Sometimes, a powerful threat is prolonged, as in a hostage incident, a kidnapping, some assaults, and some rapes. Many natural disasters—a flash flood or hurricane—may place an individual in mortal danger for hours rather than seconds or minutes. Short, deadly traumas include gunshots, explosions, earthquakes, and fires. When extreme stress is prolonged for days or weeks, adaptive mechanisms collapse. In such cases, in animal experiments, mammals suffer hemorrhagic necrosis of the adrenal gland—literally, a bloody death of that organ and, soon after, death of the organism itself.

In contrast, humans in states of prolonged catastrophic stress enter a second stage of adaptation. Hans Selye (1997), a physiologist whose stress studies guided the modern era, called this a stage of resistance following a stage of shock. During prolonged, catastrophic stress, the organism enters a state of high gain, accustomed to the increased flow of adrenaline, consciously appraising what had previously been grasped automatically. For example, at this point, a crime victim knows that he or she is a victim, although the person may still be thinking, "This can't be happening to me." At this point, details become evident, particularly to the trained observer. In group hostage situations, there is often a ritual calm, when confusion and feelings of threat diminish. This may be the time when negotiations may be successful.

Disaster workers recognize a heroic phase, a second stage after the initial bedlam, when all is shock and confusion. In the second stage, people help one another, lives are saved, lost children are found. Hope and exhilaration coexist with fear and grief. Eventually, there is a return to some equilibrium in the body, the mind, and the community. This may be a time of depression and demoralization. The high energy condition is gone. There is debris, loss, and pain. Reality sinks in. This is also the time when the press leaves. A survivor who might have been annoyed by too much attention now could feel abandoned and forgotten.

A journalist may want to consider the particular sequence of stages or phases that an interviewee has experienced, where that person is, and how each stage affects his or her perception of events. A discussion of stages may help the interview process, without actually "leading the witness." The reporter might consider saying, "Sometimes people go through a stage when they act without thinking, when they don't even know what is happening," and the reporter may elicit an interesting narrative. Some people need to be reminded that they acted instinctively. Then they can recall what occurred just before that phase and right afterward.

The victim who was thrown to the floor by the "cooler bandit" recalled, months later, that she hid her wedding ring under a shelf as she lay in the fetal position, expecting to be shot. She forgot that particular event during the time she was experiencing fear and shame and all of the diagnostic PTSD symptoms. Of special note was her instinctive protection of a valuable symbol, her refusal to yield that icon to her assailant. This woman was full of self-blame for not sounding the secret alarm, for behaving as a coward. Her therapy required a diligent search for evidence to the contrary, proof that would convince *her.* The therapist in this case was already certain that she had done what any reasonable person would have done to survive an armed robbery. She recalled hiding her ring as she talked about the instinctive, automatic things that some people do and finally agreed that her instincts were correct.

THE HUMANITARIAN ROLE OF THE REPORTER

Journalists and therapists face similar challenges when they realize that their subjects are at risk of further injury. Techniques may differ, but objectives are the same: to inform about sources of help. A therapist is not a lawyer or a security consultant but a battered woman and an abused child need to know that shelters, restraining orders, and a network of advocates are available. Therapy includes such referrals. The reporter is not responsible for individual referrals, but could include sidebars about community resources when interviewing individuals who typify the kinds of victims who would benefit from such resources.

Journalists can also mobilize colleagues in the helping professions when they come upon problems that appear neglected. Ed Chen, a reporter for the *Los Angeles Times,* called this author twice in recent years, not just for quotes about PTSD, but for help with neglected problems. Ed also covered the Gulf War. Before becoming the Dhahran bureau chief, he interviewed wives of prisoners that had been used as human shields. Many of these women were Middle Eastern and were sent for resettlement and asylum to cities in the United States where they had no family, friends, or resources. Their mental health needs were considerable, and there was no federal agency equipped to help them. Several therapists, inspired in part by Ed's reporting and his requests, established an ad hoc charity, USA Give (Leslie Kern, PhD, Director). Fifty trauma experts donated free care to eighty individuals through this charity. Ed benefited also. He had a place on the plane when a delegation of "wives of shields" flew to Baghdad to petition Saddam Hussein for the release of their husbands.

SECONDARY TRAUMATIC STRESS DISORDER

Journalists are candidates for secondary traumatic stress disorder, an empathic response, which occurs when professional detachment is overwhelmed by certain life events. For example, images of dead children leave an indelible mark. Firefighters, who would rather not admit that they have tender feelings, find themselves vulnerable to the haunting memories of a burnt child or the sight of a tiny form in a body bag.

The sheer numbers of unexpected dead in one place will penetrate the defenses of hardened rescue workers. Plane crashes rank among the most difficult assignments for American Red Cross workers who normally handle floods, earthquakes, and fires. At an air disaster, there is a concentration of death images that few doctors, nurses, or ambulance drivers have ever seen.

In writing about journalists covering Rwanda, Roger Rosenblatt mused (1994):

> Most journalists react in three states. . . . when they are young, they respond to atrocities with shock and revulsion and perhaps a twinge of guilty excitement. . . . In the second stage, the atrocities become familiar and repetitive . . . . If you have seen one loss of dignity and spirit, you've seen them all. . . . Embittered, spiteful, and inadequate to their work. . . they hate the people on whom they report. . . . they don't allow themselves to enter the third stage in which everything gets sadder and wiser, worse and strangely better.

CONCLUSIONS

In one or two decades, PTSD will be universally recognized, destigmatized, and well-treated. To be dazed at first, then haunted by horrible memories, and made anxious and avoidant is to be part of the human family. When deliberate criminal cruelty is the cause of PTSD, journalists and others often neglect the victim and become captives of collective outrage, focusing attention on crime and criminality and those who are to blame. Discussing PTSD disarms PTSD. Discussing does not prevent it but it does minimize its degrading, diminishing effects. Discussing (and reporting) PTSD helps victims become survivors, and helps those survivors to regain dignity and respect.

REFERENCES

Rosenblatt, R. (1994). *The New Republic, 210*(4142), June 6, pp. 14-16.

Selye, H. (1997). Foreword. In *The Stress Doctor*, p. 1, Available online: <stress@stressdoctor.com>.

Chapter 18

Relating to Journalists As Trauma Clinicians and Researchers

Richard Hébert

Researchers and clinicians face quite distinct challenges when relating to journalists. Researchers need to get journalists interested in what journalists are learning about people's reactions to trauma; clinicians probably wish they could be left alone to work with patients, especially when entire communities are traumatized and journalists are out looking for someone from whom to get a sound bite. Some research scientists believe that their duty ends when they have done their work meticulously, submitted it to peer review, and published it in a worthy journal. They believe that they have no continuing responsibility to talk to reporters about that work. However, both researchers and clinicians need to think about the mass media as an ally. Whether a researcher or a clinician, the goal is to get what one knows about human reactions to traumatic events reported to the public—reported accurately so that people can make informed decisions about their own health and about public health policies.

WHY COOPERATE?

Why should clinicians and researchers cooperate with journalists who are, after all, only going to misquote them, quote them out of context, get the information all confused, and totally miss the point of what has been told to them? Timothy Ferris, in *The Informal Science Review* (May-June 1997) summarizes just why traumatologists should be talking with journalists about what they do. He says it is important to encourage scientists to communicate to the general public. Taxpayers supporting scientific research have the right to know. Also, when scientists popularize themselves through ordinary language, more people can understand what they are doing. Ernest Rutherford admonished that a theory that cannot be explained to a bartender "is probably no damn good" (Ferris, 1997).

The following are further reasons why cooperation is desirable:

1. *The public wants good health information.* More than that, the public is *hungry* for information, especially in an area that affects them personally—their health. Look at all the health magazines on newsstands and at checkout counters, health reports on TV and radio talk shows, and weekly health sections in most large daily newspapers. People should be getting good health information, not quackery or pop psychology. But if those who have the knowledge don't share it, pop psychology is all that the public will get.

2. *The public pays for most research with tax dollars.* Taxpayers are owed an accounting of what is being done with their money.

3. *Continued research funding depends on public support.* If research is not explained in the open market of ideas, researchers cannot expect to compete effectively in that same marketplace when it comes time to ask for increased, or even sustained, investment in that research.

4. *Researchers have a stake in accurate reporting.* Do not expect journalists to "get it right" if those who know the material best—researchers and clinicians—do not take the time to explain it to them. Reporters come in all flavors, from downright awful to excellent, but most of them would at least meet Garrison Keillor's definition of the children of Lake Wobegon—above average. Yet just think what story some below-average reporter would write if he or she did not have the benefit of knowledge from clinicians and researchers.

5. *No paper ever saved a life sitting on a dusty shelf.* Promoting the findings of research is a critical step in the health care process. The more that people know about how to restore and maintain their health, the better armed they will be to be active partners in their own health care.

Journalists can offer clinicians a pulpit to educate and calm an entire community after a tragic event, and to redirect its anguish and painful cries for revenge and blame-placing into more benign and even positive channels. If reporters do not come to clinicians after the bombing of a federal office building or the demolition of a city by a hurricane or an earthquake, clinicians should seek out the journalist to offer calming knowledge and insights. Clinicians might even write a letter to the editor or a commentary for the op-ed page of the local newspaper.

RECOGNIZING NEWSWORTHINESS

Not every research finding and not every clinician's comment is a news story. So the question arises: how to recognize newsworthiness? What makes one piece of knowledge worth telling in a newspaper or on TV? The following rules and basic elements are important when the journalist makes that decision.

Rule number one is *never lose sight of what the reporter wants.* Reporters are trained to ask three things and three things only. They find a thousand ways to ask them, but it still boils down to these questions:

1. What is the problem?
2. What needs to be done about it?
3. So what? What does this mean to people—to the readers and/or viewers?

To help determine whether the research has news value, consider this simple list of the basic elements of news.

Is it personal?

News affects people's lives or pocketbooks; the more people it affects and the greater the effect it has on them, the more news value it has. This is why wars and crime waves are news, and reporters want traumatologists to talk when something awful happens in the community. What the traumatologist has to say at times such as these is news because it professionally touches people's lives. News can also be personal in a way that touches people's emotions. This is why health-related news stories so often start with a heart-wrenching account of someone who is suffering or has triumphed over the condition being reported.

Is it controversial?

Most news stories are about controversy. The hotter and more public the controversy, the hotter the news.

Does it involve victims and devils?

The victim is always the little guy; the devil is always a Goliath. Although it is always wrong to generalize, what is prevalent in the media today is an assumption that government—that all large institutions—will screw up and hurt little people. This is part of journalistic cynicism. Big is impersonal and, therefore, likely to do damage. This condition has now helped turn the United States into a nation of distrusting cynics.

Is it unusual?

The unexpected outcome is newsworthy. The predictable is not. People committing suicide to join a comet-tailing UFO, microbes on Mars, Hillary's chats with Eleanor (an astrologist), Nancy Reagan's astrologer: these stories made headlines because they were far from what was expected.

Is it new?

News is new. It is something that just happened or, better yet, is about to happen. It is a breakthrough finding. Here, behavior and health research have a bit tougher time because so much of what is done and learned is incremental and inferential. Typically, psychosocial factors are "associated with" and don't "cause" diseases. They are hard to pin down. That is why some of a clinician's/researcher's best friends are three little words: "Preliminary findings suggest . . ."

Is it timely?

Is the finding related to something already "in the news"? If so, it can get timeliness by association. The bigger the news hook, the more timeliness a story derives from that hook. When reporters call clinicians for comment, it is probably all too tragically timely because something terrible has just happened. That is when a traumatologist can truly serve humanity by allying himself or herself with the media and using that alliance as an opportunity to heal.

Does it involve a celebrity?

If a colleague goes for a jog and then jumps into the local river in a sweatsuit, it may be bizarre behavior but it doesn't generally land as a story in the local paper. Tipper Gore did it in Chicago several years ago and it was a national story. Obviously, not all elements of newsworthiness have to be rational.

Is it news you can use?

This category of news is everywhere these days: in checklists on how to stay healthy—everything from weight loss to exercise, from positive thinking to getting a good night's sleep. You name it, and there is a reporter out there trying to assemble a checklist of "do's and don'ts." Men's magazines, women's magazines, and parenting magazines, even TV news shows now routinely include health tips.

NEXT STEP: THE NEWS RELEASE

Once a traumatologist has become expert at recognizing news value, the "next step" is to draft a news release. This is a fairly simple task—that is, far easier than writing an original research article—and it does not have to pass a peer review.

In writing the release, the first and most important task is to frame the story. What will capture attention? Where does the finding impact people's lives? What is the most interesting thing found? What is the one thing to tell a nonscientist friend at a cocktail party to get his or her attention?

The next topic is how to answer the "So what?" question. What does the new knowledge tell the world about what should happen next? Should physicians change their ways? Should patients change behaviors? Should public health departments change policies?

Next, send the written news release to the media, an editor, or to a campus public information officer, for example. If the clinician or researcher works for a university, ask that institution's public information officer to distribute the release. In general, an institution will be thankful for the release; staff members may rewrite it, but they'll appreciate the effort. The release just saved them a bundle of work and, at the same time, told them that they are appreciated.

The Center for the Advancement of Health

In May 1997, the editors and managing editors of fourteen behavior and health research journals attended a workshop. Those in attendance decided to create a news release pool. As a result, each month, the editors who have a journal coming out the following month identify one or two articles they considered newsworthy. A news release on each article is prepared and sent to the Center. After some editing and consulting, professional quality news releases are developed. The Center then prints those releases on the letterheads of their respective journals and mails them to about 800 health reporters in the country with a cover sheet.

Reporters get the releases in advance and are expected to respect their embargo dates—the dates the journals will be mailed. Although reporters can do interviews and write their stories before that date, they are asked not to print or air them. The releases are also posted on the Internet at a highly respected Web site for reporters called EurekAlert, a Web site run by the

American Association for the Advancement of Science. AAAS allows news releases to be posted two weeks before their embargo dates. More than 1,000 health reporters are registered to use the Web site and promise to abide by the embargo dates. They are assigned a special password that allows them to see the embargoed information. This system has several advantages:

1. The releases are alongside other releases from some of the most prestigious science organizations in the world, including research centers such as the CDC, the AMA, AAAS, and *Science* magazine. This gives the releases and the research behind them greater standing, added stature, and credibility among the media.
2. Reporters get the extra, preembargo weeks to prepare their stories, rather than race into print on the day of release. Presumably, this makes for more careful, more accurate reporting.
3. On the date that the embargo is lifted for each release, the release reverts to the Center's Web site and a newsroom where all the releases are archived. They continue to be listed and summarized on the AAAS Web site but, when reporters click on a headline, it automatically bumps them over to the full release on the Web site of the Center. Gradually, the site will familiarize health journalists with all of the other behavioral health sciences research posted on the Center's site.

Once the release is written, it is on the Internet and in the mail. If everything is done correctly, the researcher/clinician may get a phone call. The traumatologist should not despair if she or he does not get any calls at all. A release is but one of hundreds, possibly thousands, that went out that same day. Sometimes, legitimate news is ignored. However, more often than not, the competition from world tragedies and political events simply overpowers the release's newsworthiness. The clinician/researcher should persist in getting research findings publicized. There is no substitute for persistence in trying to get the media's attention.

And if the reporter calls, then what?

Talking/interviewing with a reporter gives clinicians an opportunity to discuss and provide information. The issue is no longer trying to attract media attention; instead, it is what to do when the media call to ask about people's reactions to some traumatic event. This gives clinicians a chance to influence public reactions to a major tragedy, to be the public healer, to calm the injured community, and to reassure it. If one clinician does not respond to a reporter's request, be assured that someone else with less knowledge will or, worse, that no one will. Ignorance or, at best, nonpsychology, will triumph. Therefore, it is extremely important to become an ally of the media in these situations. This is the time for clinicians to do the work that brought them into the field to begin with.

HOW TO HANDLE THE INTERVIEW

The following section provides suggestions about how to handle an interview, whether as the clinician called upon to calm a community or to explain its anguish, or as the researcher with a newsworthy piece of new knowledge. First, the clinician should ask what questions the reporter wants to ask him or her. It is not rude and most reporters will oblige. After all, the clinician is not the object of the investigation but merely the source of information which the reporter needs. Then, the clinician should try to defer the interview for an hour or two—not longer than that—to prepare and decide on what information to give out. How will what is known change people's lives? A good rule of thumb is to pick two points, or at most three, to make clear. Write those points on one side of a 3 × 5 card. Remember to talk as if explaining an exquisite finding to a friend at a cocktail party, a setting that is well-known for short spans of attention. Memorize what is written on the card and then place it in your pocket.

The following sixteen rules can help guide the clinician/researcher in an interview:

1. The reporter is not an audience but a conduit. An interview is an opportunity to make a case to the public, not to the reporter.
2. Focus on the key points written on that index card, the memorized sound bite.
3. If the interview is being taped for radio or TV, ask the reporter what the first question will be, then take a few seconds to think about how to use that question to get in the key point of the interview.
4. Keep answers brief. Short answers are much less likely to be edited, twisted out of context, and misunderstood.
5. Avoid technical and professional terminology, jargon, and acronyms.
6. Make your points early and often. Some helpful language to divert the interview to that point, even when asked something else includes:

   - "The real issue here is . . ."
   - "I can't speculate about that, but we do know for a fact that . . ."
   - "That's not exactly correct. Let me clarify for your viewers/readers . . ."

7. Evoke images with words. Make the audience "see" what you are talking about. Keep verbs in the active voice.
8. Do not ramble. An interview is not a social conversation. Be wary of reporters who remain silent to get information you did not plan to divulge. It is human nature to want to fill in the silence.
9. There is no such thing as "off the record."
10. Never lie. An interviewer gets only one shot. After that, it is credibility that is shot.
11. If you do not know the answer, say so. Promise to find it out and get back to the reporter. Then keep the promise.
12. Never say "no comment" or walk away. This will be perceived as hiding something.
13. Be personable and friendly, but don't be steered away from the key points.
14. Ask how to reach the reporter with information you may think of later.
15. If the reporter asks for documents, have them faxed, couriered, or mailed by overnight service as soon after the interview as possible. Getting the documents to the reporter depends on how many documents are involved, the reporter's deadline, and the distance between clinician/researcher and reporter.
16. A clinician/researcher must make himself or herself available to reporters. Word gets around. A trusted resource will get far more considerate treatment, even from other reporters. When the reporters are needed later, they will be more likely to respond if you were there when they needed you.

The Center for the Advancement of Health believes that it is important to build relationships with health reporters. Staff members go to great lengths to convince reporters that the Center is their best resource. Staff members also go out of their way to connect reporters with the best minds identified in the Center's field of interest—the mind-body connection and psychosocial interventions. Subscribing to ProfNet helps in this process. ProfNet is a Web site that links reporters to expert sources. Several times a day, ProfNet e-mails to its subscribers, including the Center, a list of queries posted by reporters who are looking for experts to interview for various stories. Some days, the Center receives as many as 100 such queries. Each day at least a few queries are appropriate for the Center. When one seems appropriate, the Center then searches a database of researchers who have said they are willing to talk with the media about their areas of expertise. After a call to make sure that the researcher is willing and available, the Center contacts the reporter and passes along the information, along with a pitch for the reporter to use the Center as a continuing resource. Recent queries have come from health magazines, parenting magazines, *Reader's Digest, Redbook, U.S. News & World Report,* Dr. Bob Arnot on NBC, and Dr. Timothy Johnson on ABC. The Center hopes to succeed in giving part of the health care system the prominence and currency it deserves in the media and, through the media, among the general public and within the health care community. When this happens, all those involved will become equal partners with biomedicine.

CONCLUSIONS

In conclusion, clinicians/researchers might want to follow these suggestions:

1. *Be an opportunist.* As a clinician, look for opportunities in the news to respond to and offer public health advice. When tragedy strikes—and it will—the clinician/researcher has the opportunity to write a letter to the editor, call the local reporters covering the story, and offer services to help them inform the community about what it can do to heal emotionally. The researcher can get to know the local health reporters by introducing himself or herself through a letter or phone call. The researcher can let the reporter know what he or she is working on and the importance of that work to health and well-being. Reporters will appreciate these efforts.
2. *Take time to talk to a reporter who calls.* Clinicians/researchers should keep the list of interview tips in this chapter handy to refresh their memory before going into an interview.
3. *Look for opportunities to praise reporters for good work.* Reporters generally look for praise (or expect it, if it comes at all) only from their peers in the media. Surprise them once in a while and write a letter to their editor (and "cc" it to the reporter) praising them for a well-done article. In this effort, it might be possible even to add a new perspective, as long as the effort starts out by praising them.

Being a dependable, reliable source of good health information will make friends in the media who will be on the side of the clinician/researcher when it counts most.

Chapter 19

Working with Survivors
and the News Media

Janice Maxson
Roger Simpson

INTRODUCTION

A traumatic event is never expected. Individuals who had never thought about the possibility, in an instant, become victims or survivors. Police, firefighters, and trauma personnel arrive on a scene, followed by, and sometimes preceded by, reporters and photographers. People who many times are barely beginning to absorb the shock of trauma are often pressed to answer journalists' questions and offer their images for the viewing of the entire community. In some cases, the media siege may last for days or weeks.

In the months and years following a traumatic event, the news media continue to seek out survivors. Interviews, photographs, and old video footage pulled from the files are shown without warning and may well reopen old wounds and raise new problems for survivors. In some cases, anniversaries prompt requests for interviews. In cases involving continuing investigations of crimes such as murder, survivors and family members may be called every time any new development in a case "breaks." Trials severely test all those affected. The mother of a serial-murder victim described that experience. She said that when the media did not have enough information to report, but decided a suspect was interesting, they would telephone her to ask her opinion (Guillen, 1990).

This chapter describes how trauma professionals can help victims understand and respond constructively to the demands and methods of the news media. The planning and effective actions that can be taken immediately after a traumatic event and in the ensuing recovery period are described. First, it must be emphasized that some unconventional assumptions have been made. For example, it is rare for therapists and other trauma professionals to act as intermediaries between victims and the press. It also is rare for mental health professionals to cooperate in citywide or regionwide programs to help victims respond to media. Needless to say, such individual and community efforts are encouraged, and these suggestions are offered as a blueprint for such initiatives.

Many trauma professionals have encountered insensitive reporters or viewed harsh and hurtful news coverage. Furthermore, it is disconcerting when the news media pay too little attention to survivor recovery and too much attention to trauma-causing events and perpetrators of violence. The news media can help both victims and communities face trauma and loss. Some reporters and editors are bringing about major changes in their newsrooms in the interests of victims and survivors. The active interest of mental health professionals in how the news media report about trauma and victims will spur even more positive change.

REPORTERS AND ADVOCATES AS PARTNERS

The first question one may ask is "Why talk to the press at all?" Although reporters' questions may intrude on the grieving or recovery process, sometimes they help in the healing of survivors. Widows of military personnel who have been killed in the line of duty speak well of sharing with reporters the wonderful qualities of their husbands. Joe Hight, managing editor of *The Daily Oklahoman,* notes that families of the 1995 Murrah Federal Building bombing victims used newspaper articles to create memorial scrapbooks.

The relationship between the press and survivors can become adversarial. As Jack R. Hart, a managing editor at *The Oregonian* in Portland, states, in a time of tragedy, "just the fact that media representatives are there is offensive to the community." He sees the occasional disconnect between a shocked community and its local media as inevitable: "News coverage is intrusive, and grief demands privacy," Hart explains (Burroughs and Gyles, 1997, p. 36).

Bruce Shapiro, a contributing editor for *The Nation* magazine, has been both a reporter and a victim and understands how press concerns sometimes come into conflict with survivor interests. Shapiro, who was stabbed in a coffeehouse, points out that "as reporters, we talk about getting the interview as though it were a commodity. Victims feel intruded upon and harassed by us. And many people see this exploitation as a lack of press credibility; this need not be the case." He adds, "At a certain level, victims and reporters are partners. Reporters are storytellers and victims have stories to tell" (Stein, 1996, p. 13). Reporters, victims, and their advocates should all find value in the news story. Some news coverage helps victims and helps pass provictim legislation. Other stories direct community members to needed resources. Most stories have the potential to educate and inform readers and viewers.

A student who lost friends in the 1988 Pan Am jet explosion in Lockerbie, Scotland, points out media strengths as well as weaknesses:

> I think all of you know where and when you stepped over the line. But it's also important that you were there not only for those of us who experienced grief, and needed to share their feelings, but for the rest of the world to share our experiences. (Deppa, 1994, p. 179)

Deni Elliot encourages "media and official sources [to] form partnerships in times of crisis" (Elliot, 1989, p. 162). Media attention to relief efforts in the wake of Hurricane David in Dominica in 1981 was important to devastated communities. Also, in the aftermath of the Oklahoma City bombing in 1995, there were so many selfless community acts that the city's newspaper, *The Daily Oklahoman,* assigned one editor exclusively to document what the newspaper called "acts of compassion." The editor made sure that the newspaper included all the kindnesses that followed the bombing and outlined survivor needs that volunteers might address.

Janet Horne, an editor at *The Seattle Times,* speaks from the journalist's point of view:

> I have seen reporters, after they have been assigned a difficult story, sit at their desks, frozen, steeling up the courage to make calls to the family. It's a hard job. I just had a police reporter come and say—"I can't do this anymore." . . . When I was a little girl, my brother was hit by a car and killed. Within an hour, the reporters started to call. My mother was horrified that they would call and ask how she felt. I will never forget my mother's feelings and I think about that whenever I send a reporter out on a story like that. (Horne, interview, 1997)

Reporters, victims, and their advocates can work together toward constructive, healing outcomes. This has happened in many cities. The proposals that follow are designed to help clinicians and those for whom they advocate reach that goal.

NETWORK RESPONSE BEFORE A CRISIS

The formation of local or regional networks of people who can be helpful to victims at the time of a crisis is strongly encouraged. Such a network may include public safety representatives, trauma specialists, and mental health professionals, as well as victim advocates. Members of the network should be prepared to help when a crisis occurs.

Draft a master plan.

Cooperative preparation of a master emergency plan is encouraged. This should identify areas such as: situations in which members might try to be present, needs of victims and family members, and likely requests and actions by news media personnel. In addition, the master plan should identify local, regional, and national media and provide the names, and telephone and facsimile numbers for key personnel.

Establish a contact network.

A list of names and contact numbers of people who can help victims with media contacts should be prepared. It should include agencies, organizations, and individuals willing to speak to the media about victim and trauma issues. Formulating a list or plan can be useful to the process of beginning, mentally, to plan for disaster. An ideal outcome would be an "alert network" with someone available to respond quickly in any circumstance, and someone able to coordinate contacts.

AFTER THE EVENT

The technology of news gathering allows reporters to be "on the scene" within minutes of an event. Computer databases enable news organizations to pinpoint names, home addresses, and telephone numbers quickly. A reporter assigned to a serial-murder case recalled using city directories, real estate records, department of motor vehicle lists, voting records, and funeral home notices as a means of finding people. If that failed, he would go to the last listed address and talk to neighbors. This type of quick response has resulted in the need for protective, immediate interventions. In other words, networks should be prepared to intervene quickly; by the time you have been called for help, reporters may already be at the scene.

Some assistance to help victims should be in place to deal with press contacts. Migael Scherer, a rape survivor and victim advocate, asserts that the first personal contact a victim has after a trauma also has an important impact on recovery (Scherer, 1996). A journalist could be the first person who interviews a trauma survivor. This awareness may position the clinician to help survivors in a range of circumstances, who, if properly prepared, could be the ideal counterpoint to the press presence.

Response-network participants need to take the time to learn about news-gathering, media deadlines, and key contact people at newspapers, and television and radio stations. Just as police and rescue workers have jobs to do, so must the press find a way to gather information and report on the story, usually while up against tight deadlines.

Encourage families to use answering services to filter calls.

The use of answering machines or answering services, which appear to be obvious and necessary buffers to shield family from media intrusions, may not seem so obvious to a person in shock. The delay in time provided by an answering machine or service provides a survivor the chance to decide when to respond to reporters' questions, if at all.

Cover options with survivors, regarding interviews, statements, and photographs.

Assure clients that they have a right to say "no" to any and all interviews, and give assurances that it is all right to change their mind and to call a halt to an interview at any point. It is also important to let survivors know that they should refuse or postpone interviews that disrupt personal or family routines. Reporters will not necessarily think about family mealtime, the need for rest, periods of emotional stress, and the illnesses that accompany trauma. Likewise, the press may not understand the necessity for medical bed rest.

Recognize that some survivors will not be prepared to speak to the press. Provide a contact person, other than a survivor, to answer questions, relay requests. In high-awareness cases, twenty-four-hour access may be necessary.

Family members or friends should be asked to designate a spokesperson for all those affected. By appointing a spokesperson, the family may be able to express concerns while maintaining privacy for grieving, discussions, and movement. Editors and reporters usually will respect such a decision. Burroughs and Gyles advise reporters that, if they are refused an interview, they should ask for a spokesperson and offer to be available when the time is right (Burroughs and Gyles, 1997).

A designated spokesperson should realize that media calls can come any time of the day or night. After the explosion of Pan Am Flight 103, when some organizations refused to give information to the press, reporters, working on deadlines, sought it from inappropriate sources (Deppa, 1994). It is in the survivors' interest to keep control over information. You can help the spokesperson by deciding upon the kinds of information that will be provided, the timing of responses, and any conditions desired for interviews or photographs.

Map out and inform the media of a grief zone in which survivors will not deal with reporters and photographers: the home, morgue, etc.

Although some reporters are sensitive to the needs and privacy of victims and survivors, this is not always the case. Sadly, funerals are favorite places for the press to gather. Therefore, it may be wise to make it clear that the family desires privacy at such moments. When the family's wishes are clearly explained, the burden is on the press to respect those wishes. For instance, the drowning of three Coast Guard rescue personnel near the quiet Native American community of La Push, Washington, in 1997, created a flood of media attention. While some residents felt that the coverage was intrusive, several Coast Guard personnel recalled later that, during a private ceremony when flowers were scattered in the water as a tribute to those who had died, the press chose not to film the obviously emotional moment.

On the other hand, examples abound of less sensitive press behavior. In some cases this has been the result of the absence of a clear statement from the family about places and activities that are off limits. In coverage of a Seattle serial-murder case, reporters staked out homes, focused cameras on doorways, were present at funerals, and intruded on a family's visit to the morgue to identify a victim. In the wake of the Springfield, Oregon, school shootings in 1998, students constructed barriers and wrote signs which read: "Media Free Zone—Leave Us To Grieve In Private." In fact, communities in other countries hit by tragic incidents have sometimes successfully defined a zone into which the media were not to intrude. Although the declaration to the media in Springfield may have been the start of a trend, most American cities and towns have been unwilling or unable to enforce such limits.

Create a directory of experts who are experienced in working with the media.

Trauma workers can help the press gain an understanding of victim concerns by preparing a list of community agencies and individuals as referral sources. For instance, therapists could refer those who are reporting on a rape victim to the local sexual assault programs. The same list could be offered to the press to be printed as a sidebar to news reports.

THE ROLE OF INTERMEDIARY

Expect to be asked for a good picture of the victim; find one, make copies, and request that the pictures be returned.

Usually, reporters will request a color 8 × 10 photo of the victim. Family members often prefer that a favorite photograph be used by the press and their wishes should be honored. Write a clear identification on the back of the photograph and include or attach a name, address, and phone number for return of the picture.

Make sure names are spelled correctly.

Survivors have said that among the distressing outcomes of news coverage is seeing their own names or the names of loved ones misspelled. Errors hurt and anger survivors, which fosters a loss of confidence in the press. An advocate should print out names and other information to be given to the press at the time of the interview. Journalists understand the importance of this detail. After the Oklahoma City bombing, one editor was assigned the duty of making certain that all victims' names were spelled correctly.

Understand deadlines.

Television reporters are always mindful of the next news broadcast. Deadlines influence what they do. Frequently, reporters and photographers are dispatched to a home, accident site, or hospital for a live report. In such cases, expect that the news crew will have limited time to set up and that you have little chance to discuss conditions for interviews. Be prepared with written information. Live reports invariably occur at times when one expects privacy for meals, family gatherings, and sleep.

Newspaper reporters may appear to be less harried, but they also have to work against deadlines. Those working for morning papers face deadlines running from mid-afternoon to late in the night; afternoon newspapers often have early to mid-morning deadlines. It should be understood that delays in providing information, obtaining photographs, or granting interviews affect the day's coverage. In some cases, a family's failure to respond on the day of the media request means that by the next day the story will no longer be covered.

The reporter likely will not tell the story the way the survivor would tell it.

When the victim/survivor is willing to speak with the press, the resulting story may be disappointing. A reporter may omit details that the survivor felt were important. Editing, usually by someone other than the reporter, may result in information being left out or mishandled. The reporter may have nothing to say about the headline or photographs used with the story. Space and time may affect what is included in the report. A frank discussion about this will help survivors handle the ensuing news coverage.

Help the survivor to plan the interview.

The following guidelines are suggested for trauma survivors who agree to press interviews. An advocate should discuss these points before the interview begins.

- Ask the reporter what the focus of the story will be. Think about the relative merits of stories regarding consequences of a newsworthy event, such as public policy changes, and stories that appear to satisfy curiosity about "how it feels" to suffer a traumatic event.
- Explain what will and will *not* be discussed. A survivor may have thoughtful opinions on issues raised by an event; speculation on matters such as how someone died or the cause of an accident will help neither the public nor the survivor.
- Set a time limit on the interview. Twenty minutes to half an hour might be a reasonable time.
- If possible, have a support person available during the interview. Arrange beforehand to interrupt if the interview becomes difficult.
- Establish rules about speaking "on" and "off" the record. Not everything said needs to be included in an article.
- Stop the interview if necessary, or go on to another question if the one raised causes discomfort. Expect that speaking about the traumatic incident may bring unwanted memories. Expect emotions that can't be controlled. Have tissues handy; reporters rarely think to bring them to an interview.
- Be prepared for the possibility that someone may ask the question "How do you feel?" or others similar in tone. It may be wise to decide beforehand whether an answer to that type of question will be given. Some survivors say they have been hurt, even reminded of the trauma, by "how do you feel?" questioning; others are insulted by the vagueness of it; some victims have responded thoughtfully to that type of question when asked in a caring, sincere way.

- Determine at the end of the interview (if the reporter doesn't ask) if there is anything else that should be included.
- After the interview, think carefully about whether to read a newspaper account or watch a television broadcast. Interviews, especially if they appear to distort what was said or intended, may increase the stress of the trauma.
- *Understand it's a job.*

A favorite press request is for the survivor to share the last conversation he or she had with the lost relative or friend. This is bound to raise painful memories. However, the reporter is essentially trying to flesh out the story of a victim who has died. If the survivor is able, he or she can contribute to the story so that others may understand more about this person. Reporters may also request copies of letters and additional photographs. It is helpful to remember that the reporter's job is not to violate privacy, it is to tell the story. Requests for personal items should be discussed openly with those most affected.

Obtain a copy of "A Media Code of Ethics" from the National Organization for Victim Assistance (NOVA, 1998) and review its provisions with the person being helped. The Code can be usefully employed to set limits for interviews. The Code's opening paragraph identifies the risks of interviewing survivors:

> crime and trauma victims who are most of interest to the media deserve to be treated as innocent victims; are likely to be in a state of crisis; are likely to say and do things in that vulnerable state which they later consider undignified and embarrassing; are not likely to have had any experience in working with the media; are therefore vulnerable to "second injuries" by inaccurate, intrusive, or unfair press coverage; and may, in later times, re-experience their trauma if their stories are republicized without warning. (NOVA, 1998, pp. 1-2)

COVERAGE IN THE FIRST FEW WEEKS

Plan how best to frame issues in interviews, press conferences, and news releases. Prepare for interviews, anticipate that stories may reflect a different event. Recognize that news stories may be neither neutral nor objective.

Frank Ochberg, a psychiatrist who has influenced the press to cover trauma victims more humanely, describes the initial shock of a traumatizing event, and its second stage, which some call a heroic phase in which "hope and exhilaration co-exist with fear and grief." In the next stage, Ochberg adds, the victim and community return to some equilibrium after the event: "There is loss. There is pain. Reality sinks in." By that point the ubiquitous media have moved on to other assignments. "A survivor who might have been annoyed by too much attention could feel abandoned and forgotten," (Ochberg, 1996, pp. 25-26). In general, this is a time when it is possible for an advocate to help a victim understand and react constructively to conditions that will range from no press attention at all to dismaying kinds of coverage.

Be aware that the coverage may actually include information that is surprising or in bad taste. For instance, a Canadian widow was displeased to read an article about her husband's death. In it a reporter colleague of her deceased spouse recounted what he considered to be "funny" stories about her husband's newsroom pranks. She considered the stories to be a violation of her privacy.

Learn what makes a story newsworthy. Recognize, also, that many stories are framed by official sources, such as police, prosecutors, or public officials whose intentions may affect the nature of a story in ways a victim will not expect. It may be possible to anticipate how the news media will handle the story and provide a reporter with an alternative theme. Background on a victim's volunteer work, hobbies or interests, for instance, may balance a focus on the way a crime was committed. Think about the stages of reporter and community interest: At first, what happened? Then, who are the victims? Then, for some time, why did this happen?

For interviews, encourage meetings in settings other than homes.

Victims and survivors may see the interview as a further violation of the grieving process. Migael Scherer tells about being asked by a television reporter to allow an interview at her home. Scherer turned the request around and proposed that the interview be in the reporter's home. The reporter admitted later that she was up at 5 a.m. cleaning her house and that she also began to understand that the news media can be intrusive when they seek interviews (Scherer, 1996).

Inform the media that the family and survivors will not respond each time there is a suspect.

Plan a response for the eventual filing of charges. Consider a press conference or issuing a press release instead of giving several media interviews. As the case proceeds, create press information, including a sheet of relevant facts, names and numbers of contacts, and previous and current statements by survivors.

A fact sheet may shield the family from repetitive questions and a press release will keep the family or survivor interest clearly focused. After media attention has cooled, a survivor may wish to keep an unsolved crime or an injustice in the public eye. In this case, the goal may be to seek press aid in gaining public attention for the case.

If a perpetrator is at large, survivors and witnesses may want to use a silhouette in TV interviews.

The advocate can be helpful in dealing with broadcast media also. Interviews may be delayed, thus increasing anxiety. Lighting may not adequately protect a person who does not wish to be identified. Carefully planned interview responses may be turned into a sound bite of a few seconds. These outcomes should be considered beforehand. The value of giving an interview still could outweigh the difficulties.

Identify reporters who show sensitivity; let them know you appreciate their work through letters and calls.

One victim explained how attuned she was to sensitive and insensitive news coverage of her case. Subsequently, she decided to make a special effort to acknowledge journalists who show concern for victims and survivors.

Identify reporters and media who do not show sensitivity.

Do not hesitate to ask that a distasteful photo or descriptive term or personal reference not be used. Challenge the use of graphic descriptions of how a person was killed or how a body appeared.

Editors in all media, sensitive to how poor editorial decisions translate into lost readers and viewers, take public complaints about inappropriate coverage seriously.

LONG-TERM CONCERNS

Often, the press loses interest in a case while the survivor is only beginning to face recovery. If new information on the case develops, support survivors should seek out an editor or journalist who had previously expressed interest in the story.

It may be helpful to know, however, that reporters who have followed stories closely, may, themselves, have difficulty leaving them behind. Joe Hight, of the *The Daily Oklahoman,* has recognized the bonding that may occur between victims and reporters. He has even found it necessary to counsel reporters who have developed friendships with victims.

Dealing with a Trial

In the event of a trial, a new set of concerns emerge. One is that the trial, and the media attention that surrounds it, set back the recovery process. Victims who testify in trials describe an emotional roller coaster in which press coverage one day may focus on victim concerns and the next entirely focus on the defendant. News stories may reflect trial procedures that appear more concerned with the defendant than with victims. Victims may be shattered by reports of testimony that appear to emphasize the assertions or accusing questions of a defense attorney. Depositions and pretrial publicity will also create stress for the survivor. An effective means of support at such times is to offer to speak to reporters, handle arrangements, and be available to explain what is happening.

Anticipate six-month, one-year, and subsequent anniversaries. Challenge the use of file footage and photos.

Responses might include statements, but not interviews. Ask the media to refrain from doing anniversary stories and using file photos or footage showing injured victims, scenes of the incident, bodies, or body bags. Television newsrooms regularly pull up archival video to illustrate continuing stories. A Seattle television station showed a body-bag recovery numerous times over a several-year period to the dismay and anger of a victim's mother. A stabbing victim was startled to see video taken at the time of the attack used months later to illustrate a story about a legislative anticrime action.

Be especially alert about approaches from radio and television talk shows.

Producers of network and syndicated shows are often able to convince a survivor that it is in her or his interest to appear on a program. One rape survivor, willing to speak about her experience, found that the invitation was really contingent on her husband's appearance on the show with her. The couple wisely turned the producers down.

As the case raises issues of concern for survivors, contribute letters to editors and offer to write articles for local magazines and newspaper editorial sections.

Although trauma specialists are often interviewed by the media about events that gain national attention, such as a bombing or school shooting, few interviews allow the professional to say much about the nature of trauma and its effects on victims. Many editors welcome offers of essays that, in 300 to 500 words, clarify and explain trauma. A short letter outlining the proposed piece may be sent by facsimile to the editor of the local newspaper editorial page.

Cooperate with those who are trying to change media responses to violence: journalism schools, advocacy groups, victim groups, trauma practitioners, medical centers, the International Society for Traumatic Stress Studies, etc.

Journalism schools at Michigan State University and the University of Washington assure that every graduate knows about trauma's effects and has thought about how to sensitively interview victims. Other schools are adopting the techniques used at those schools, and journalism groups are paying more attention to trauma issues.

CONCLUSION

Even as more young journalists enter the field knowing about trauma, and as victim advocates assume a greater role in shaping news coverage of violence, news-industry trends continue to undermine these gains. The need for compelling images drives television news producers to skirt the ethical considerations outlined in this chapter. Tensions between the media and those who work on behalf of victims has increased in some places and dissipated in communities where constructive planning and dialogue has taken place.

Constructive activism on the part of those who work for victims can usefully affect news coverage. Victims have not had advocates for a very long period of time. In many communities, therapists have not played a major role in public advocacy for victims. Dialogue between the press and victim advocates is a necessary step toward journalism that helps, rather than hurts, its community.

REFERENCES

Burroughs, E. and Gyles, B.Z. (1997). "Truth and Trauma." *Presstime,* September, 35-41.

Deppa, J. (1994). *The Media and Disasters: Pan Am 103.* New York: New York University Press.

Elliot, D. (1989). "Tales from the Darkside: Ethical Implications of Disaster Coverage." In L. M. Walters, L. Wilkins, and T. Walters, (Eds.), *Bad Tidings: Communications and Catastrophe,* (pp. 161-170). Hillsdale, NJ: Lawrence Erlbaum.

Guillen, T. (1990). "Privacy and the Media Amid the Serial Killer Phenomenon: A Case Study of the Green River Serial Murders." Unpublished master's thesis, University of Washington.

National Organization for Victim Assistance (1998). "A Media Code of Ethics." Washington, DC: Author.

Ochberg, F. (1996). "A Primer on Covering Victims." *Nieman Reports,* Fall 1996, 21-26.

Scherer, M. (1996). "Why I Turned Down Oprah Winfrey." *Nieman Reports,* Fall 1996: 1(3):35-36.

Stein, M.L. (1996). "Sensitizing Reporters." *Editor and Publisher,* April 20, 1996.

SECTION VII:
CONCLUSION

Chapter 20

Some Final Thoughts on Competence

Mary Beth Williams
John F. Sommer

For those who have worked in the field of trauma for any length of time, the faces of trauma are many. Personal and professional experiences with traumatic events have led some to conclude that the numbers and range of events which could be defined as traumatic gets more and more extensive as time passes, and that the course of treatment and healing for individuals who have experienced Type I (one time) and Type II (chronic) traumas is becoming more distinct. Each new client/patient brings challenges and variability in presentation as well as course of treatment.

The primary editor of this book has had the privilege of being a member of the faculty of the first trauma training program for therapists in Finland. Over the course of a three-year period, approximately twenty experienced therapists have become trained traumatologists. This program, under the sponsorship of Raile Rinne, the Finnish Association for Mental Health/ Institute for Advanced Training, and Paivi Saarinen of the Center for Post-trauma Therapy and Trauma Education, combines lectures, experiential exercises, internats (extended retreats combining both educational and recreational experiences for self-care), EMDR, practicum, supervision, and personal work. Trauma experts from the United States, Israel, Norway, Finland, and other countries provide instruction, experiential involvement, and EMDR. Although the Finns take this training very seriously and work exceptionally hard during training sessions, they also recognize that it is essential to provide for self-care to combat vicarious traumatization and to diffuse trauma overload. Whether cross-country skiing, dancing, downhill skiing, going to sauna, or listening to the fantastic guitar playing of Duo Mennen, these professionals take care of themselves and their own mental health. What they put in practice is an essential part of professional (and personal) competence.

As this concluding chapter took form, the word "competence" kept coming to mind, just as it had as a key concept in the title of the book. Just what constitutes competence for the traumatologist? The competent therapist believes that he or she can make a difference by offering help to the client. The competent therapist has self-worth and self-confidence, both as a professional and as a human being. That individual constantly seeks training and keeps in close contact with professional peers both for information about trauma and for personal support. The competent professional is able to admit mistakes. That individual stays present, to the greatest extent possible, during sessions and is first and foremost a model of a safe, trustworthy human being.

Much of what is now being written in the trauma field puts the same message in new packages. The goal of this conclusion is to again present some fundamental "truths" in simple, forthright language. Philosophically, some adhere to certain truths as guides to life and practice. Perhaps the most inclusive of these is the phrase "It Can Be Done," the motto of Mary Beth Williams' father, the Reverend John Calvin Little. In the face of trauma and disaster hope still remains and, with hope comes a future. All of the authors in this book, whether educator, researcher, clinician, veterans' advocate, retired FBI agent, police psychologist, freelance science writer, reporter, professor, political advocate, public school employee, or physician promote the goal of competent practice. Just as traumatic events take many shapes and forms, so do the paths to healing. Exposure to a traumatic event does not necessarily lead to pathological outcomes. To be sure, the road to healing and resilience is often long and arduous. Some individuals will never be able to return to a level of salutogenic functioning. Some will remain frozen in time, locked in their memories and flashbacks. Others will avoid, turning into heads of cabbage—closed in, tight, and cold, with many facets and folds. But many will fight for some modicum of control—some measure of integrity.

Perhaps words from several clients express this path best:

> A definition of healing is to live fully in the present, when the past no longer has any power over the present. What helped most [in this healing] is [my] dogged determination to more than just survive. (JCT)

But what guides the clinician in this quest? The following principles of competence must be taken into account if one is to help survivors "go beyond" the pain of the present toward the face of a manageable future.

The competent clinician is ethical.

The competent clinician adheres to and believes in a set of values that frame clinical practice; the competent clinician also adheres to a trauma-based code of ethics. One code that incorporates this value system is the Code of Ethics of the Association of Traumatic Stress Specialists (ATSS)

(1995). That particular code will not be presented here in its entirety; however, some of its major principles are included.

Values lie at the foundation of any ethical statement, including the following:

- Do no harm (nonmaleficence).
- Promote human welfare (beneficence).
- Be fair (justice).
- Fulfill commitments to clients (fidelity).
- Strive to model empathic, engaged, responsive interaction and a high degree of professionalism.
- Engage in acts to assist in the normative healing processes of trauma recovery through multiple levels of interaction.
- Use sensitive and respectful interventions.
- Recognize that the primary obligation of the clinician is to the physical, emotional, and spiritual safety of the client/patient, whether individual, family, group, workplace, and/or community.
- Assume an advocacy role for nonempowered survivors.
- Obtain informed consent.
- Maintain confidentiality unless indicated by law not to do so.
- Avoid any retraumatizing actions, to the greatest extent possible.
- Keep the welfare of the client paramount.
- Assure delivery of services if at all possible.
- Place the needs of clients primary in the work setting.
- Operate within personal level(s) of training, expertise, education, and experience.
- Seek to be culturally sensitive and attempt to operate within the cultural norms of the population they are serving to the fullest extent possible.
- Share information and knowledge about trauma and its impact with victims, colleagues, organizations, communities, and nations.
- Keep client safety primary above all else, including research.
- Self-monitor personal capacity to do "the work."
- Take regular and ongoing actions to insure self-care and enhance the ability to deliver quality services.
- Join similar organizations and obtain regular, continuing education.

The competent clinician recognizes that trauma survivors are stuck in the freeze-frame present of trauma.

On one hand, trauma is a sensory experience. It leaves its legacy of associated sights, sounds, and smells. For instance, it may be the smell of rotting, decaying bodies left unattended in the graveyard, and the sight of the streets of Quang Tri after the Tet offensive of 1968. It may be the sound of a child crying/screaming to the Vietnam veteran who ordered the air strike on a Viet Cong stronghold, only to soon realize that the "stronghold" contained an orphanage with over 240 bodies and countless other maimed and wounded children. It may be the image of hooded figures in a movie that reminds a survivor of satanic abuse experienced as a child and sends her into agonizing nights of flashbacks.

That is the one face of trauma. On the other hand, trauma is a meaning-challenging experience that takes away the sense-making capacity of life (Williams-Rosenbloom). The competent clinician, therefore, must take into account both of these aspects of trauma and provide individualized, differentiated treatment for each and every survivor, whether that survivor has experienced a Type I, one-time catastrophic event (e.g., a rape) or is a survivor of chronic, ongoing trauma (e.g., sexual abuse from ages four through twenty). That single-incident trauma may be initially approached with a combination of critical incident stress management and debriefing techniques combined with EMDR (Horn).

The competent clinician knows trauma theory.

The theoretical basis of practice is continuously (and continually) changing and expanding and modifying. This theory is both practice and research-based. Some proponents of treatment stress that it is important (and necessary) for the survivor to work though (at least) some of his or her traumatic experiences in order to heal. According to David Foy (1999), Vietnam veterans need to do just that. In a research project, in a group setting, veterans chose one or more traumatic scenes that needed resolution, and then discussed those scenes in detail with group members for a twenty- to thirty-minute period of time. The telling was repeated for between nine and twelve times, until it became boring, nonemotional, and was systematically desensitized to be removed from the freeze-frame present and was put into the more distant past. Other practitioners seek to avoid such processing and believe that revisiting trauma in this way is destructive.

According to Foa and her colleagues, trauma survivors, particularly those with complex PTSD, have lost the normal capacity for self-regulation and have incurred a weakening of identity. They also have a diffusion of the self-boundary with others (Tinnin et al.). Schiraldi (2000) lists seven principles of healing:

1. Healing starts by applying skills to manage PTSD symptoms of arousal, anger, and intrusion.
2. Healing occurs when traumatic memory is processed or integrated, assimilated, digested, metabolized so that the client comes to terms with what happened.

3. Healing occurs when confronting replaces avoidance.
4. Healing occurs in a climate of safety and pacing.
5. Healing occurs when boundaries are intact.
6. Healing is aided by kind awareness and acceptance.
7. Healing is work and requires balance in life.

The competent clinician keeps up to date with the newest trauma-related research.

How is this possible? For example, the clinician may be a member of the ISTSS and receive the *Journal of Traumatic Stress.* The clinician may attend conferences and annual meetings and listen to presentations that are research-based or provide research findings. The clinician may spend a great deal of nonsession time perusing the ever-growing trauma literature. The competent clinician reads recently published materials that include books, articles, and workbooks. The competent clinician is familiar with online trauma resources including the Web pages of the ISTSS, the Association of Traumatic Stress Specialists (ATSS), Hope Morrow (hopefull@earthlink. net), David Baldwin's Trauma Information Pages (www.traumapages.com), and the PILOTS database for publications about PTSD based at Dartmouth University under the direction of Dr. Fred Lerner.

An example of an article a clinician should read is "Effects of Mode of Writing on Emotional Narratives" (Brewin and Leonard, 1999). Subjects in this study wrote about their stressful (though not always a Criterion-A traumatic) experience over a three- to five-day period for between fifteen and thirty minutes daily. Writing was done in longhand as a means to help clients elicit and confront painful memories as part of systematic exposure and cognitive restructuring. Although the writing of the ninety-seven students in the study was associated with greater negative affect, it also was associated with greater disclosure and greater perceived benefit.

The competent clinician recognizes that it is important to gather a complete trauma history or (if not all traumas are readily accessible to historical memory) as complete a history as possible. Then, the competent clinician must look at the nature and dimension(s) of the event(s) included in that history.

Numerous instruments are available to record traumatic events. However, one of the most detailed has been developed by the Traumatic Stress Institute in South Windsor, Connecticut.

The clinician, additionally, should recognize that many factors influence client vulnerability including fantasy versus reality caused by negative beliefs; imagination caused by negative thoughts of worst case scenarios;

and/or exposure to horrific traumas/extreme incidents in the past (Horn). Also important to understand are the subjective experiences of the traumatized individual based on experience, culture, and personality; cognitive style; present perception and appraisal; and the culture and nature of the recovery environment (Turnbull). In addition, it is important to look at the neurochemical and neurophysiological experience of the trauma.

Frequently, other diagnoses accompany the PTSD diagnosis. The survivor may be depressed, bipolar, anxious, or otherwise impaired or impacted. A psychosocial history of the individual also looks at the person's strengths within the life span as well as the ideographic manifestations of the trauma (Flack, Litz).

The clinician should recognize that certain types of traumatic events tend to lead to more serious expressions of the phenomenology of the disorder. Combat trauma, exposure to atrocities, or experiencing serious bodily harm can be included within this caveat (Hendin and Haas, 1991). However, perceiving those events as damaging, disenchanting, disheartening, or debilitating can make the outcome even more distinctive and disturbing.

In taking the trauma history, the clinician should recognize that nonverbally communicated information about the trauma and its impact also provides information. Sometimes this information reveals even more than unconsciously motivated reenactments.

**The competent clinician knows that a well-designed treatment plan
is crucial to effective treatment (Lindahl).**

Ideally, treatment begins with assessment. However, overwhelming the client with papers to fill out and tests to complete during the initial treatment sessions can be negative in impact and can diminish the development of initial rapport. Furthermore, some clients immediately begin to relate their stories or emote the pain of what happened to them without giving the clinician time to gather a history. When this happens, assessment and differential diagnosis is incorporated into the treatment sessions themselves.

The competent clinician helps the client evaluate his or her need for, and gain access to, appropriate medication. It is absolutely essential that the clinician develop good working relationships with competent psychiatrists who are aware of the impacts of trauma on the individual as well as the appropriate trauma-based course of treatment. As Liber-

zon and colleagues note, the four goals of pharmacological treatment are to

1. provide immediate relief for overt symptoms;
2. reduce core symptoms so that the client can become more able to participate in therapy;
3. treat comorbid symptoms and syndromes; and
4. attempt to correct, temper, or restore alterations of neurobiological symptoms.

Furthermore, the clinician knows it is not possible to cure PTSD through pharmacological interventions alone.

The competent clinician uses a biopsychosocial approach to treatment (Turnbull) to facilitate flexible management of PTSD and its multifaceted nature.

This approach begins with initial assessment through explanation of and education about PTSD theory. This approach recognizes that, in general, the trauma survivor is part of a family whose members have their own idiosyncratic secondary trauma responses. How the family members assimilate or accommodate to a trauma is of major concern. Harris, in describing the work of Figley (1989), states that the competent clinician should recognize that the key to family integration of trauma is information processing, adaptation to change, organization, maintenance, and regulation through communication.

The competent clinician validates, appreciates, and tries to understand the client's experiences during the traumatic event(s) (Flora). Treatment helps the victim tell the story of the traumatic event(s) before, during, and after their occurrence. This process anchors the victim to the traumatic experiences and memories so that he or she can embed them with the life narrative. The systematic recovery and talking through of traumatic memories, therefore, is an emotion-controlling linking of current symptoms with actual traumatic experiences. As this recovery occurs, the victim also contains, organizes, and discharges potentially overwhelming trauma-related emotions. Within this process, the key to healing is connection and listening. Listening to trauma, whether in the office setting or in the classroom (e.g., as Mabe writes), must be combined with reverence for the trauma survivor's experiences, and should offer safety and "honored seriousness."

The competent clinician recognizes that treatment promotes emotional processing of the traumatic event.

The client must make fear-relevant information available to activate fear memory and to form new memories that can be integrated into the evoked memory structure. The clinician helps the client diffuse anger. This emotional processing can be done through exposure, cognitive restructuring, or a combination thereof using education, breathing retraining, and/or imaginal and in vivo exposure (Zoellner, Foa, et al.). The process allows the client to become less of a victim to the mind's remembering. The clinician's role during exposure to the traumatic event is to help modulate distress. Cognitive restructuring reduces dysfunctional thoughts the client holds about the world, others, and the self. Challenging beliefs through a variety of techniques, including those related to CSDT (Rosenbloom and Williams), is very helpful in this process.

The competent clinician recognizes that the goal of treatment is processing of the trauma information, including disclosure.

There are three principal components to that treatment:

1. Processing and coming to terms with the experience
2. Controlling and mastering biological stress reductions
3. Reestablishing social connections and interpersonal efficacy (van der Kolk)

Active engagement in adaptive action to neutralize emotional arousal is a major aspect of the phase-oriented treatment process. This examines and challenges the way victims view themselves, others, and the world through an examination and realignment of schemas, emotions, and situations (van der Kolk, Williams, and Rosenbloom). By deconditioning memories and lessening excessive arousal, the victim/survivor is better able to acquire new information and regain a sense of safety and mastery (van der Kolk). Thus, gaining access to the traumatic memory to develop a verbal narrative frees the ego state that has been frozen in time so that trauma memory can transform into historical memory (Tinnin).

The competent clinician also recognizes that the outcome(s) of treatment is significantly impacted by the use of the self by the therapist and the therapeutic relationship. The client must have at least a beginning level of trust in the clinician's motives, acceptance, knowledge, and (at times) credentials. The competent clinician must provide an atmosphere and physical setting of safety and respect, modeling appropriate interaction, listening, disclosure, and humanity (Mabe). Whatever the theoretical approach, however, the clinician should approach the client with flexibility and creativity (Nurmi).

The competent clinician recognizes that talking with responsible journalists can help provide their profession and the public with good, relevant information about the trauma(s), information that can touch their lives and emotions (Hébert).

This can be done through a news release, an interview, or a statement or op-ed piece. A reporter is a conduit between clinician and audience, and medical professionals and other interested, "need to know" parties. The clinician is also responsible to arrange for appropriate reporters to attend some official functions. It is the responsibility of the therapist to make sure that others are helped to translate words into images so that the audience can "see" what trauma is, does, and leads to. The competent clinician, therefore, is someone who adheres to the motto "carpe diem" (seize the day) and also gets assistance in facing the trials and tribulations of everyday work.

The competent clinician knows that exposing survivors to media can be disastrous, unless media interviews are conducted by individuals aware of the nature of trauma. Media representatives must approach victims/witnesses/practitioners with respect in a safe, comfortable setting, if at all possible (Ochberg). Ethically speaking, the reporter should give the interviewee as much control and foreknowledge as possible. The reporter also has the opportunity to refer interviewees to community resources when he or she is aware of appropriate referral sources. The competent clinician can serve as an intermediary between client and reporter, helping the survivor plan the interview or, at times, mopping up thereafter (Simpson).

The competent clinician frequently assumes many roles other than the role of therapist while treating trauma survivors.

Among those roles are the following:

1. *Advocate:* a spokesperson for the client, presenting and arguing the client's cause to achieve therapeutic objectives. In this role, the competent clinician does not take a neutral stance. Instead, that clinician negotiates, argues, and/or manipulates the environment for and on behalf of the client.
2. *Broker:* a facilitator directing the client to utilize the system to obtain services that are of the most benefit. In this role, the therapist links elements of the service delivery system to the client. It is important for all

system providers to communicate, perhaps within the context of an interdisciplinary team staffing.

3. *Mobilizer:* in this role, the clinician assembles and energizes existing groups, resources, organizations, and structures or creates new ones to help in solving problems within the client's life or to aid in the prevention of future trauma-related problems.

4. *Enabler:* as an enabler, the clinician helps clients find coping strengths and resources within themselves to accomplish tasks and goals and effect change. The enabler is also a teacher and information provider, *not* an advice giver. The enabler helps the client alter his or her environment to achieve those goals.

5. *Mediator:* a neutral negotiator between systems helps the client avoid situations in which winning and/or losing are paramount issues. In this role, the clinician assists the client and another individual (partner, spouse, child, employer) to uncover common interests as negotiations proceed.

The competent clinician respects and encourages resilience.

The clinician should not allow for the client to accept a victim mythology as a way of life, to be resigned to a vegetative existence, and fearful of approaching doom and gloom (Tinnin). To discover the meaning of resilience to clients, the clinician should listen to the clients' words as guidelines for practice. Some survivors say:

- "Healing is allowing yourself the possibility of joy in your life . . . it is waking up one day and choosing life."
- "Healing is releasing pain through processing the components of the feelings associated with the source within myself. . . to release, have closure."
- "Normal is a cycle on the dryer."
- "What has helped is releasing the pain by processing through understanding and recurring therapist guidance and detached input enables me to see more clearly what has actually happened to me . . . to realize how my thought processes contribute to the amount of pain I experience."

The competent clinician recognizes the need for self-care and the warning signs of that immediate need.

The clinician should avoid isolation from professional peers. She or he should recognize that spacing out and dissociating on a regular basis during sessions are indicators that the need for self-care is long overdue. For example, when the therapist experiences a sudden reevaluation of personal foundations and values that leads to increased feelings of vulnerability, it is time for self-care. What can be done?

1. Schedule alone time.
2. Schedule time for fun.
3. Seek out new experiences and develop new interests.
4. Work out, exercise, or do some other form of physical activity.
5. Be respectful of your body and make good lifestyle choices.
6. Expand your mind and engage in self-renewal.
7. Set reasonable self-expectations and problem solve when you have less control than you would like to have.
8. Say "no" and then mean it when too many requests are made of you.
9. Develop new, quality relationships that are lasting, not temporary, to bring you social support.
10. Spend more time living in the present moment.
11. Keep your sense of humor.
12. Get your own therapy when you need it and find alternative ways to heal that fit your beliefs (reiki, massage).
13. Seek to develop a spiritual self (McDermott and Fellbaum, 2000).

These thirteen guidelines can help the traumatologist immensely both professionally and personally. The impact on trauma on the clinician extends far beyond the therapeutic setting. At times, the clinician may need to turn to a personal "bag of tricks" to control personal thoughts—through thought stopping, diversion of cognitions to more positive and productive thoughts, and reinterpretation/reprioritization of thoughts. The clinician as well as the client must use strategies to enhance personal self-esteem, personal resources for support, and reinterpretations of thoughts as cues to recall those thoughts that are most useful. Through these and other cognitive restructuring processes, and through challenging of the five basic psychological needs and their accompanying beliefs, the clinician will "survive to wage war against the demons haunting his/her clients" another day. In other words, only through awareness and action will the competent clinician find peace and tranquility.

REFERENCES

Association of Traumatic Stress Specialists (1995). *Code of ethics.* Irmo, SC: ATSS.

Brewin, C. R. and Leonard, H. (1999). Effects of mode of writing on emotional narratives. *Journal of Traumatic Stress, 12*(2), 355-361.

Figley, C. (1989). *Helping traumatized families.* San Francisco, CA: Jossey-Bass.

Foy, D. (1999). "Trauma focus group therapy for chronic PTSD." Paper presented at Fifteenth Annual Meeting of the International Society for Traumatic Stress Studies, Miami, FL, November 14.

Hendin, H. and Haas, A. P. (1991). Suicide and guilt as manifestations of PTSD in Vietnam combat veterans. *American Journal of Psychiatry, 148,* 596-591.

McDermott, W. V. and Fellbaum, G. A. (2000). "Some days . . . the dragon wins; Helping wounded healers heal." Paper presented at the ATSS Annual Conference, San Antonio, TX, March 2.

Schiraldi, G. R. (2000). *The post-traumatic stress disorder sourcebook: A guide to healing, recovery, and growth.* Los Angeles, CA: Lowell House.

Index

abreaction, 141
  in others, 171
  as a treatment, 34
accommodation, 121, 393
Accommodation Phase, 303
Achilles heel, 313-314
adaptation, 140
ADD (attention deficit disorder), 222
addictive behavior, 312
adrenaline, 358
adrenergic agents, 64
affect regulation, 29, 31
affirmations, positive, 175, 200
Alarm Phase, 302, 305
alexithymia, 102, 121
alienation, from feelings, 131
allegations, credible, 220
altered state of consciousness, 110
alters, 178
  how formed, 192
  identified, 191
amnesia, 29, 352
anamnesis
  art, 110
  art therapy, 107
  dissociative imagery, 107
  recursive, 100-101
anniversary, as trigger, 192
anticonvulsants, 60
antidepressants, 50, 64
antikindling (anticonvulsant), 49
antipsychotic agents, 62
  anxiety as, 37, 82, 93, 103, 153
  Anxiety Management Training,
    AMT, 154
  and increased catecholaminergic
    functioning, 49
  inventory, Beck, 16, 86
  levels, 52
  management, 78
  seen in PTSD, 49
  separation, 226

antipsychotic agents *(continued)*
  similarity between behavioral
    and physiological
    manifestations, 49
  and tachycardia, 49
arousal
  autonomic, 29
  increased, 49, 93
  levels, 153
  PTSD symptoms, 49
art therapy, 103, 107, 109
assault, 93
assertive communication, 173
assessment, 9, 392
assimilate, 393
assumptions, 121
  core, 223
  "shattered," 152
  unrealistic, 84
  veterans', 335
ATSS (Association of Traumatic Stress
    Specialists), 388-389, 391
attachment, 36
autobiographical history, 109
autonomic
  arousal, 29
  hyperarousal, 147
  nervous system, 141, 142
autonomous ego function, 109
auxiliary ego function, 109
avoidance, 94
  reaction, 140
avowal, 113

barbiturates, replaced, 61
Bargaining Phase, 303
basic need(s)
  five, 119, 126
  self, 119
Beck Anxiety Inventory, 16, 86

399

Beck Depression Inventory, 16, 86, 145
behavior, addictive, 312
behavioral manifestation, of anxiety, 49
belief(s)
    systems and schemas, 170
    testing one's, 126-127
beneficence, 389
benzodiazepines, 57, 61, 62, 147
biofeedback, 78
biopsychosocial approach, 147, 393
biphasic nature of human response, 331
bombing, Oklahoma City, 315, 318,
        354, 373
Bonnie and Clyde (movie), 314
boundaries, 11, 18, 103, 123, 171, 175,
        176
brain chemistry, 120
brofaromine, 52, 53
bupropion, 59
buspirone, 59
"buying time" process, 302

capacity for evil, human, 225
CAPS-DX (Clinician-Administered
        PTSD Scale), 14, 145
carbamazepine, 60
catecholaminergic functioning in
        anxiety, 48
catharsis, 141
CBCL (Child Behavior Checklist), 217
CDI (Children's Depression Inventory),
        217
central nervous system (CNS), 26, 31
ceremony, social and ritual, 336
characterological changes/distortions,
        227
"check in," 170
checklist, PTSD, 15
chronology of events, 220
Churchill, Winston, 321
CIRT (Critical Incident Response
        Teams), 320
CISD (Critical Incident Stress
        Debriefing), 33, 150, 271
CISM (Critical Incident Stress
        Management), 315, 316, 321
CITES (Children's Impact of
        Traumatic Events Scale), 217
clinical interview, 266

clinician overidentification, 346
clonidine, 147
Closing Phase, 304
clozapine, 62
code of ethics, ATSS, 388, 389
cognitive
    avoidance, 90
    -behavioral techniques, 76
    distortions, 224
    errors, 172
    restructuring, 84, 85, 87, 88, 89, 91,
            92, 175, 394
    reworking, 224
    schemas, 223
    theory, 143
co-leaders, 169
Columbine, CO, 278
combat, 4
    neuroses, 141
command hallucinations, 114
commitment, 173
communication
    assertive, 173
    interpersonal, 291
    skills, 172
community of peers, 181
compassion fatigue, 230
competence, 387
complex PTSD, Type II, 115
    defined, 104, 159
    development, 227
    traumatic experiences, 159
confidentiality, 11
confrontation, 82
connection
    as key to healing, 393
    with oneself (and others), 119
containment, 128, 175
continuity, 250
control, 119, 126
coping, 31, 91, 122, 125
    mechanisms, 174
    responses, 142
    skills, 176
core
    assumptions, 223
    problem, 25
countertransference, 180
CPTSDI (Children's Post-Traumatic
        Stress Disorder Inventory), 217

credible allegations, 220
CRF (corticotrophin releasing factor), 65
crisis
    intervention, 39, 181
    plan, 246
    teachers in, 242
Crisis Management International, Inc., 271
Criterion A, of DSM-IV PTSD
    definition, 138
    "Gatekeeper Criterion," 138, 153, 154
Criterion B, first cluster, reexperiencing cluster of symptoms, 139
Criterion C, second cluster, avoidance and numbing, 139
Criterion D, third and last cluster, hyperarousal, 139
critical incidents, 245, 299
    Program, FBI, 319
    Response Teams, CIRT, 320
    seminars, post-, 316
    situation, 301
    stress debriefing, 250
    stress management, 321
CST (Contextual Self-Development Theory), 126

debriefed, 305
    culture, 336
debriefers, primary, 146
debriefing
    critical incidents stress, 250
    cumulative traumatic stress, 255
    "the debriefers," 252
    psychological, PD, 151, 250, 252
    Red Cross volunteer, 356
    routine, 272
    rules, 251
deconditioning, fostering, 50
defusing
    failures, 246
    hostility, 245
dehumanization, 353
delayed traumatic stress, 7
depression, 94, 335
    inventory, 16, 145

DES (Dissociative Experiences Scale), 100, 102, 104, 107
desensitization, and fragment intrusion, 34
development
    psychological, of traumatized children, 226
    spiritual, 230
developmental distortions, 226
Devereux Scales of Mental Disorders, 217
diagnosis, 4, 10, 176
DID (Dissociative Identity Disorder), 165, 166, 171
didactic teaching, 153
direct therapeutic exposure, 18, 37
disclosure, 142
dissociated traumatic memories, 99
dissociating, 221
dissociation, 4, 30, 36, 102, 108, 115, 117, 177
dissociative imagery anamnesis, 107, 110
    PTSD, 108
dissociative states, 221
dissociative symptoms, 168
distortions, 153
    characterological, 227
    developmental, 226
distraction, 78
dominance, parental, 263
DRS (Dissociative Regression Scale), 100, 104
DSM-III, 139
DSM-IV, 138, 332
duration of traumatic events, 353
dysthymic disorder, 335

3-E Formula, 272
EAP (employee assistance programs), 320
education component, 81
effects, simultaneous, 264
efficacy, interpersonal, 394
ego function
    autonomous, 109
    auxiliary, 109
ego regression, 103, 109
ego state, 115

Einstein, Albert, 313
EMDR (eye movement desensitization
        and reprocessing), 78, 270,
        317, 318, 319, 387
emergency master plan, 374
emergency service personnel,
        personality profile, 311
emotional
    attachment, 39
    construction, 28
    distance, 111
empathy, 12, 39, 230
Employee Assistance Unit, FBI, 316,
        318
endogenous opioids, 49
entitlement, 117
environments
    healing, 229
    safe, 332
epidemiological data estimate lifetime
        prevalence, of PTSD, 75
ethics, 356, 395
evaluation, 216
    functional approach programs, 76
exposure, 82
    direct, 18, 34, 37
    in vivo, 394
externalized dialogue, 114, 117

FACES (Family Adaptability and
        Cohesion Scale), 268
false allegations, 220
False Memory Association, 181
familiarity, 250
family
    reintegration, 157
    relationship work, therapeutic, 344
    system, 263
    therapy, 272, 340, 341
    trauma, intra, 264
fatigue, compassion, 230
fear structure, 143
feature story, 355
FBI (Federal Bureau of Investigation),
        301
    Critical Incident Program, 319, 321
    Employee Assistance Unit, 316, 318
    integrated response, 319
    Peer Support Team, 321

FBI (Federal Bureau of Investigation)
        (continued)
    Post-Critical Incident Seminars,
        314, 316, 317
feedback, positive, 172
fidelity, 389
Finland, Police College, 300
First Step Program, 168
fixation, to trauma, 25
"fixed idea," 112
flexibility, 263
"flooding" techniques
    effects of, 34, 36
    procedures, 37
fluoxetine, 55, 57
fluvoxamine, 56, 57
focal psychotherapy, 101, 116
Freud, 4, 5, 6, 24
frozen in time, 115
futility, 106

GABAergic system, 61
"Gatekeeper Criterion," Criterion A,
        PTSD, 138, 153, 154
general systems theory, 261, 262
GHQ-28, General Health
        Questionnaire, 145
grief reactions, 140
grounding strategies, 173, 192
group
    activities, 144, 149
    cohesion, 149
    contagion, 174
    psychotherapy, 146
    socialization, 178
    treatments, 144
Group Treatment Programme for
        PTSD, 137
guilt (and shame), 94, 116, 130
    survivor, 153
Gulf War, 137, 144, 146, 148, 359

hallucinations, 114
healing
    defined, 388
    environments, 229
    key to, 393
    principles, 390

healthy touch, 229
heart and soul, of police officers, 314
helplessness, learned, 142
heroic phase, 358
histamine, 51
Holocaust Memorial, Jerusalem, 41
homeostasis, 262
homework, 107, 113
hopelessness, 106
hostage negotiations, 299
hostility defusing, 245
House-Tree-Person Projective Drawing
      Technique, 217
HPA (hypothalamic-pituitary-adrenal
      axis), 49
human capacity for evil, 225
human response, biphasic nature of,
      331
"human shield," Iraqi, 149
hyperalertness, 169
hyperventilation, 82
hypnosis, 110
hypnotic anamnesis, 110
hysteria, 4, 5

*ICD-10 Classification of Mental and
      Behavioral Disorders*, 138
identity, 103
imaginal
      exposure, 76, 77, 83, 84, 87
      reliving, 89, 90
imagination, Albert Einstein, 313
imipramine, 63
Impact of Event Scale, 15
implosive therapy, 37
in vitro experiences, in office, 222
in vivo exposure, outside office, 76, 77,
      82, 87, 222, 394
      exercises, 90
inescapable shock, 142
informed consent, 357
inpatient treatment, 195
integration, as key element of PTSD,
      34
intelligence, 122
intensity of traumatic events, 353
interpersonal efficacy, 394
intervention teams, 249
interview, 14

interview *(continued)*
      clinical, 266
      how to handle, 16 rules, 367, 368
      journalist, 355
      as a Red Cross volunteer, 355
      structured, for PTSD, 15
intimacy, 126, 131, 132
interpersonal communication, 291
intervention plans, school, 246
intrafamily trauma, 264
intrusive symptoms, 7
invulnerability, 116
irritability, 141
"irritable heart," 47
ISSD (International Society for the
      Study of Dissociation), 165
ISTSS (International Society for
      Traumatic Stress Studies)
      Practice Guidelines of, *xix, xxi*
      Standards of Care Committee, 261,
            270
      treatment guidelines, 165, 166

Janet, Pierre, 4, 25, 47
Journal of Traumatic Stress, 391
journalist/reporter, 351

key to healing, connection and
      listening, 393

lactic acid, 29
ladder exercise, 156
law enforcement, 311
learned helplessness, 142
*Life After Trauma: A Workbook
      for Healing,* 119
Life Experiences Screening, 268
Life Status Review, 267
limbic system, 49
line-of-duty death, 215
lines exercise, 155
listening
      formula, 280
      as key to healing, 393
lithium, 59, 60, 148
Lockean theory, 6
Lockerbie, Scotland, 373

MAOIs (Monoamine Oxidase
    Inhibitors), 52, 54, 53, 55, 57
master emergency plan, 374
meaning
    challenging, 390
    making, people as, 50
    to suffering, 117
    of traumatic events, 122
media, 307, 371
"Media Code of Ethics," NOVA, 379
medical model of informed consent,
    357
memories
    child's, 219
    fear of, 394
    intrusive, 7
    repressed, 152
    retrieval of, 40
Miranda warning, equivalent, 357
mirtazapine, 58, 59
Mississippi Scale, 15
MMPI (Minnesota Multiphasic
    Personality Inventory scale),
    16
MMPI PTSD subscale, 145
moclobemide, 52
monitoring, 151, 308
monoamine levels, 52
mood stabilizers, 64
mourning, 227
Mowrer, Two Factor Learning Theory,
    140
Multiple Personality Disorder/
    Dissociative Identity
    Disorder, MPD/DID, clients,
    165
Murrah Federal Building, Oklahoma
    City, 372
"myth of invulnerability," 152
mythology, victim, 396

nalmefene, 64
narcissism, 225
nefazodone, 58
negotiation process
    Accommodation Phase, 303
    Alarm Phase, 302, 305
    autonomic, 357
    Bargaining Phase, 303

negotiation process *(continued)*
    central, 26, 31
    Closing Resolution Phase, 304
neuroendocrine systems, 49
neuroleptics/antipsychotic agents, 62,
    63, 65
neuromodulation, 27
neuroses, traumatic, 25
NLP (Neuro-Linguist Programming)
    techniques, 193
nonmalficence, 389
noradrenergic, 57
normalize reactions, 241
NOVA (National Organization for
    Victim Assistance), 271, 379
NVVRS (National Vietnam Veteran
    Readjustment Study), 23, 75
numbing, 352

"observer mode," 110
Oklahoma City bombing, 315, 318,
    354, 373
olanzapine, 63
opiate antagonists, 64
opioids, endogenous, 49
outcomes, transformative, 230
overidentification, by clinician, 346

Pan Am
    Flight 103, 375
    1988 explosion, Lockerbie,
        Scotland, 373
paradigms, treatment, 269
    "person-in-environment," 328
paroxetine, 57
pathological cognitions, 80
PCIS (Post-Critical Incident Seminars),
    316
PD (psychological debriefing), 151,
    152, 252
peer support, 315, 321
Penn Inventory, 15
personal audit, 155
personal power, 129
Personal Shield, 130
personalization, 313
"person-in-environment," 328

pharmacological treatment of PTSD, 50
phenelzine, 52, 53, 54, 55
PILOTS database, 391
Piper Alpha disaster, 152
plane crashes, 274
Police College of Finland, 300
police officers, 314
positive affirmations, 175, 200
positive feedback, 172
Post-Critical Incident Seminars, FBI
  Academy, 314, 316, 317
posttraumatic reactions, 4
postwar readjustment, 327
power, 126, 129
power therapies, *xx*
powerlessness, 224
POW/MIA, 336
presynaptic alpha-2 autoreceptor, 59
prevention
 primary, 243
 secondary, 248
 tertiary, 254, 255
 violence, 244
primary
 prevention, 243
 protection against emotional
  attachment, 39
 trauma, 328
problem solving, 173
processing, information, 141
progressive relaxation, 110
prolonged exposure, 77
propranolol, 63, 147
PSS-I (PTSD Symptom Scale-
  Interview), 86
psychoanalysis, 5
psychoeducational group, 182
psychogenic amnesia, 352
psychological development of
  traumatized children, 226
psychometric instruments, 9
psychotherapy, 35
psychotraumatology, 241
PTSD
 checklist 15
 comorbidity of, *xxi*
 complex, 103, 104, 105, 107, 108, 115
 core problem, 25
 defined, 104
 dissociative, 108
 drop-out rates of study, 57

PTSD *(continued)*
 DSM-IV, 332
 epidemiological data estimate
  lifetime prevalence of, 75
 etiological theories for, 139
 future of, 65
 goals, 50
 Gulf War, 137
 MAOI/TCA, 57
 overt symptoms, 50
 pharmacological, 50, 51
 phenomenology, 102
 placebo trials, 53
 PTSD/SSRI, comparison, 57
 RAF Wroughton Programme,
  England, 137
 startle response, 49
 symptoms, 25
 Ticehurst House Hospital, 137
 war related, 345
PTSD-RI (Post-Traumatic Stress
  Disorder Reaction Index), 217

RAF Hospital Wroughton, 143
RAF Wroughton Programme, England,
  137
randomization, 65
"rap" groups, 144
rape victims, female, 56
RCMAS (Revised Children's Manifest
  Anxiety Scale), 217
Read Out teaching tool, 283-287, 289,
  292
readjustment, postwar, 327
rebuilding, 33
reconnecting, the veteran, 335
recursive, anamnesis, 100, 101
review, 88, 107, 110
Red Cross volunteer, 355, 356
reenactments, transference-bound, 333
reexperiencing trauma, 93
regression, ego, 103, 104, 109
regroup, 175
rehabilitation, 159, 327
reintegration, family, 157
relationship
 building a, 10, 175
 with self, 123
  progressive, 110

relationship, with self *(continued)*
   therapeutic, 229
     therapist and child, 229
   therapeutic, 24
relaxation, 76, 78, 174
reliability, 219
reporter/journalist, 353
repressed memories, 152
research, sleep and dreaming, 143
resilience, *xx,* 396
response
   somatic, 26, 36
   startle, 49
restlessness, 141
restructuring, cognitive, 394
retraumatize the self, 175
retreating, traumatized child, 229
reworking, cognitive, 224
risperidone, 62, 63
ritual and social ceremony, 336
Roberts Apperception Test, 217
role of therapist, 395
Rorschach Inkblot Technique, 217
Rotter Incomplete Sentence Blank, 217
Royal Air Force, 137, 321

safe environment, 332
   one step removed, 221
safe place, 174, 175
safe room, 199
safety, 11, 24, 35, 39, 105, 117, 119,
     126, 127, 182, 192, 193, 195,
     223, 245
   commitment to, 196
   issues, 204
   mechanisms, 172
   nets, 157
   objects, 175
   plans, 194, 197, 207
   and trust, 171
schemas, 35, 38, 39
   and belief systems, 170
   cognitive, 223
school intervention plans, 246
SCID (Structured Clinical Interview
     for the DSM-IV), 16, 86
SCL-45, 100
Scotland Yard, 301
secondary trauma, 328

security, 33, 127
   psychological, 277
sedation, 100
self
   -abusive behavior, 195
   -blame, 92
   -boundary, 103, 390
   -care, 396, 397
   -concepts, healthy, 277
   -destructive, 201
   -efficacy, 39
   -esteem, 130
   five basic needs, 119
   -harm, 204
   -help, 117, 204
   -loathing, 124
   -mutilating, 179
   -mutilation, 30, 114
   -mutilatory, 175
   -regulation, 33, 390
   relationship with, 123
   -responsibility, 173
   -state, 115
   -worth, 119
Selye, Hans, 358
separation anxiety, 226
serotonin, 34
sertraline, 56, 57
sexual abuse, grooming process, 224
shame, 94, 116, 123, 130
"shattered assumptions," 152
shock, 358, 379
simultaneous effects, 264
SIT (stress inoculation training), 78
sleep and dreaming research, 143
social ceremony and ritual, 336
social skills techniques, 78
socialization, group, 178
somatic response, 26, 36
South Vietnam, 319
spiritual development, 230
spiritual sense, of connection, 133
spirituality, 124
splitting, 108
SSRIs (Selective Serotonin Reuptake
     Inhibitors), 55-57, 64, 147
stabilization, 40
staff support, 248
stigmatization, 166
Stockholm Syndrome, 306
stress, *xix,* 153

Stressful Life Experiences Screening, 267-268
Structured Interview, for PTSD, 15
subjective interpretation, of threat, 141
SUDS (Subjective Units of Discomfort Scale), 83, 84, 88, 89, 268
suffering, 117
suicide attempts, 114
support, 176
    groups, 166
    peer, 315
"survivor guilt," 153
systemic therapy, 268

tachycardia, 49
TAT (Toronto Alexithymia Scale), 100
TCAs (Tricyclic Antidepressants), 50-52, 54, 64
teachers in crisis situations, 242
temperament, 353
tertiary prevention, 254-255
testing, one's beliefs, 126, 127
TFS Archetype, 266, 269, 273
TFT (Thought Field Therapy), 270
"therapeutic community," 144
therapeutic family relationship work, 344
therapeutic stance in group, 173
therapies, power, *xx*
therapist, role of, 395
therapy, systemic, 268
"thousand-yard stare," 110
"thwarted intention," 112
Ticehurst PTSD Group Treatment Programme, 143
"time out," 169
timing, 354
TIR (Traumatic Incident Reduction), 270
T-LTT (Time-Limited Trauma Therapy), 270
torture, 130
trance, 110
transference-bound reenactments, 333
transformative outcomes, 230
trauma
    in the classroom, 277
    defined, *xix*
    dissociative, 107
    fixation to, 25

trauma *(continued)*
    history, 392
    intra-family, 264
    membrane, 39
    memory, 39
    multiple, 108
    narrative, 110
    phobia, 103
    profile questionnaires, 101
    re-experiencing, 93
    rehabilitation services, 327
    related thoughts, 84
    Type I, one time, *xix*, 219, 387
    Type II, chronic, *xx*, 107, 387
    work, 103
traumatic events
    accommodated, 50
    assimilated, 50
    complex, 159
    complex PTSD development, 227
    duration of, 353
    intensity of, 353
    memories, dissociated, 99
    neuroses, 25
    Type I, *xix*, 219
    Type II, chronic, ongoing, *xx*, 219
traumatic stress
    delayed, 7
    disorder, secondary, 360
Traumatic Stress Institute, 391
traumatization, vicarious, 180
traumatized child, retreating, 229
trazodone, 58
treatment, 79, 269
    guidelines, ISTSS, 166
trigger, 169, 176, 178, 179, 193, 194
    anniversary issues, 192
trust, 119, 126, 128, 346
    and safety, 171
"trustworthy," 128
TSCC (Trauma Symptom Checklist for Children), 217
TSI (Traumatic Stress Institute), 126
Two Factor Learning Theory, Mowrer, 140
Type I, traumatic events, *xix*, 219
Type II, traumatic events, *xx*, 219

validation, 182
valproic acid, 60

values, 177, 389
venlafaxine, 59
venting, 153
verbal
    fluency, 306
    symbolization, 103
veteran, 325, 327, 335
veteran's war, 325
vicarious traumatization, 180
"victim mentality," 174
victim mythology, 396
video
    assisted focal psychotherapy, 99,
        107
    dialogue, 99, 102, 103, 107, 108,
        114, 115, 117
    technology, 99
    therapy, 103, 113, 116
Vietnam, 314, 334, 390
    South, 319
    War, 139, 144
Vietnam Veterans Memorial, 41, 337
"views of the world," 95, 105
violence prevention, 245
visualization, 109, 110

VKD (Visual Kinesthetic Dissociation),
    270
vulnerability, 397
VVAW (Vietnam Veteran's Against
    the War), self-help, 144

war-related PTSD, 345
WISC-III (Weschler Intelligence Scale
    for Children-Third Edition),
    216
WJ-R (Woodcock-Johnson
    Psychoeducational Battery-
    Revised), 216
working-through phase, 345
World War II, 321
worldview, 105
WRAT-R (Wide-Range Achievement
    Test-Revised), 216
writing, 230, 282
    curriculum, 290

Yohimbine injections, 29

THE HAWORTH MALTREATMENT AND TRAUMA PRESS®
Robert A. Geffner, PhD
Senior Editor

SIMPLE AND COMPLEX POST-TRAUMATIC STRESS DISORDER: STRATEGIES FOR COMPREHENSIVE TREATMENT IN CLINICAL PRACTICE edited by Mary Beth Williams and John F. Sommer Jr. (2002). "A welcome addition to the literature on treating survivors of traumatic events, this volume possesses all the ingredients necessary for even the experienced clinician to master the management of patients with PTSD." *Terence M. Keane, PhD, Chief, Psychology Service, VA Boston Healthcare System; Professor and Vice Chair of Research in Psychiatry, Boston University School of Medicine*

FOR LOVE OF COUNTRY: CONFRONTING RAPE AND SEXUAL HARASSMENT IN THE U.S. MILITARY by T. S. Nelson. (2002). "Nelson brings an important message—that the absence of current media attention doesn't mean the problem has gone away; that only decisive action by military leadership at all levels can break the cycle of repeated traumatization; and that the failure to do so is, as Nelson puts it, a 'power failure'—a refusal to exert positive leadership at all levels to stop violent individuals from using the worst power imaginable." *Chris Lombardi, Correspondent, Women's E-News, New York City*

THE INSIDERS: A MAN'S RECOVERY FROM TRAUMATIC CHILDHOOD ABUSE by Robert Blackburn Knight. (2002). "An important book. . . . Fills a gap in the literature about healing from childhood sexual abuse by allowing us to hear, in undiluted terms, about one man's history and journey of recovery." *Amy Pine, MA, LMFT, psychotherapist and co-founder, Survivors Healing Center, Santa Cruz, California*

WE ARE NOT ALONE: A GUIDEBOOK FOR HELPING PROFESSIONALS AND PARENTS SUPPORTING ADOLESCENT VICTIMS OF SEXUAL ABUSE by Jade Christine Angelica. (2002). "Encourages victims and their families to participate in the system in an effort to heal from their victimization, seek justice, and hold offenders accountable for their crimes. An exceedingly vital training tool." *Janet Fine, MS, Director, Victim Witness Assistance Program and Children's Advocacy Center, Suffolk County District Attorney's Office, Boston*

WE ARE NOT ALONE: A TEENAGE GIRL'S PERSONAL ACCOUNT OF INCEST FROM DISCLOSURE THROUGH PROSECUTION AND TREATMENT by Jade Christine Angelica. (2002). "A valuable resource for teens who have been sexually abused and their parents. With compassion and eloquent prose, Angelica walks people through the criminal justice system—from disclosure to final outcome." *Kathleen Kendall-Tackett, PhD, Research Associate, Family Research Laboratory, University of New Hampshire, Durham*

WE ARE NOT ALONE: A TEENAGE BOY'S PERSONAL ACCOUNT OF CHILD SEXUAL ABUSE FROM DISCLOSURE THROUGH PROSECUTION AND TREATMENT by Jade Christine Angelica. (2002). "Inspires us to work harder to meet kids' needs, answer their questions, calm their fears, and protect them from their abusers and the system, which is often not designed to respond to them in a language they understand." *Kevin L. Ryle, JD, Assistant District Attorney, Middlesex, Massachusetts*

GROWING FREE: A MANUAL FOR SURVIVORS OF DOMESTIC VIOLENCE by Wendy Susan Deaton and Michael Hertica. (2001). "This is a necessary book for anyone who is scared and starting to think about what it would take to 'grow free.' . . . Very helpful for friends and relatives of a person in a domestic violence situation. I recommend it highly." *Colleen Friend, LCSW, Field Work Consultant, UCLA Department of Social Welfare, School of Public Policy & Social Research*

A THERAPIST'S GUIDE TO GROWING FREE: A MANUAL FOR SURVIVOR'S OF DOMESTIC VIOLENCE by Wendy Susan Deaton and Michael Hertica. (2001). "An excellent synopsis of the theories and research behind the manual." *Beatrice Crofts Yorker, RN, JD, Professor of Nursing, Georgia State University, Decatur*

PATTERNS OF CHILD ABUSE: HOW DYSFUNCTIONAL TRANSACTIONS ARE REPLICATED IN INDIVIDUALS, FAMILIES, AND THE CHILD WELFARE SYSTEM by Michael Karson. (2001). "No one interested in what may well be the major public health epidemic of our time in terms of its long-term consequences for our society can afford to pass up the opportunity to read this enlightening work." *Howard Wolowitz, PhD, Professor Emeritus, Psychology Department, University of Michigan, Ann Arbor*

IDENTIFYING CHILD MOLESTERS: PREVENTING CHILD SEXUAL ABUSE BY RECOGNIZING THE PATTERNS OF THE OFFENDERS by Carla van Dam. (2000). "The definitive work on the subject. . . . Provides parents and others with the tools to recognize when and how to intervene." *Roger W. Wolfe, MA, Co-Director, N. W. Treatment Associates, Seattle, Washington*

POLITICAL VIOLENCE AND THE PALESTINIAN FAMILY: IMPLICATIONS FOR MENTAL HEALTH AND WELL-BEING by Vivian Khamis. (2000). "A valuable book . . . a pioneering work that fills a glaring gap in the study of Palestinian society." *Elia Zureik, Professor of Sociology, Queens University, Kingston, Ontario, Canada*

STOPPING THE VIOLENCE: A GROUP MODEL TO CHANGE MEN'S ABUSIVE ATTITUDES AND BEHAVIORS by David J. Decker. (1999). "A concise and thorough manual to assist clinicians in learning the causes and dynamics of domestic violence." *Joanne Kittel, MSW, LICSW, Yachats, Oregon*

STOPPING THE VIOLENCE: A GROUP MODEL TO CHANGE MEN'S ABUSIVE ATTITUDES AND BEHAVIORS, THE CLIENT WORKBOOK by David J. Decker. (1999).

BREAKING THE SILENCE: GROUP THERAPY FOR CHILDHOOD SEXUAL ABUSE, A PRACTITIONER'S MANUAL by Judith A. Margolin. (1999). "This book is an extremely valuable and well-written resource for all therapists working with adult survivors of child sexual abuse." *Esther Deblinger, PhD, Associate Professor of Clinical Psychiatry, University of Medicine and Dentistry of New Jersey School of Osteopathic Medicine*

"I NEVER TOLD ANYONE THIS BEFORE": MANAGING THE INITIAL DISCLOSURE OF SEXUAL ABUSE RE-COLLECTIONS by Janice A. Gasker. (1999). "Discusses the elements needed to create a safe, therapeutic environment and offers the practitioner a number of useful strategies for responding appropriately to client disclosure." *Roberta G. Sands, PhD, Associate Professor, University of Pennsylvania School of Social Work*

FROM SURVIVING TO THRIVING: A THERAPIST'S GUIDE TO STAGE II RECOVERY FOR SURVIVORS OF CHILDHOOD ABUSE by Mary Bratton. (1999). "A must read for all, including survivors. Bratton takes a lifelong debilitating disorder and unravels its intricacies in concise, succinct, and understandable language." *Phillip A. Whitner, PhD, Sr. Staff Counselor, University Counseling Center, The University of Toledo, Ohio*

SIBLING ABUSE TRAUMA: ASSESSMENT AND INTERVENTION STRATEGIES FOR CHILDREN, FAMILIES, AND ADULTS by John V. Caffaro and Allison Conn-Caffaro. (1998). "One area that has almost consistently been ignored in the research and writing on child maltreatment is the area of sibling abuse. This book is a welcome and required addition to the developing literature on abuse." *Judith L. Alpert, PhD, Professor of Applied Psychology, New York University*

BEARING WITNESS: VIOLENCE AND COLLECTIVE RESPONSIBILITY by Sandra L. Bloom and Michael Reichert. (1998). "A totally convincing argument. . . . Demands careful study by all elected representatives, the clergy, the mental health and medical professions, representatives of the media, and all those unwittingly involved in this repressive perpetuation and catastrophic global problem." *Harold I. Eist, MD, Past President, American Psychiatric Association*

TREATING CHILDREN WITH SEXUALLY ABUSIVE BEHAVIOR PROBLEMS: GUIDELINES FOR CHILD AND PARENT INTERVENTION by Jan Ellen Burton, Lucinda A. Rasmussen, Julie Bradshaw, Barbara J. Christopherson, and Steven C. Huke. (1998). "An extremely readable book that is well-documented and a mine of valuable 'hands on' information. . . . This is a book that all those who work with sexually abusive children or want to work with them must read." *Sharon K. Araji, PhD, Professor of Sociology, University of Alaska, Anchorage*

THE LEARNING ABOUT MYSELF (LAMS) PROGRAM FOR AT-RISK PARENTS: LEARNING FROM THE PAST—CHANGING THE FUTURE by Verna Rickard. (1998). "This program should be a part of the resource materials of every mental health professional trusted with the responsibility of working with 'at-risk' parents." *Terry King, PhD, Clinical Psychologist, Federal Bureau of Prisons, Catlettsburg, Kentucky*

THE LEARNING ABOUT MYSELF (LAMS) PROGRAM FOR AT-RISK PARENTS: HANDBOOK FOR GROUP PARTICIPANTS by Verna Rickard. (1998). "Not only is the LAMS program designed to be educational and build skills for future use, it is also fun!" *Martha Morrison Dore, PhD, Associate Professor of Social Work, Columbia University, New York, New York*

BRIDGING WORLDS: UNDERSTANDING AND FACILITATING ADOLESCENT RECOVERY FROM THE TRAUMA OF ABUSE by Joycee Kennedy and Carol McCarthy. (1998). "An extraordinary survey of the history of child neglect and abuse in America. . . . A wonderful teaching tool at the university level, but should be required reading in high schools as well." *Florabel Kinsler, PhD, BCD, LCSW, Licensed Clinical Social Worker, Los Angeles, California*

CEDAR HOUSE: A MODEL CHILD ABUSE TREATMENT PROGRAM by Bobbi Kendig with Clara Lowry. (1998). "Kendig and Lowry truly . . . realize the saying that we are our brothers' keepers. Their spirit permeates this volume, and that spirit of caring is what always makes the difference for people in painful situations." *Hershel K. Swinger, PhD, Clinical Director, Children's Institute International, Los Angeles, California*

SEXUAL, PHYSICAL, AND EMOTIONAL ABUSE IN OUT-OF-HOME CARE: PREVENTION SKILLS FOR AT-RISK CHILDREN by Toni Cavanagh Johnson and Associates. (1997). "Professionals who make dispositional decisions or who are related to out-of-home care for children could benefit from reading and following the curriculum of this book with children in placements." *Issues in Child Abuse Accusations*

Printed in the United States
by Baker & Taylor Publisher Services